HEART SURGERY IN CANADA

Memoirs, Anecdotes, History and Perspective

Second Edition

HEART SURGERY IN CANADA

Memoirs, Anecdotes, History and

Perspective

Bernard Goldman, M.D., F.R.C.S.(C.)

Susan Bélanger, B.A., M.L.S.

To order additional copies of this book, contact:
Xlibris Corporation
1-888-795-4274
www.Xlibris.com
Orders@Xlibris.com
26018

CONTENTS

DEDICATION

I wish to dedicate this anthology to the surgical residents in cardiac training programs, those that I was fortunate to teach and those from whom I learned. Their professional lives are based on the history and stories related herein, and their own achievements will enrich the contributions of Canadian heart surgery.

ABOUT THE AUTHORS

Bernard S. Goldman, MD, BSc, Med FRCS(C), trained in Toronto with Wilfred G. Bigelow and William T. Mustard, true pioneers of heart surgery in Canada. After twenty years at Toronto General Hospital, he opened the cardiac surgical unit at Sunnybrook and Women's in 1989 and was later chief of surgery at that hospital. His professional life represents a generation intermediate between the founders of heart surgery in Canada and contemporary surgeons in practice. His own practice began with the advent of heart transplantation and coronary bypass. He was Editor of the *Journal of Cardiac Surgery* until 2008 and is Professor Emeritus of Surgery at the University of Toronto. His interest in surgical history stems directly from the influence of his mentors Wilfred Bigelow and Ronald Baird, both humble men of great achievement and fiercely dedicated to our Canadian heritage. He will soon retire from active surgical practice, but remains a consultant to the Ontario Ministry of Health, the Pacemaker Clinic at Sunnybrook, and the Toronto Rehabilitation Institute.

Susan Bélanger, BA, MLS, is research coordinator and administrative assistant to the History of Medicine Program, Faculty of Medicine, University of Toronto. A graduate of the University of Toronto, she spent several years as bibliographies editor for the *Dictionary of Canadian Biography / Dictionnaire biographique du Canada.* Since 1994 she has pursued her interest in health-related research and writing with the History of Medicine Program.

CONTRIBUTORS

Victor Aldrete, BSc, MD, FRCS(C), FACS, Staff Surgeon retired, Holy Cross Hospital, Calgary, Alberta

Ronald Baird, MD, FRCS(C), Professor Emeritus, University of Toronto, former Chairman University Division of Cardiac Surgery and Head, Cardiac Surgery Toronto General Hospital

Clare Baker, MD, FRCS(C), Professor of Surgery, University of Toronto, former Head, St. Michael's Hospital

Jaroslaw Barwinsky, MD, FRCS(C), Professor Emeritus, University of Manitoba

Pierre Bédard, MD, FRCS(C), Cardiac Surgeon, Ottawa Heart Institute, Associate Professor, University of Ottawa

Wilfred Bigelow†, MD, FRCS(C), Professor Emeritus, University of Toronto, former Chairman University Division of Cardiovascular Surgery and Head, Cardiac Surgery, Toronto General Hospital

André Brassard, MD, FRCS(C), Staff Surgeon, Complexe Hospitalier de la Sagamie, Chicoutimi, PQ

Lawrence H. Burr, BA, MSc, MD, FRCS(C), Clinical Associate Professor Emeritus, University of British Columbia

Ed Busse, BA, MD, FRCS(C), LLD (h.c.), Former Chief of Cardiovascular and Thoracic Surgery and Director, Mosaic Heart Centre, The Regina Qu'Appelle Health Region, Regina, Saskatchewan

Paul Cartier, MD, FRCS(C), Cons. Hôpital Ste.-Justine, Ass't Surg., Centre Hospitalier de l'Université de Montréal-Pavillon Hôtel-Dieu

Claude Chartrand, MD, FRCS(C), former Head of Cardiac Surgery, Ste-Justine Hospital

Ray Chu-Jeng Chiu, MD, PhD, FRCS(C), Professor of Surgery and Past Chairman, Division of Cardiothoracic Surgery, McGill University, Montreal

Robert Cossette, MD, FRCS(C), Professor of Surgery, Université de Montréal, Head, Cardiac Surgery, Hôpital du Sacré-Coeur de Montréal

Tirone David, MD, FRCS(C), Head, Cardiovascular Surgery, Toronto General Hospital, Professor of Surgery, University of Toronto

Kathy Deemar, Chief Perfusionist, Sunnybrook Health Sciences Centre

Nimesh Desai, MD, Former resident in CV Surgery, University of Toronto, Assistant Professor, University of Pennsylvania, Philadelphia, PA

Anthony Dobell, MD, FRCS(C), Professor Emeritus, McGill University, Montreal, former Head of Cardiovascular and Thoracic Surgery, Royal Victoria Hospital

Lee Errett, MD, FRCS(C), Head, Cardiovascular Surgery, St. Michael's Hospital, Toronto, Assistant Professor, University of Toronto

Shafie Fazel, MD, Resident in CV Surgery, University of Toronto

Paul Fedak, MD, PhD, Former resident in CV Surgery, University of Toronto, Cardiac Surgeon, Foothills Hospital, Calgary

Stephen Fremes, MD, MS, FRCS(C), Head, Cardiac and V ascular Surgery, Sunnybrook Health Scienes Centre, Professor of Surgery, University of Toronto

Martin Goldbach, MD, FRCS(C), Cardiac Surgeon, London Health Sciences Centre, Associate Professor of Surgery, University of Western Ontario, London, Ontario

Bernard Goldman, MD, FRCS(C), Professor Emeritus, University of Toronto, Sunnybrook Health Sciences Centre, former Head of Cardiovascular Surgery and Surgeon-in-Chief, Sunnybrook and Women's Health Sciences Centre

Claude Grondin, MD, FRCS(C), Cardiovascular Surgery, Montreal Heart Institute, St. Luke's Hospital, Cleveland, Ohio

Harpreet Grover, MD, Research fellow, Division of Cardiovascular Surgery, Toronto General Hospital

Ray Heimbecker, MD, MS, FRCS(C), Professor Emeritus, University of Western Ontario, former Head, University Hospital, London, Ontario

Teresa Kieser, MD, FRCS(C), Associate Professor, University of Calgary, Foothills Hospital, Calgary

Arvind Koshal, MD, FRCS(C), Clinical Professor and Director of Cardiac Surgery, University of Albera, Head, Cardiac Surgery, University Hospital, Edmonton

Gabriel Laberge, MD, FRCS(C), Centre Hospitalier Universitaire de Sherbrooke-Hôpital Fleurimont, PQ

Léo La Flèche, MD, CM, FRCS(C), Centre Hospitalier Universitaire de Montréal (Notre Dame Hospital), McGill University Hospital Centre (Montreal Chest Hospital— Division of Royal Victoria Hospital)

David Latter, MD, FRCS(C), Cardiovascular Surgery, St. Michael's Hospital, Associate Professor, University of Toronto

Michel Lemieux, MD, FRCS(C), Institute de Cardiologie, Hôpital Laval, Sainte-Foy, PQ

James MacDonald, CPC, CCP, Chief, Clinical Perfusion Services Cardiac Care Program, London Health Sciences Centre, London, Ontario

Neil McKenzie, MB, ChB, FRCS, FRCS(C), Cardiac Surgeon, London Health Science Centre, Professor of Surgery, University of Western Ontario, London, Ontario

Avdesh Mathur, MD, FRCS(C), former Chaief of Cardiovascular and Thoracic Surgery, Sudbury Memorial Hospital, Sudbury, Ontario

Kevin Melvin, MD, FRCS(C), Chief of Cardiac Surgery, Health Sciences Centre, St. John's NL

David Murphy, DVM, MD, FRCS(C), BFA, Professor of Surgery, Dalhousie University, Halifax, NS

Jean Morin, MD, FRCS(C), former Head, Cardiovascular Surgery, Royal Victoria Hospital, Montreal

Arthur Pagé, MD, FRCS(C), FACS, Honorary Professor, Faculty of Medicine, Université de Montréal, Hôpital du Sacré-Coeur de Montréal

Normand Poirier, MD, FRCS(C), Head, Department of Cardiovascular and Thoracic Surgery, Centre Hospitalier de l'Université de Montréal—Hôpital Notre-Dame, Professor Université de Montréal

Zlatko Pozeg, MD, Former resident in Cardiac Surgery, University of Alberta, Edmonton, AB, Cardiac Surgeon, Southlake Hospital, Newmarket, ON

Vivek Rao, MD, FRCS(C), Surgical Director of Cardiac Transplantation and Mechanical Circulatory Support at Toronto General Hospital, Associate Professor of Surgery, University of Toronto

Guy Roberge, MD, FRCS(C), Cardiac Surgery, St. Luc Hospital, Montreal

Tomas Salerno, MD, FRCS(C), Tenured Professor of Surgery, University of Miami, Chief, Cardiothoracic Surgery, Jackson Memorial Hospital, Miami, FL, USA

Bertrand Scalibrini, MD, FRCS(C), Cardiovascular and Thoracic Surgery, Centre Hospital, Universitaire de Sherbrooke—Hopital Fleurimont, Associate Professor Surgery and Chief of Cardiovascular and Thoracic Services, Université de Sherbrooke

Gilbert Tang, BA, MD, Resident in CV Surgery, Toronto General Hospital, University of Toronto

Javier Teijeira, MD, FRCS(C), Centre Hospitalier Universitaire de Sherbrooke—Hôpital Fleurimont, Cons. Centre Hospitalier Universitaire de Sherbrooke—Hôpital Hôtel-Dieu, Professor, Université de Sherbrooke

George Trusler, CD, MD, BSc, MS, FRCS(C), FACS, Professor Emeritus of Surgery, University of Toronto, former Head, Cardiovascular Surgery, Hospital for Sick Children, Toronto

Richard Weisel, MD, FRCS(C), Professor and Chair, Division of Cardiac Surgery, University of Toronto, Toronto General Hospital

William G. Williams, MD, FRCS(C), former Head, Division of Cardiovascular Surgery, University of Toronto and the Hospital for Sick Children

INTRODUCTION AND ACKNOWLEDGEMENTS

Bernard S. Goldman

This book is an anthology of the events and the people that created, nurtured and sustained heart surgery in Canada from the earliest days to the present. The book is a collection of memoirs, anecdotes, interviews, and surgical perspective contributed by colleagues from across the country. It is not a detailed historical review of heart surgery in Canada, although some chapters do summarize the entire fifty years since 1952 in particular institutions. There is considerable material on the early development of heart surgery in Canada as remembered by some of the pioneer surgeons as well as current thoughts and reflections provided by contemporary surgeons and residents.

My interest in compiling this work came from my position as editor of the *Journal of Cardiac Surgery*. Larry W. Stephenson of Detroit, Michigan, is a prolific surgical historian with numerous published articles, chapters, and texts. As a member of my editorial board, he suggested that the journal commemorate the fiftieth anniversary of open-heart surgery using an extracorporeal circuit with a series of articles from the major centres of that era. Writing about the early Toronto experience ("Thinned Blood, Monkey Lungs, and the Cold Heart"—Fazel, Williams, Goldman) stimulated me to reflect further on Canadian contributions over the same period. I soon realized that, with few exceptions, many of the early surgeons were alive and available. Subsequent inquiries revealed similar interest and considerable enthusiasm from numerous colleagues across Canada: advice and information came from Wilfred Bigelow (since deceased), Donald Wilson, John Callaghan (since deceased), Beverly Lynn (since deceased), and Pierre Grondin (since deceased) as well as wonderful memories from Ronald Baird, Raymond Heimbecker, Clare Baker and George Trusler. Phil Ashmore, Anthony Dobell and David Alton Murphy wrote compelling chapters; Kevin Melvin had already presented a history of heart surgery in Newfoundland to the local historical society; Jean Morin was preparing the history of heart surgery in Quebec; Claude Grondin literally burst out of retirement to provide a detailed history of the Montreal Heart Institute and Wilbert Keon had prepared a summary of the Ottawa Heart Institute as he prepared to step down as director. Thus, chapters and contributors readily fell into place.

Although I am neither historian nor writer, I recognized, as an editor, that more was needed to capture the flavour and impact of a full half century on the growth and development of heart surgery in Canada. I was gratified at the response to subsequent requests, and these chapters all make for interesting reading: *Women in Heart Surgery* (Kieser); *Perfusion History* (MacDonald and Deemar); *Transplantation* (Rao); *Research at McGill* (Chiu); and the *View from the U.S.* (Salerno). I was especially pleased with the contributions from surgical residents: *The Edmonton Heart Institute* (Pozeg); *Current Status of Heart Surgery in Canada* (Fazel); *Origins of Heart Surgery* (Desai); *Training Programs* (Tang); and *Future Directions* (Fedak). I am grateful for their interest and efforts and admire their talents.

The true impetus for this anthology was in all likelihood personal reflections on my professional life as I approach retirement. Like so many other surgeons of my generation (Yao, Miyagishima, Tyers, Gelfand, Morin, etc.), we have all played a part in the evolving history of heart surgery and have bridged the period between the "true pioneers" and the current practitioners. We have been fortunate to have been both observers and participants in the transition from a new discipline with high mortality to one that is commonplace with high volume procedures performed daily at low risk and with superb outcomes. This incredibly rapid progress mirrored the technology revolution throughout medicine. Nonetheless, the leap from cold immersion (hypothermia) for rapid closure of an atrial septal defect (Bigelow) to robotic construction of a mammary-coronary bypass (Boyd) is impressive and similar to the progress and achievements made in the space program over the same period. It was pure serendipity that put me in practice at the time of the most significant clinical explosions in heart surgery—I was in Bristol, United Kingdom, doing thoracic surgery with Ronald Belsey when Barnard performed his first heart transplant and in Boston, learning about coronary flow, left ventricular function, and intraaorrtic balloon pump assist shortly before the first coronary bypass surgeries were reported. This set the stage for an exciting and satisfying career in heart surgery.

Although the remarkable achievements in heart surgery over the past fifty years have been international in origin, Canadian contributions have indeed been significant. Nonetheless aside from the seminal work of Bigelow and Mustard in the past, and perhaps David currently, many milestones and achievements have been diluted or neglected by American and European colleagues. Indeed present-day cardiologists, nurses, surgical trainees, and

the lay public have little appreciation or understanding of
the unique Canadian contributions: to coronary surgery,
to the correction of congenital defects, to myocardial
protection or valve reconstruction. Who today is aware
of the efforts of Edouard Gagnon and Arthur Vineberg
in Montreal or Gordon Murray in Toronto? Murray
reported on valve reconstruction as early as 1938 and
had performed almost six hundred heart operations on
infants, children, and adults by 1951 as well as performing
the first human aortic valve transplant in 1955. Surgical
residents in Canadian training programs today do not
appreciate the landmark understanding of saphenous
vein graft patency and attrition (Fitzgibbon, Bourassa,
Grondin), myocardial preservation (Tyers, Weisel,
Salerno, Lichtenstein, Fremes), or valve performance
(Christakis, Desmunils, Cartier, David) and numerous
other major contributions.

Few have questioned the problems of timely access to
innovative procedures or new technology in a chronically
underfunded public health care system. How has cardiac
surgery in Canada, based primarily in university hospitals
that face chronic deficits, remained "cutting edge" with
excellent outcomes despite constant competition for
scarce resources from other important disciplines? How
have Canadian surgeons delivered the same quality
of patient care and important research as their U.S.
counterparts who work in a more affluent and lavishly
endowed health care system?

Cardiac surgery has been at the forefront of incorporating
an interdisciplinary approach to basic research and
clinical application. In the years since 1952, cardiac
surgery stimulated marked progress in other related
fields: anaesthesia, hematology and transfusion, critical
care and vascular surgery. Cardiac surgeons have been

leaders in many surgical departments throughout the country. However, they were not all giants, nor heroes, nor great researchers. Many were simply dedicated, talented, innovative, and resourceful clinicians who worked long hours as they perfected their craft in a rapidly evolving field—and some succumbed to the stress and pace and ultimately left. Most however had the courage and tenacity to create a rapidly expanding new discipline, despite the challenges of numerous clinical trials, disappointing early results and often reluctant support.

The purpose of this book then is to document where possible the difficulties and the achievements of heart surgery in Canada in the years 1952-2002, from the beginning of extracorporeal circulatory support to current practice. There is no particular style or effort at continuity. I can only apologize for repetition or redundancy; contributing authors had the freedom to incorporate material that best reflected their interest or experience, and their writing style and thoughts vary greatly. I apologize also to those enthusiastic authors who provided so many photographs, newspaper clippings, etc. It was simply not feasible nor technically possible to include them all, and it was necessary for me to be somewhat selective. I am grateful for the advice and guidance provided by Edward "Ned" Shorter, Hannah Professor of History of Medicine in the Faculty of Medicine at the University of Toronto, and in particular, for "loaning" his research assistant Susan Bélanger who has edited each chapter with meticulous verification of referenced events, dates and persons.

As this project evolved. I came to realize that my mentors and teachers had themselves recognized the historical impact of the many dramatic events that marked the clinical progress of heart surgery during their own careers. In retrospect, each of them intuitively understood that the slow and painstaking application of their innovations would ultimately become milestones in the course of cardiac surgery. They exposed and introduced me to other early contributors from around the world and always instructed me to understand and incorporate the efforts of these great surgeons as being landmarks in the evolution of our discipline.

I was trained by Bill Bigelow and Bill Mustard. Bigelow cautioned me to approach the wonders of our field and the accompanying respect and adulation it created, with a degree of humility. Mustard taught me perseverance and to see humour in ourselves and the world around us—the better to cope with the rigours and disappointments of heart surgery at that time.

Raymond Heimbecker and Ronald Baird, teachers and later colleagues and friends, were particularly cognizant of the historical roles that they and other Canadians played in heart surgery, and I am grateful for their wise counsel and contributions to my career and this book. I was also influenced by Seymour Furman (since deceased), the noted pacemaker expert, for his discipline and dedication to creating a historical record of the evolution of intracardiac rhythm devices for NASPE, the North American Society of Cardiac Pacing and Electrophysiology.

The book is printed by Xlibris, publishers in Philadelphia, Pennsylvania, and the material maintained in an electronic database. Thus, it is readily available for updates or further contributions, which will be accessible almost as a continuum rather than a defined second or subsequent edition. This allows me or my successors to input new information from centres or surgeons not represented at this time or to permit existing reflections on early development to be expanded to include present accomplishments. Finally, I am grateful to both my secretary Shirley Combeer and Susan Bélanger for their hard work bringing this effort to completion. I particularly wish to acknowledge the significant financial contribution provided by Medtronic of Canada Inc., and I especially thank Medtronic's longstanding and recently retired president Donald Hurley, whose support of heart surgery projects in Canada has been constant, important, and appreciated. Edwards Laboratories, Sulzer Medica and St. Jude Medical were also generous in their support. I wish also to note that the Schulich Heart Centre at Sunnybrook and Women's College Health Sciences Centre provided personal support through a Tana Schulich Research Award.

I appreciate the encouragement and interest of the Canadian Society of Clinical Perfusion, through its present president, Mr. Paul Murphy, the Canadian Cardiovascular Society, through presidents Dr. Pierre Pagé and Dr. David Johnson, and especially the Canadian Society of Cardiac Surgeons, Drs. Jim Dutton, president; and Tim Latham, secretary treasurer; and it is to the latter society that all rights and royalties from this book have been assigned.

Toronto, Canada, September 2004.

EDITOR'S COMMENTS ON A SECOND VERSION

Heart surgery in Canada, indeed throughout the Western world, has undergone significant and possibly existential change since this book was first published in 2004. The most profound change, with perhaps the greatest impact of course, has been that of the decline of coronary bypass graft surgery. The dramatic decrease in case numbers has been accompanied by an equally dramatic increase in the overall patient risk profile. In many centres this change in patient volume and demographic has affected resident training, research and recruitment. On the other hand valve surgery is on the increase, particularly mitral repairs for ischemic mitral regurgitation and aortic surgery for calcific aortic stenosis in the elderly. Exciting developments in endovascular therapies for thoracic aortic pathology and/or replacement of the aortic valve provide constant stimulation. In some centres surgery for heart failure, including mechanical circulatory assist devices, has also made tremendous progress.

Cardiac surgery, as this text has shown, is rarely static. While every specialty goes through cycles of advancement, retrenchment and reevaluation as new technologies and innovative approaches arise, the changes in cardiac surgery have been disconcerting to say the least. This second version of "Heart Surgery in Canada" attempts to capture some of these changes in both a historical and contemporary context. Cardiac surgeons are by nature busy folks and few answered the call to revisit or revise their original contribution. However some material has been deleted and significant new chapters inserted. One of the "missing" chapters concerns heart surgery at Queen's University in Kingston, Ontario. Dr. Bev Lynn was asked to prepare this chapter, but he unfortunately passed away before doing so, and there was no response from the current cardiac staff. Dr. Lynn did remind me, however, of the contributions of Ed Charrette, Tomas Salerno, John Pym and Stephanie Brister, all of whom trained at Queen's and are herein acknowledged. His note also mentioned the first open heart cases in Saskatoon in 1955 and the first successful removal of a right atrial myxoma in 1958. Bev Lynn was indeed one of Canada's great cardiac pioneers.

I hesitate to call this a Second Edition because it is really an electronic process wherein we can produce a different version of the original book whenever enough material is accumulated: thus I have labeled it a "Second Version". Approximately 300 copies of the initial text are in circulation and hopefully cardiac surgeons, surgical residents and fellows, nurses and others involved in the care of heart surgical patients will continue to find this an interesting look at the past, the present and perhaps a glimpse into the future.

The costs of production of this "Edition" have once again been generously supported by Medtronic of Canada and I am grateful to Neil Fraser, President and CEO of Medtronic Canada for his continued enthusiasm and encouragement. The royalties from distribution will once again be forwarded to the Canadian Society for Cardiac Surgery.

My hope is that young surgeons and others in fields related to cardiovascular surgery will read and learn how this fascinating discipline evolved in this country, who were and are the contributors to progress and excellence and thus take pride in our collective accomplishments in the past and deal with the challenges in the future ahead.

Toronto, Canada, Februrary 2009

CHAPTER 1

HISTORY OF HEART SURGERY I

Nimesh Desai

Throughout recorded history, scholars, philosophers, and physicians contemplated the moral implications and scientific possibilities of touching man's heart. This introductory chapter provides a brief synopsis of the personalities and technical achievements that led to the modern era of heart surgery. It begins with an explanation of the often hostile environment in which heart surgery pioneers first attempted to develop and apply their craft and culminates with medicine's greatest invention—the heart-lung machine.

The pioneers of heart surgery often had to endure the scorn of their physician colleagues, the media, and the general public. Fuelled by the urgency to save their patients, the drive for innovation, or simply unabated hubris, these surgeons attempted heroic and often misadventurous operations under the close scrutiny of their peers. The opposition to surgery on the heart by philosophers and scientists date back to the finality in the words pronounced by Hippocrates in the fourth century BC, "A wound in the heart is mortal."[1] Later, Aristotle asserted, "The heart alone of all the viscera cannot withstand injury. This is to be expected because when the main source of strength is destroyed there is no aid that can be brought to the other organs which depend on it."[2]

Many centuries later, the famed sixteenth-century French battlefield surgeon Ambrose Paré proclaimed, "The heart is the chief mansion of the soul, the organ of vital faculty, the beginning of life, and the fountain of the vital spirits, and so consequently the continued nourisher of the vital heat, the first to live and the last to die."[3] Such sentiments continued to echo throughout recorded history and continued even well into the nineteenth century when the preeminent surgeon of the era, Theodor Bilroth, pronounced that, "A surgeon who tries to suture a heart wound deserves to lose the esteem of his colleagues."[4]

Understanding of Cardiovascular Physiology

The courage to attempt operative repair on the heart came only after better understanding of the structure and function of the heart and observations that the heart could withstand injury and recover its function.

Hippocrates (460-355 BC) first described that the palpable pulse was due to the flow of blood through vessels, which he traced back to the heart.[5] The great physician, Galen (AD 130-200), ignored Hippocrates' unproven suggestions and speculated that while the venous system contained blood, the arterial system in fact contained air.[6] He envisioned that the air, purified by the lungs mixed with blood, entered the pulmonary artery and crossed over to the left side of the heart via holes or pores in the interventricular sepum.

The Arabian physician Ibn-An-Nafis (1210-88) was the first to suggest that there were in fact two parallel circulations: pulmonary and systemic. However, his texts were not accepted widely and nearly three hundred years passed until Servetus (1509-53) independently described the same concept of parallel circulations.[7]

The first detailed anatomic drawings of the heart were created by Leornardo da Vinci (1452-1519). Da Vinci's work, although lost within Windsor Castle for centuries, questioned Galenic dogma and was well ahead of its time, providing detailed explanations for the mechanism of aortic valve leaflet closure.[8] While much of da Vinci's work on the structure and function of the heart was never seen by subsequent scholars, the Paduan physician Andreas Vesalius (1514-1564) openly defied Galen's explanation of the circulation based on detailed pathologic dissections.[9] He refuted Galen's claim that pores existed between the ventricles and observed that organs were supplied by arteries and veins, which he believed was a convenient arrangement for the ebb and flow of blood. Servetus, a contemporary to Vesalius, rightly identified the parallel circulations but his critical views of Calvin and the Reformation movement led him to be burned at the stake.

English physician William Harvey (1578-1657) ushered in the modern understanding of circulatory physiology.[10] He described that the heart ejected blood during systole and passively filled in diastole. He also discovered that the valves found in veins were responsible for ensuring unidirectional flow and he definitively described the parallel circulations. The knowledge of circulatory physiology incrementally gained by these great historical figures paved the way for future pioneers to attack cardiac lesions.

Wounds of the Heart

Accounts of physicians observing traumatic injuries to the heart date back to the observations of Galen, physician to the court of the Roman emperor Marcus Aurelius. Galen, as surgeon to the bloody gladiator matches of the second century AD, observed that the heart could continue to beat after being completely torn from the body.[11]

The first scientific observation that humans could survive a penetrating heart wound was by Barthelemy Cabrol of Montpelier, France in 1604.[12] He described healed scars found in the heart muscle, known as myocardium, of two criminals hung for their crimes. Later that decade, William Harvey, observed that a deer shot in the heart on the estate of King Charles I did not die immediately. Harvey, at the behest of his king, also examined the son of the Viscount of Montgomery, who had suffered from multiple infected abscesses of his chest wall.[13] The boy was left with a residual hole in his left chest wall through which Harvey could feel the surface of his heart. He observed that the surface of the living heart was insensitive to touch.

Over the next two centuries, isolated autopsy reports suggested that there were occasional instances of people surviving penetrating injury to the heart. The Paduan pathologist Morgagni collected detailed autopsy reports and concluded that collection of blood in the pericardial sac led to compression and arrest of the heart.[14, 15] In 1884, Berlin surgeon Edmund Rose coined the term "Herztamponade" to describe this condition.[16]

In 1820, the French surgeon to Napoleon, Baron Larrey, endeavored to drain the pericardium of a French soldier who had stabbed himself in the heart.[17] The soldier had survived the initial injury but nearly forty-five days later presented with symptoms of cardiac tamponade. Larrey proceeded to insert a flexible catheter into the pericardial sac and the patient initially survived, but died later of septic complications.

George Fischer published a monograph in 1868 that documented a 10 percent recovery rate in 452 patients with heart wounds.[18] This report indicated that heart wounds did not necessarily result in certain death. Investigators began to explore the possibility of surgical intervention in heart wounds. In 1882, Block reported creating stab wounds in rabbits and then repairing them. He suggested attempts in patients.[19]

The first reported case of successful operative management of a heart wound was performed in 1893 by a pioneering African-American surgeon in Chicago named Daniel Hale Williams, who treated a young man with a stab wound in the chest.[20] He removed the knife and managed the wound without surgery since he assumed it was superficial. After the patient deteriorated overnight, Williams opened the young man's chest and found that there was a one-and-one-quarter-inch tear in the sac covering the heart, known as the pericardium, and a small nick in the muscle of the right ventricle about a half inch to the right of the left anterior descending coronary artery. Williams determined the heart itself was not bleeding and did not touch the heart wound. He sutured closed the pericardial sac and tied off bleeding vessels in the chest wall.[21] Although the patient needed a second operation to drain fluid around the heart, he survived for over twenty years after the operation. Nearly two years earlier, surgeon Henry C. Dalton, of St. Louis, performed a similar operation, but the patient died soon after discharge from the hospital.[22]

Around this time, Stephen Paget, in *The Surgery of the Chest*, wrote: "Surgery of the heart has probably reached the limits set by Nature to all surgery. No method, no new discovery, can overcome the natural difficulties that attend a wound of the heart."[23]

However, in combination with experiments in animals and the pioneering work of Wells and Morton in anaesthesia, Lister in aseptic technique, and Roentgen in X-ray imaging, the frontiers of what was possible had been pushed forward.

The first surgeon to successfully place sutures on the heart was Ludwig Rehn, a surgeon in Frankfurt, Germany.[24] In 1897, he daringly opened the chest of a twenty-two-year-old man stabbed in the fourth intercostal space during a fencing match. The patient slowly bled from his chest for over twenty-four hours and then developed severe shock.

> *I decided to suture the heart wound. I used a small intestinal needle and silk suture. The suture was tied in diastole. Bleeding diminished remarkably with the third suture, all bleeding was controlled. The pulse improved. The pleural cavity was irrigated. Pleura and pericardium were drained with iodoform gauze. The incision was approximated, heart rate and respiratory rate decreased and pulse improved postoperatively . . . I hope this will lead to more investigation regarding surgery of the heart. This may save many lives.*[25]

Despite a subsequent empyema, the patient eventually made a full recovery. News of Rehn's accomplishment prompted tremendous interest in operatively managing heart wounds, and within a decade of his original operation, Rehn compiled a summary of 124 known cases.[26] In most instances, the principles of management included removal of foreign bodies, suturing of the heart wound, and closure of the pericardium and chest wall. Overall survival was 40 percent in this first series of operations with most deaths occurring due to infection or pneumothorax.

The first case of successful North American heart suturing was performed by Dr. Luther Hill in Montgomery, Alabama, in 1902.[27] The patient, a thirteen-year-old boy named Henry Myrick, had been stabbed five times in the chest. Hill performed the operation in the middle of the night aided by six other physicians. The surgery took place on the patient's kitchen table in a rundown shack, and lighting was provided by two kerosene lamps borrowed from neighbors. One stab wound had perforated into the left ventricle resulting in cardiac tamponade. Hill closed the hole in the ventricular muscle with two catgut sutures. The boy made a complete recovery. Ironically, in 1942, at the age of fifty-three, the same patient got into a heated argument and was again stabbed in the heart and died from the wound.

Management of penetrating cardiac injuries continued to advance during the First and Second World Wars with improvements in anaesthetic care, surgical instruments, allogenic whole blood transfusion and penicillin. In early 1944, U.S. Army surgeon Dwight Harken, a disciple of Elliott Cutler, was stationed at a base hospital for American troops in the United Kingdom, the 160th General Hospital in Cirencester.[28] Several days after D day, the Allied invasion of Normandy on June 6, 1944, great volumes of casualties began to arrive at Cirencester. The hospital and its surgeons became reputed for ceaselessly operating day and night to treat the nonstop flow of wounded soldiers. In addition to his duties at Cirencester, Harken would often travel with a team of surgeons and nurses to other hospitals to perform operations. In this setting, Harken perfected techniques of operative management of cardiac wounds. He used fluoroscopy to precisely localize intrathoracic foreign objects and then removed them, even if they were deep within cardiac structures. Massive blood transfusions facilitated open exploration of cardiac chambers. He would often inject penicillin directly into the pericardial sac. During the war, Harken successfully removed 134 intracardiac missiles with no deaths.[29] The operating team decided not to operate on only fifteen patients with cardiac penetrating trauma. Among foreign objects removed, thirteen were from myocardium, seventeen from pericardium, thirteen from heart chambers, and seventy-eight from the great vessels. Such outcomes were remarkable given the extreme conditions under which these operations were performed.

Surgical Treatment of Pulmonary Embolism

Pulmonary embolism is a potentially fatal condition in which blood clots, usually from the large veins in the leg and thigh, embolize into the pulmonary circulation via the inferior vena cava, right atrium and right ventricle. Blood clots form within the veins as a result a triad of factors described by the nineteenth-century pathologist Virchow: injury to the lining vein wall, prolonged periods of stasis of blood within the vein, and abnormal blood-clotting tendency (hypercoagulability). These clots, depending on their size, can cause sharp chest pain, progressive shortness of breath, and eventually circulatory collapse and death. After nine deaths from pulmonary embolism at his hospital in Leipzig, German surgeon Frederic Trendelenberg began experimenting with cadaveric operations to remove clots from the pulmonary arteries. He developed a technique in which he passed a rubber tube through the transverse sinus to encircle the great vessels. He would place tension on the rubber tube to stop all blood flow and, with only seconds to work, open the right ventricular outflow.[30] He evolved from early experiences trying to suck the clot with a suction catheter to opening the pulmonary artery directly and removing the clot with forceps. Unfortunately, all attempts were unsuccessful and fatal until 1924 when the German surgeon Kirschner, for the first time, successfully removed such clots from a man's pulmonary artery using instruments and the technique developed by Trendelenberg.[31] It is reported that John Gibbon, inventor of the first heart-lung machine, was inspired to create the device to attempt to improve the result of the pulmonary thrombectomy. Interestingly, the development of the anticoagulant heparin (discussed later in this volume) and thrombolytic (clot-busting) medications has subsequently relegated pulmonary thrombectomy to a historical footnote.

Extracardiac Operations for Congenital Heart Disease

Patent Ductus Arteriosus

The era of congenital cardiac surgery began with an operation to address patent ductus arteriosus. Untreated, this condition was associated with a high incidence of heart failure, bacterial endocarditis, and early death. Boston surgeon John Streider first successfully interrupted a patent ductus arteriosus in 1937.[32] As the posterior wall of the ductus was very adherent to the right pulmonary artery, he used plicating sutures. The patient become septic and died on the fourth postoperative day. At autopsy, bacterial vegetations extended from the ductus to the pulmonary valve. In 1938, surgical resident Robert Gross, at Boston Children's Hospital, operated on a seven-year-old girl with his surgical mentor John Hubbard.[33] Gross described the ductus as seven to eight millimeter in diameter and five to six millimeter in length. A single no. 8 braided silk suture was placed around the ductus, and the vessel was occluded for a three-minute observation.

The blood pressure rose from 100/35 to 125/90. He decided to ligate the ductus permanently and the patient made an uneventful recovery. Gross later reported a technique for successfully dividing the ductus.

Coarctation of the Aorta

Untreated aortic coarctation is associated with aortic dissection, endocarditis and heart failure. In 1943, Clarence Crafoord, in Stockholm, Sweden, while attempting to ligate a patent ductus arteriosus, accidentally tore a large hole in the aorta.[34] He gained hemostatic control by clamping the proximal aorta and took nearly thirty minutes to complete his repair. The patient recovered without dreaded lower limb paralysis. This prompted Crafoord to attempt operative repair of coarctation, which required clamping of the descending thoracic aorta. He performed the first repair, an excision of the coarctation and end-to-end aortic anastomosis, in October 1944. Robert Gross, who had been working on a coarctation model in the laboratory, first operated on a five-year-old boy with this condition in June 1945. The patient died in the operating room. One week later, Dr. Gross operated on a second patient, a twelve-year-old girl. This patient's operation was successful.[35] Dr. Gross had been unaware of Dr. Crafoord's successful surgery several months previously, presumably because of World War II.

The Blue Baby Operation

Tetralogy of Fallot is a devastating congenital heart malformation in which there is a narrowing at or just below the pulmonary valve, a hole between the two ventricles of the heart; the aorta is positioned over the ventricular septal defect instead of in the left ventricle, and the right ventricle is more muscular than normal. This life-threatening condition is often signaled by a bluish or cyanotic cast to the skin, hence the term "blue baby." Helen Taussig, pediatrician in charge of the children's cardiac clinic at Johns Hopkins University, noticed that children with tetralogy of Fallot who had associated persistent patent ductus arteriosus fared better than those who did not.[36] She also noticed that on fluoroscopy, children with tetralogy had small and relatively nonpulsatile flow in their pulmonary arteries. These two observations led her to believe that the major problem in tetralogy was poor pulmonary blood flow. She speculated that an artificial ductus or connection between the systemic and pulmonary circulation would increase pulmonary blood flow and prevent cyanosis. She discussed her theories with Robert Gross in the late 1930s, who did not feel such an operation would be feasible. Perhaps serendipitously, Dr. Alfred Blalock was appointed to the surgical staff at Johns Hopkins in 1941. Blalock had previously reported experimental work connecting the subclavian artery to the pulmonary artery as a treatment for pulmonary stenosis at Vanderbilt University. After persistent persuasion, Helen Taussig convinced Blalock of the potential benefits of improving pulmonary blood flow in tetralogy patients and he began experimental work with the aid of gifted African-American assistant Vivien Thomas. Together, they developed a shunting technique in which the left subclavian artery was joined to the left pulmonary artery. Vivien Thomas developed the fine suturing techniques required to join the two arteries and performed many successful surgeries on animals. In November 1944, Blalock with first assistant William Longmire, and Vivien Thomas and Helen Taussig offering guidance, attempted the first shunt in humans. In the weeks leading up to the surgery, there was tremendous resistance from the medical community at Johns Hopkins for such a risky and unproven procedure to be attempted on a small child.[37] The first patient was a gravely ill eleven-month-old girl named Eileen Saxon. The left subclavian artery was joined to the left pulmonary artery. Almost immediately, the baby's blue complexion turned healthy pink. The baby's postoperative course was complicated, but she eventually was discharged two months postoperatively. Unfortunately, a second shunt procedure was required six months later and the child eventually died. Longmire later described the procedure,

> We lacked the modern vascular instrument and really had little but the professor's determination to carry us through the procedure . . . It was amazing to see the professor gently but blindly insert the right angle clamp into the mediastinum and after dissecting over his index finger, pull out the innominate artery . . . Vivien Thomas stood in back of Dr. Blalock and offered a number of suggestions in regard to the actual technique of the procedure.[38]

Two additional successful cases were done within three months of the first patient and the procedure came to be known as the Blalock-Taussig shunt.

Valve Operations before Cardiopulmonary Bypass

Before antibiotic medicines became widely used, rheumatic fever was the single biggest cause of valve disease. Rheumatic fever is a condition that is a complication of untreated group A streptococcal infection and is likely the result of an unregulated autoimmune response which may lead to rheumatic heart disease. Rheumatic heart disease acutely produces a pancarditis, characterized by endocarditis, myocarditis, and pericarditis. Endocarditis is manifested as mitral and aortic valve insufficiency. Severe scarring of the valves develops during a period of months to years after an episode of acute rheumatic fever, and recurrent episodes may cause progressive damage to the valves. The mitral valve is affected most commonly and severely (three-fourths of patients); the aortic valve is affected second most commonly (one-fourth of patients).

The French surgeon Tuffier, guided by his friend Alexis Carrel, attempted to open a stenotic rheumatic aortic valve in 1912. Tuffier grasped the heart and, using his index finger, invaginated the flaccid aortic wall and attempted to push through the stenotic aortic valve orifice.[39] The twenty-six-year-old patient returned home to Belgium twelve days later in good condition. Although it is unclear how much the patient benefited from this valve dilatation, the operation was the first successful attempt at heart valve repair.

After the First World War, Evarts Graham and Duff Allen, of St. Louis, invented the cardioscope, a mirrored device designed to allow the surgeons to visualize the intracardiac structures on which they were attempting to operate.[40] They successfully used the cardioscopy technique on many dogs to visualize the mitral valve through either the left ventricle or atrium and incised the valve using a knife blade introduced beside the cardioscope. Unfortunately, their first patient, a thirty-two-year-old woman with severe mitral stenosis, died on the table and they never attempted the operation again.

Elliott Cutler, a student of Harvey Cushing, performed the first successful mitral valve surgery in 1923.[41] He reasoned that mitral regurgitation was better tolerated than mitral stenosis and showed this in multiple animal experiments where he created moderate regurgitation with a tenotome knife. His first patient was an eleven-year-old girl. He started through a median sternotomy incision and, after opening the pericardium, inserted the tenotome knife through the left ventricle. The girl lived for over four years after the operation, although her symptoms were not greatly improved. Autopsy revealed that there was indeed an orifice-enlarging incision in the valve! Cutler's next six patients all died within a week of their operation. In his final report of these cases, Cutler lamented that the median sternotomy, transventricular approach may have been too invasive for the extremely sick patients to endure.

Another breakthrough in mitral surgery came in 1925, when British surgeon Henry Souttar attempted an approach through the left atrium.[42] The patient was a fifteen-year-old girl with a history of fulminant rheumatic endocarditis of the mitral valve. She developed severe congestive heart failure with hemoptysis, and in a last ditch attempt to save her life, surgery was considered. Souttar approached the heart through a thoracotomy below the fourth rib, opened the pericardium, and placed ligature sutures around the left atrial appendage. He incised the appendage and placed his right index finger through the appendage and into the mitral valve orifice. Here, he manually dilated the orifice with his index finger, rather than incising it with a blade. The patient made an uneventful recovery. Despite his success, his colleagues refused to send him any other mitral cases and it was twenty-one years until this approach was used in the operating room again. In Souttar's own words, "Although my patient made an uninterrupted recovery, the physicians declared that it was all nonsense and in fact the operation was unjustifiable. In fact, it is of no use to be ahead of one's time."[43]

It was Charles Bailey, a surgeon in Philadelphia, who finally developed a reproducible operation to address mitral stenosis with a reasonable operative mortality.[44] He reckoned that there was a tremendous need for an answer to the problem of mitral stenosis due to its frequency and devastating effect on life expectancy. Bailey, after many animal experiments, attempted to open the mitral valve of three patients between 1945 and 1948. The first died on the operating room table; the second, forty-eight hours after operation; the third, five days after operation. While examining the mitral valve of the second patient at autopsy, Bailey observed that fusion of the commissures at either end of the valve was responsible for the obstruction to flow. He speculated that freeing these commissures would relieve stenosis without cutting into the valve leaflets themselves. Given his three operative mortalities, Bailey knew that only a dramatic success would allow him to continue operating in Philadelphia, where he was given the cruel nickname "the butcher of Hahnemann Hospital." He devised a daring scheme in which he arranged for two mitral valve operations at the same day in different hospitals. He knew that if word got out about a fourth death, his career and reputation would be destroyed so he arranged to perform the first mitral case in the morning at one hospital and perform the second at a different hospital. He reasoned that if the first operation was a failure, he would rush over to the second hospital and perform the second case before anyone knew about the first failure. His gamble paid off. Indeed, the first patient died on the operating table and Bailey quickly went over to the second hospital to perform his second mitral operation. The second operation was a success, and ten days later, Bailey shocked the audience of the American College of Chest Physicians by presenting the patient, in excellent condition, to his colleagues. Soon thereafter, Dwight

Harken, now in Boston, and Lord Brock in London performed successful mitral commissurotomy and the era of closed mitral commissurotomy was born![45, 46]

Bailey would later perform the first successful aortic valve commissurotomy, spurred on by the death of his surgical colleague Horace Smithy, who succumbed to aortic stenosis at the age of thirty-four.[47] The first successful pulmonary valvulotomy was performed by Thomas Holmes Sellers in 1947.[48] The patient had severe tetralogy of Fallot and advanced bilateral pulmonary tuberculosis. A systemic-pulmonary artery shunt was planned on the left side, but Sellers felt a firm structure pushing through the pulmonary trunk during ventricular systole. Suspecting an imperforate pulmonary valve, Sellers used a tenotomy knife, which he passed through the infundibulum to perform a valvulotomy. The patient made a good recovery.

Artificial Heart Valves

The first foray into implantation of an artificial heart valve was performed by Toronto surgical pioneer Gordon Murray. Several years preceding Bailey's successful commissurotomy, Murray attempted to resect the lateral portion of the posterior leaflet of the mitral valve by using a valvulotome and inserting a sling of inverted cephalic vein filled with the palmaris longus tendon across the valve orifice.[49] He positioned two pieces inside the ventricle such that during diastole, the slings allowed blood to enter the ventricle from the atrium. In systole, the slings would occlude the mitral orifice, thereby preventing regurgitation. Although clear records of these operations were not kept, potentially seven of nine cases were performed successfully. The success of Bailey's commissurotomy completely overshadowed Murray's work, and it was not until 1952 that implantation of a heart valve was attempted again.

Charles Hufnagel, in the 1940s, began working on artificial substitutes for large arteries. He developed hollow tubes using the polymer methyl-methacrylate (used in Plexiglas), which was fairly easy to work with and had a low propensity for clot formation. Building on his experimental work with artificial arteries, he eventually set out to devise an artificial heart valve. The valve consisted of a hollow Plexiglas ball caged within a hollow Plexiglas tube. He experimented on over a hundred dogs trying many valve designs in multiple positions, including the ascending and descending aorta. After deciding on the safer descending thoracic aorta position, Hufnagel first implanted his valve into a radiology technician with aortic regurgitation, who recovered and even returned to work.[50] In 1954, Hufnagel reported a series of twenty-three patients starting September 1952 who had this operation, among which there were four deaths in the first ten patients and two deaths in the next thirteen. Late complications included ball dislodgement and thrombosis. The noise created by Hufnagel's caged-ball valve was very loud and easily audible from several meters' distance. It is said that patients with arrhythmias would call Dr. Hufnagel and place the phone to their chest so that he could diagnose their arrhythmia. Progression of heart failure occurred in many patients after Hufnagel's valve implantation in the descending thoracic aorta since the native valve at the aortic annulus remained incompetent. While the era of cardiopulmonary bypass was rapidly approaching and would soon allow open repair and replacement of heart valves within their native annulus, Hufnagel's design inspired many future valve designs, including the Starr-Edwards valve designed by surgeon Albert Starr and retired engineer Lowell

Edwards in 1958.[51] Gordon Murray would soon implant an aortic valve homograft in the descending aorta (described later).

Coronary Surgery before Cardiopulmonary Bypass

Future Nobel Laureate Alexis Carrel, in 1910, performed the first coronary bypass surgery on a dog. He used a length of carotid artery to join the descending thoracic aorta to a circumflex coronary artery branch. In his words:

> *I attempted to perform an indirect anastomosis between descending aorta and the left coronary artery. It was for many reasons a difficult operation. On account of the continuous motion of the heart, it was not easy to dissect and to suture the artery. In one case, I implanted one end of a long carotid artery, preserved in a cold storage, on the descending aorta. The other end was passed through the pericardium and anastomosed to the pericardial end of the coronary near the pulmonary artery. Unfortunately, the operation was too slow. Three minutes after the interruption of the circulation fibrillary contractions appeared, but the anastomosis took five minutes. By massage of the heart, the dog was kept alive, but he died less than two hours afterwards. It shows that the anastomosis must be done in less than three minutes.*[52]

In the 1930s, Claude Beck, in Cleveland, observed in a postmortem examination that a patient with totally occluded right and left coronary arteries had developed dense adhesions around his heart, which Beck believed arose as a response to augment myocardial blood flow from adjacent tissue. Based on this observation, he set out to design experiments in which adjacent tissues including pericardium, pericardial fat, pectoralis muscle, and omentum were mobilized and wrapped around the heart. Postmortem examination showed that anastomotic vessels did develop between these tissues and the myocardium. In the first patient, Beck roughened the outer surface of the heart with a burr and then sutured a pedicle graft of pectoralis muscle to the left ventricular wall.[53] The patient made an uneventful recovery and was angina free after the operation. Beck performed this operation, known as the Beck I, on sixteen patients with only four deaths. Dwight Harken in Boston and others attempted similar procedures. Harken, believing the epicardial layer prevented collateral formation, used 95 percent carbolic acid to remove it.[54] Beck later speculated that the coronary veins may be able to carry oxygenated blood back to myocardial tissue. Beck used a length of brachial artery to join the aorta with the coronary sinus and then ligated the coronary sinus where it enters the right atrium to prevent blood from flowing back into the atrium instead of forward into the coronary veins.[55] In 1950, Canadian Arthur M. Vineberg, based at McGill University, reported implanting the internal mammary artery through a tunnel into the myocardium.[56] He did not actually anastomose the left internal mammary artery to a coronary artery but placed the graft directly into the muscle. Vineberg previously observed in animals that although direct arterial implantation into skeletal muscle lead to the formation of large hematomas in heart muscle, this was not the case, and it acted more like a sponge with the blood distributed into channels within the muscle itself. While many surgeons disputed this concept, Vineberg was able to show that many patients with disabling angina were able to return to their normal lives, angina free. Mason Sones, inventor of coronary angiography, later validated Vineberg's concept by demonstrating communications between the graft in the myocardium and the coronary system by angiography in two patients operated on five and six years earlier.[57] The first coronary bypasses were performed in humans in 1964 by Soviet surgeon V. I. Kolessov.[58] Operations were performed through a left thoracotomy without extracorporeal circulation or preoperative coronary angiography. In 1968, American surgeons George Green and Charles Bailey separately published case reports in which the internal mammary artery was used for coronary artery bypass in patients.[59,60] Bailey and Hirose carried out the anastomosis on the beating heart while Green advocated using cardiopulmonary bypass and fibrillatory arrest. Rene Favaloro performed the first saphenous vein graft aortocoronary bypass in 1968.[61] W. Dudley Johnson furthered efforts to standardize coronary surgery by applying a disciplined approach which could be reliably taught to others. Johnson stated when presenting his paper,

> *Our experience indicates that five factors are important to direct surgery. One: Do not limit grafts to proximal portions of large arteries . . . . Two: Do not work with diseased arteries. Vein grafts can be made as long as necessary and should be inserted into distal normal arteries. Three: Always do end-to-side anastomosis . . . . Four: Always work on dry, quiet field. Consistently successful fine vessel anastomoses cannot be done on a moving, bloody target . . . . Five: Do not allow the hematocrit to fall below 35.*[62]

The road to the development of heart surgery was riddled with controversies and dramatic characters. The following section describes the development of cardiopulmonary bypass, the enabling technology that made heart surgery routine and safe in the modern era.

Notes:

1. Aristotle, *De Partibus Animalium*, Lib III, Cap 4 (Opera Edidit Academia Regia Borussica), 3: 328 quoted from Claude S. Beck, "Wounds of the heart: The technic of suture," *Arch Surg* (1920), 13: 206.

2. Ibid.

3. *The Works of Ambrose Paré*, quoted from Balance, Charles, "Bradshaw Lecture on surgery of the heart," *Lancet* (1920), I, I.

4. R. Nissen, "Billroth and cardiac surgery," *Lancet* (1960), 2: 250.

5. R. G. Richardson, *The Surgeon's Heart* (London: William Heinemann Medical Books Ltd., 1969), chapter 4, p. 43.

6. Ibid.

7. S. Westaby, *Landmarks in Cardiac Surgery* (St. Louis: Mosby-Year-Book Inc., 1997), p. 3.

8. R. G. Richardson, Opus cited, Ref. # 5.

9. Ibid.

10. Ibid.

11. S. Westaby, Opus cited, Ref. # 7, p. 4.

12. Ibid., p. 3.

13. Ibid., p. 8.

14. J. B. Morgagni, "De Sedibus et Cuasis Moroburum" (Lipsiae sumptibus Leopoldi Vossli, 1829), quoted from C. S. Beck, Opus cited, Ref. # 1: 209.

15. S. Westaby, Opus cited, Ref. # 7, p. 12.

16. E. Rose, "Herztamponade" (Ein Beitrag zur Kerchirgurgie), *Deutsche Ztschr Chir*, 20: 329, quoted from C. S. Beck, Opus cited, Ref. # 1: 213.

17. R. G. Richardson, Opus cited, Ref. # 5, chapter 1, p. 13.

18. G. Fischer, "Die Wunden des Herzens und des Herzbeutels," quoted from C. S. Beck, Opus cited, Ref. # 1: 210.

19.   Block, "Verhandlungen der Deutschen Gesellschaft
      fur Chirurgie," quoted from Ibid.: 210.
20.   D. H. Williams, "Stab wound of the heart and
      pericardium—suture of the pericardium—recovery-
      patient alive three years afterwards," *Med Rec* (1897)
      51: 439.
21.   C. W. Lillehei, commentary on Daniel Hale Williams
      in C. H. Organs and M. M. Kosiba, eds. A *Century
      of Black Surgeons: The USA Experience* (Norman,
      Oklahoma: Transcripts Press, 1987), pp. 332-34.
22.   H. C. Dalton, "Report of a case of stab wound of
      the pericardium, terminating in recovery after
      resection of a rib and suture of the pericardium,"
      Ann Surg (1895), 21: 147.
23.   S. Paget, *Paget's Surgery of the Chest*, 1897.
24.   L. Rehn, "On penetrating cardiac injuries and
      cardiac suturing," *Arch Klin Chir* (1897), 55: 315.
25.   J. W. Blatchford 3rd, "Ludwig Rehn: The first
      successful cardiorrhaphy," *Ann Thorac Surg.* (May
      1985), 39(5): 492-95.
26.   L. Rehn, "Zur Chirurgie des Herzens und des
      Herzbeutels," *Arch Klin Chir* (1907), 83: 723; quoted
      from C. S. Beck, Opus cited, Ref. # 1: 212.
27.   L. L. Hill, "A report of a case of successful suturing
      of the heart, and table of thirty seven other cases
      of suturing by different operators with various
      terminations, and the conclusions drawn," *Med Rec*
      (1902), 2: 84.
28.   S. L. Johnson, *The History of Cardiac Surgery* (Johns
      Hopkins Press, 1970), p. 11.
29.   D. E. Harken, "Foreign bodies in and in relation to
      the thoracic blood vessels and heart, I: techniques
      for approaching and removing foreign bodies
      from the chambers of the heart," *Surg Gynecol Obstet*
      (1946), 83: 117.

30. F. Trendelenburg, "Zur Operation der Embolie der Lungenarterie," *Dtsch Med Wochenschr* (1908), 34: 1172; quoted from L. W. Stephenson, "History of Cardiac Surgery," in *Cardiac Surgery in the Adult*, 2nd edition, L. H. Cohn and L. H. Edmunds Jr., eds. (New York: McGraw-Hill, 2003), 329.

31. M. Kirschner, "Ein durch die Trendelenburgische Operation geheiter fall von Embolie der art. Pulmonalis," *Arch Klin Chir* (1924), 133: 312.

32. A. Graybiel, J. W. Strieder, and N. H. Boyer, "An attempt to obliterate the patent ductus in a patient with subacute endarteritis," *Am Heart J* (1938), 15: 621.

33. R. E. Gross and J. H. Hubbard, "Surgical ligation of a patent ductus arteriosus: report of first successful case," *JAMA* (1939), 112: 729.

34. C. Crafoord and G. Nylin, "Congenital coarctation of the aorta and its surgical treatment," *J Thorac Cardiovasc Surg* (1945), 14: 347.

35. R. E. Gross, "Surgical correction for coarctation of the aorta," *Surgery* (1945) 18: 673.

36. S. L. Johnson, Opus cited, Ref. # 28, p. 81.

37. A. Blalock and H. B. Taussig, "The surgical treatment of malformations of the heart in which there is pulmonary stenosis or pulmonary atresia," *JAMA* (1945), 128: 189.

38. L. W. Stephenson, Opus cited, Ref. # 30,p. 329.

39. R. G. Richardson, Opus cited, Ref. # 5, chapter 2, p. 104.

40. S. Westaby, Opus cited, Ref. # 7, p. 4.

41. E. C. Cutler and S. A. Levine, "Cardiotomy and valvulotomy for mitral stenosis," *Boston Med Surg J* (1923), 188: 1023.

42. H. S. Souttar, "Surgical treatment of mitral stenosis," *Br Med J* (1925), 2: 603.

43. R. G. Richardson, Opus cited, Ref. # 5, chapter 2,
     p. 44.
44. C. P. Bailey, "The surgical treatment of mitral
     stenosis," *Dis Chest* (1949), 15: 377.
45. S. L. Johnson, Opus cited, Ref. # 28, p. 99.
46. Ibid.
47. C. P. Bailey et al., "Commissurotomy for rheumatic
     aortic stenosis," *Circulation* (1954), 9: 22.
48. T. H. Sellors, "Surgery of pulmonary stenosis: a
     case in which the pulmonary valve was successfully
     divided," *Lancet* (1948), 1: 988.
49. S. L. Johnson, Opus cited, Ref. # 28, p. 98.
50. C. A. Hufnagel, "Aortic plastic valvular prostheses,"
     Bull Georgetown Med Cent (1951), 4: 128.
51. A. Starr and M. L. Edwards, "Mitral replacement:
     clinical experience with a ball-valve prosthesis," *Ann
     Surg* (1961), 154: 726.
52. A. Carrel, "On the experimental surgery of the
     thoracic aorta and the heart," *Ann Surg* (1910), 52: 83.
53. C. S. Beck, "The development of a new blood supply
     to the heart by operation," *Ann Surg* (1935), 102:
     805.
54. R. G. Richardson, Opus cited, Ref. # 5, chapter 2,
     p. 206.
55. C. S. Beck, "Coronary sclerosis and angina pectoris:
     treatment by grafting a new blood supply upon the
     myocardium," *Surg Gynecol Obstet* (1937), 64: 270.
56. A. M. Vineberg et al., "Myocardial revascularization
     by omental graft without pedicle: Experimental
     background and report on 25 Cases followed 6 to 16
     months," *J Thorac Cardiovasc Surg.* (January 1965),
     49: 103-29.
57. A. M. Vineberg, "Development of an anastomosis
     between the coronary vessels and a transplanted
     internal mammary artery," *Can Med Assoc J* (1946),
     55: 117.

58. V. I. Kolessov, "Mammary artery-coronary artery anastomosis as a method of treatment for angina pectoris," *J Thorac Cardiovasc Surg* (1967), 54: 535.
59. G. E. Green, S. H. Stertzer, and E. H. Reppert, "Coronary arterial bypass grafts," *Ann Thorac Surg* (1968), 5: 443.
60. C. P. Bailey and T. Hirose, "Successful internal mammary-coronary arterial anastomosis using a minivascular suturing technic," *Int Surg* (1968), 49: 416.
61. R. G. Favaloro, "Saphenous vein autograft replacement of severe segmental coronary artery occlusion," *Ann Thorac Surg* (1968), 5: 334.
62. L. W. Stephenson, Opus cited, Ref. # 30, p. 329.

HISTORY OF HEART SURGERY II

Claude Grondin

The advent of anaesthesia in the 1840s was a medical milestone. The discovery by two young New England dentists[1] of the anaesthetic properties of nitrous oxide and sulfuric ether was indeed to establish surgery as a science. The surgical trade was regarded until then as one providing a mode of therapy of last resort, forever risky and, in the eyes of many, somewhat barbaric. Death as an alternative was often what drove the patient to the surgeon! Anaesthesia—the term was coined by Oliver Wendell Holmes—also brought about the creation of surgical subspecialties, each assigning itself to a functional system of the body or to a regional group of organs. At the turn of the twentieth century, some fifty years later, it was said however that heart surgery, regrettably, had reached the limits set by nature.[2] The prediction was to prove wrong in the second half of that century as technical developments pushed back the limits and lifted nearly all obstacles.

The cornerstones of cardiac surgery were first laid in the 1940s by daredevils who pioneered closed heart operations. In the course of the next decade, medical and engineering breakthroughs would make possible correction of complex congenital and acquired heart lesions. Indeed, the development of the heart-lung machine made these corrections available to most patients and to most countries of the world. Furthermore, the second half of the century was to witness the burgeoning not only of the specialties of cardiac surgery and cardiology but also of centers devoted exclusively to the care of cardiac patients.

The Status of Cardiac Surgery in 1954

In early 1954, cardiac surgery seemed at a standstill. Closed heart procedures for mitral stenosis or patent ductus arteriosus (PDA) abounded but open-heart surgery had yet to come along. The majority of grand surgical firsts seemed dated. Closed heart procedures were indeed long in the tooth beginning with repair of PDA (Gross, Boston,[3] 1938), Blalock's anastomosis (1944[4]), commissurotomy of the mitral valve (Bailey, Philadelphia; Harken, Boston,[5] 1948), the pulmonary valve (Brock, London,[6] 1948) and the aortic valve (Bailey,[7] 1951). Valvular insufficiency appeared out of surgical reach and was wrongly believed to be harmless. Things seemed to have stalled. But, to the keen eye, events in fact were moving fast, especially south of the Canadian border.

In Canada, Gagnon had succeeded in opening the mitral[8] and the aortic valves, a few weeks before Bigelow in Toronto.[9] Indeed, the two would begin shortly to exchange through the mail the expensive aortic valve dilator bought by the Montreal Heart Institute. Meanwhile, Dubost in France (1953) and Tubbs in England (1954) developed metallic dilators for aortic and mitral commissurotomies.[10, 11] In the interim, however, interest had shifted south of the Forty-fifth Parallel, away from what shortly would be referred to as "closed heart surgery."

The First Steps Towards Open-heart Surgery

True intracardiac surgery, soon to be called "open-heart surgery" (OHS), began in fact three years earlier, on April 5 1951, at the University of Minnesota.[12] On that day in Minneapolis, Clarence Dennis and Richard Varco attempted closure of a secundum atrial septal defect (ASD) with the help of a cardiopulmonary bypass (CPB) apparatus developed by John Gibbon of Philadelphia who had been working on this project and this device for over fifteen years.[13] Dennis, a brilliant student at Harvard College and at Johns Hopkins Medical School, was Wangensteen's protégé and trainee at the University of Minnesota. He had visited Gibbon in 1945 and had brought back the blueprints of his machine. Over the years, Dennis had made significant changes to the device in his lab. Unfortunately for him and Varco that day, the patient had a complete atrioventricular (AV) canal defect and not a secundum type ASD. The two surgeons could not begin to understand, let alone fix, this complex anomaly. Diagnosis would have been easy through intracardiac angiography (the so-called goose neck deformity on the left ventriculogram) but the technique was years away. The Schönander biplane apparatus would come from Sweden much later. Already in 1938, however, someone in New York, following Gross's closure of a PDA, had begun injecting 20-40 ml of contrast through an arm vein and taking a single picture, four or five seconds later, to visualize the heart and great vessels.[14]

In the early nineteen-fifties several groups were working in the lab to build an apparatus capable of taking over oxygenation and circulation of the blood while the heart was arrested and repair of a defect was made. In addition to Gibbon and Dennis, Dodrill in Detroit, Senning in Stockholm, Kirklin in Rochester, Clowes in Cleveland, and others, whose failed attempts would never be publicized were working on this project. Someone would eventually dare to use such a device and that day would belong to Clarence Dennis.

The Minneapolis School

In 1951, following their previous failure, as mentioned, due to a misdiagnosis, Dennis and Varco succeeded in closing the defect—a true ASD, this time—but the patient succumbed a few hours later, the result of a large air embolus that had occurred earlier during CPB. These two failures would not daunt the Minneapolis group, however. Indeed, several people at the University of Minnesota Hospital were working under the same roof in separate laboratories, each approaching the problem from a different angle.

All this activity, this pioneer spirit, which favored discovery and strokes of genius, was owed to the man in charge, Owen H. Wangensteen, "The Chief," as they called him. At age thirty-one, Wangensteen had been the youngest head of a department of surgery in a U.S. university. Of Norwegian extraction like a lot of his fellow Minnesotans, Wangensteen had put his alma mater on the map with a classic treatise on bowel obstruction and with his studies on duodenal ulcers that led to the famous but short-lived technique of gastric freezing. He was also known for the "second look" operations for carcinoma of the breast, the ganglions and the intestine. On Purple surgery (his service), one did nearly everything: ample gastrointestinal surgery, to be sure, some thoracic procedures (Wangensteen did the world's second PDA in 1939[15] and was successful in eight of his first ten attempts), a tad of gynecology, and at times, some urology. He could prove the world's greatest technician one day and the total opposite the next, as wrote Norman Shumway, one of his most famous pupils.[16] But what a genius! He trained more future heads of departments of surgery than Sauerbruch, Billroth and the European masters of the nineteenth century. He showed early cardiothoracic surgery to Varco who, in turn, instructed Lillehei who was to teach all the others.

The Atrial Well Technique

In 1952, meanwhile, at the Boston Children's Hospital, Robert E. Gross who had ligated the first PDA, closed the first ASD, using a thin rubber well sewn low on the right atrium. This well allowed blood to rise above the atrial incision level without overflowing, while the surgeon grabbed the edges of the defect with a forceps and oversewed it.[17] Several surgeons began to use this technique for ASD closure, including Kirklin at the Mayo Clinic who, with Barratt-Boyes, his resident, reported a never equaled low mortality (4 percent) in seventy-one patients.[18] But the clinic had already abandoned the technique by the time the manuscript was printed in 1956. Indeed, although the heart was opened, the closure of the defect was not done "under direct vision." In fact, one could not see anything under the pool of blood. Further, surgeons would stumble on an AV canal defect or a large ASD requiring a patch of pericardium or of Ivalon. The atrial well technique could not truly allow closure of these defects.

Hypothermia And Temporary Caval Flow Occlusion

Back in Minneapolis, F. John Lewis, aware of Bigelow's experimental work in Toronto on hypothermia,[19, 20] closed an ASD under hypothermia and temporary occlusion of both venae cavae (a technique called "inflow stasis" or "inflow occlusion") again with the help of Richard Varco. Varco had been using temporary inflow occlusion—and normothermia—for pulmonary valvotomy since 1950 or '51 and would continue using it well into the seventies. With the aorta and the pulmonary artery clamped, the ASD was perfectly seen. The term "under direct vision" was coined. It constituted another first for the Minnesota group: September 2, 1952. The technique would soon spread on both sides of the Atlantic in 1953 and '54. Henry Swan, in Denver, followed suit in early 1953 and performed his hundredth case a little over a year later.[21] Bigelow would do Canada's first case in January 1954. None were carried out at the Montreal Heart Institute (see below) but Joffre Gravel would make use of the technique in Quebec City. Nevertheless, Clarence Dennis's pioneering but unsuccessful attempt to operate within the heart with the help of CPB in 1951 was not forgotten. Its time would come.

Gibbon's First Success with Cardiopulmonary Bypass

In Philadelphia, John Gibbon had heard of Clarence Dennis's failures with CPB. In 1952, he tried on his own to close an ASD in a fifteen-month-old child but the operative field became flooded with blood from an unsuspected PDA. There was no ASD. The child succumbed, once again as a result of a misdiagnosis. One year later, on May 6, in an eighteen-year-old girl, the diagnosis was the right one, and Gibbon succeeded in closing the defect.[22] News of the first successful operation with CPB spread around the world. Gibbon was to attempt and fail on four subsequent occasions before calling a moratorium on CPB.[23] He would not return to open-heart surgery. He was only fifty. Much like F. John Lewis, Gibbon could not cope with operative deaths and the loss of four consecutive patients proved too much.

Between 1951 and 1954, other attempts with CPB failed, those of Helmworth, Dodrill, Mustard and Clowes, to the point that of the first eighteen patients, Gibbon's was the only one to survive.[15] All investigators had had success with their apparatus in the lab before their clinical trial. They came to believe that the problem lay not with the machine or even the surgeon but with the patients whose damaged hearts could not cope with the surgical assault. Lillehei's cross-circulation would soon disprove this point.

Cross-circulation

In the meantime, Morley Cohen (who would later return to Winnipeg to begin OHS), C. Walton Lillehei and F. John Lewis had read a recent report in the *British Journal of Surgery*[24] to the effect that a dog's brain could sustain two hours of clamping of both venae cavae without apparent damage while the heart received only the azygos venous return. Cohen, upon Lillehei's request, repeated the experiment, measured the azygos flow and infused it through an isolated dog lobe for oxygenation.[25] The dog survived while his brain and the rest of his body were subjected to a cardiac output only 10-15 percent of normal. This meant that one could use someone else's lungs and heart for the oxygenation and pumping of blood while the patient's heart was arrested to allow repair of defects, as long as a minimal amount of well-oxygenated blood reached the patient's brain via the arterialized blood of that other person. One no longer needed the cumbersome paraphernalia of CPB: only two sets of arterial and venous lines, a pump to regulate flow and a second person—often a relative— whose blood was compatible. Cross-circulation between two persons appeared simple. Moreover, the inherent low-flow principle would help prevent flooding of the operative field which Lillehei, Lewis and Varco believed responsible for Dennis's and Gibbon's failures.[15]

On April 23, 1954, after an initial failure one month earlier, Lillehei with the help of Varco, Cohen and Herb Warden (who shortly afterwards returned to West Virginia to begin an OHS program) succeeded in closing a VSD (ventricular septal defect), with interrupted sutures, in a four-year-old girl whose father served as the "perfusor and oxygenator."[26] The picture of the little Queen of Hearts, as she was to be called, spread around the world. It was the very first closure of a VSD in a human, three years after Dennis's failure and two years after Lewis's success at the same Minneapolis hospital.[20] Both surgeons had left Minnesota by then: Lewis had gone to St. Paul and was on his way to Northwestern University in Chicago and Dennis was already in Brooklyn, and pretty much in oblivion, also. Lillehei, on the other hand, was to achieve instant fame and to remain in the limelight for years to come.

One month later, in comments on his resident's presentation on the experimental aspect of cross-circulation to the American Association for Thoracic

Surgery gathered for its annual meeting in Montreal, Lillehei stunned the crowd at the Mount Royal Sheraton by releasing the details of a few clinical cases he already had performed.[27] Even Herb Warden, the resident, was taken aback! In the next few weeks, Lillehei did several first timers with cross-circulation, including the complete correction of AV canal and of tetralogy of Fallot. In early 1955, a mother used in cross-circulation suffered a cerebrovascular accident which the critics ascribed to air embolism, a complication feared by all and which had delayed acceptance of the procedure by other centers. That was not the case. The patient had presented with a cardiac arrest following perfusion, requiring cardiac massage through a left thoracotomy. She recovered fully and was discharged on the eighth day but the critics would not relent.[14]

Resumption of Cardiopulmonary Bypass

A few months later, on July 12, 1955, Lillehei corrected a tetralogy of Fallot in a six-year-old child with the help of DeWall's bubble oxygenator.[28] Richard DeWall, a general practitioner from a small town in Minnesota who had been denied a surgical residency by the university committee, had been working for some time in Lillehei's lab on his oxygenator. The "bubbler" as it would be called was "homemade," simple to build and was about to revolutionize the field. The oxygenator part—the "bête noire" for all investigators—rested on the simple principle of gas and blood interface. It consisted of a vertical tube through which the blood flowed upwards and contained at the bottom an 18-gauge needle linked to a pressured air line that pushed O_2 through the blood column. Further along, blood streamed down a serpentine tube or helix coated with a defoaming agent to remove air bubbles. The pump at the bottom of the helix consisted of fingerlike structures that compressed the arterial line in an undulating fashion, akin to the device used by dairy farmers to milk cows! However, a few weeks before, John Kirklin, at the Mayo Clinic,[29] ninety miles south of Minneapolis, closed a VSD with a modified version of the Gibbon machine (to be called the Mayo-Gibbon apparatus). Nevertheless, both Minnesotans, as would later be known, were beaten to the wire by Clarence Crafoord and Åke Senning, in Stockholm, who, in July 1954, removed a left atrial myxoma, utilizing cardiopulmonary bypass.[30] Only, their report would appear a full three years later. The two Swedish surgeons from the Karolinska Institute had used a disc oxygenator which would serve as a model for the Kay-Cross apparatus. They also had combined hypothermia—through a heat exchanger placed on the lines (also a first)—in their 1954 operation.[30] Will Sealy, at Duke University, would get credit for this combination of techniques on this side of the Atlantic.[31]

Frederick S. Cross, a former resident in Minnesota who had scrubbed on Lewis's famous first ASD closure, had moved to Cleveland and worked on his gear in the lab at St. Luke's Hospital before his first successful clinical trial with CPB on January 18, 1956.[32] The Kay-Cross apparatus was rapidly commercialized in the United States and Canada and appealed to all who were concerned with the air bubbles potentially escaping defoaming in DeWall's system. The extensive use of the "bubbler" by Denton Cooley in Houston whose number of open-heart cases swiftly outdistanced those of everyone in the field soon dispelled those fears.[33, 34] For many years, the oxygenators of DeWall-Lillehei and of Kay-Cross were the ones most used by surgeons around the world. On the other hand, the Kay-Cross as well as the Mayo-Gibbon heart-lung machines necessitated large priming volumes and required time to clean, sterilize, mount, etc. Neither one ever became disposable whereas the DeWall was a disposable unit, beginning in 1955.[35] Ultimately, even the Mayo Clinic abandoned its Rolls-Royce and dropped it for good in 1971.[14] By the middle seventies, almost all centers had converted to a bubble type of oxygenator.

By 1956, the University of Minnesota Hosptial had become the place to learn or observe open-heart surgery. Dwight Harken, Denton Cooley, Russell Brock, John Kirklin, Henry Bahnson, George Trusler and others could be seen in attendance. Trusler, for his part, returned to Toronto following his visit to the Mecca, and convinced Mustard to abandon his use of a monkey's lung for oxygenation. Mustard had lost all his patients up until then, using a monkey's lung, and in all was to lose eighteen of his twenty-one patients.[14, 36] Lillehei, likewise, used a dog lung as an oxygenator in March 1955, in cooperation with Gill Campbell,[37] but abandoned the cumbersome technique after only four of twelve patients survived the operation. In March 1955, he also had used in a group of five small infants continuous infusion of arterialized blood, thus doing away with the oxygenator part of bypass. The blood was "arterialized" through a fifteen-minute immersion of the blood donor's arm into a basin of hot water, the morning of the scheduled operation.[38] Thus, in 1955, Lillehei tried several different techniques before settling on the heart-lung machine which he used that year in more than fifty patients.

Complete Heart Block and Pacemakers

Complete heart block was a rare but tragic complication of surgical closure of a VSD. Fortunately, most blocks were temporary as sinus rhythm usually returned before the patients' discharge but the permanent ones were associated with 70 percent mortality. The first pacemaker used for temporary postoperative pacing was developed by Vince Gott, then a resident on Lillehei's service in Minneapolis. Its first use was in January 1957.[39] The device was neither portable nor autonomous. One had to run in the halls of the hospital from one electrical outlet to the next in order to move the patient from the operating room to the intensive care unit or to the ward. Earl Bakken, the electrical engineer in charge of all equipment at the University Hospitial succeeded in building a portable pacemaker unit.[39] (He built the gizmo in his garage.) Children were then able to walk around the halls with a small box clipped to their hospital gown or hung around their neck. Cardiac surgeons around the world began copying Lillehei's technique, leaving a pair of electrical wires on the right ventricle in all OHS patients for postoperative pacing. Bakken's breakthrough (which, shortly afterwards, led him to form the Medtronic Company) had begun in Boston with Paul Zoll, a cardiologist, and, in fact earlier in Toronto, with Callaghan and Bigelow.[40, 41]

The Toronto Input

While working on hypothermia, Bigelow noted that a finger nudge on the ventricle would "pace" a heart arrested by cold. A little later, John Callaghan, on Bigelow's advice, came up with an electrical unit which provided a jolt that duplicated the finger scratch effect. He reported the matter to the annual meeting of the American College of Surgeons held in Boston in 1950.[41] Zoll, informed by his surgical colleagues, contacted the Toronto group. He was to be credited with the designing of paddles which, when applied externally to the chest of patients with bouts of sudden heart block (and Adams-Stokes syncope), would electrically jolt the patient and begin to pace his heart until a rhythm of an acceptable rate would resume. The external pacemaker was used first in 1952.[40] This technique which could be life saving in the short term was of little use in permanent adult heart block and was unsatisfactory even for temporary postsurgical block. It was painful and scared the patients, particularly the children, and, with time, would excoriate the skin. Therefore, Gott's and Bakken's surgical invention proved a real progress. Ultimately, Medtronic, with the advent of transistor circuitry, built an implantable unit. The first pacemaker implantation did not take place in Minneapolis, however, but in Sweden with Senning and Elmquist, his engineer, in October 1959.[42] The early batteries had a very short life. In fact, Senning's patient needed two changes of battery units in the first postoperative days and ultimately went home without one as his basic rate had increased. He received a permanent unit of somewhat longer duration at a later date. In the interim, Sam Hunter, a former resident in Minneapolis, now working in St. Paul, developed a bipolar electrode that required a low voltage. He implanted the first one in April 1959.[43] Medtronic had not yet perfected its implantable unit but Hunter would eventually connect the patient's electrodes to a Medtronic unit and be credited with the first implantation of a permanent pacemaker in America. As is often the case, however, with scientific discoverers and inventions, Callaghan, Zoll, Senning and Hunter could count on the subsequent discovery of one or two forerunners.

Thus, some twenty years earlier, Albert S. Hyman, in New York, had constructed a device, akin to a dynamo, which, when hand rewound, could deliver for up to eight minutes an electrical discharge of variable rate through a long transthoracic needle and stimulate the right atrium. Hyman had tried the device in the lab as well as in some patients.[44] With success? No one knows as he never published his clinical results. Hyman, who is credited with coining the term "pacemaker," did present his data—orally—at a New York medical meeting in 1932. His clinical trials and device were soon forgotten, however, much like Souttar's commissurotomy a little earlier. The film *Frankenstein* had caused quite a stir in 1931 and people associated Hyman's experience with that of the physician created by Shelley!

Some years earlier, Mark C. Lidwill, an Australian anaesthesiologist, concocted a simpler device made of a skin plate or pole and a needle insulated down to the tip, both linked to a standard electrical wall plug. The device could regulate both rate and voltage and deliver a jolt of current to the ventricle through the long needle. Lidwill used the device in stillborn babies whose heart could not be revived with intracardiac adrenalin. One day around 1925 or '26, a newborn baby's heart resumed beating after few minutes of pacing, with complete recovery. This astonishing feat was published in the proceedings of the 1929 meeting of the British Medical Association in Sydney.[45]

That both Hyman's nor Lidwill's ideas and devices received much attention should not be surprising. Heart rate, fast or slow, was of little interest at the time. So much so that Claude S. Beck, who was working on ventricular fibrillation (VF) in the late 1930s, was told by a colleague present at the surgical meeting[46] where Beck had just shown a motion picture on VF: "Claude, you work on the most screwy subjects!" The interest in heart rates rekindled in the fifties with the development of cardiac surgery. Although the pathophysiology of heart block was unclear at the time, the association between Adams-Stokes syncope and slow heart rate had long been

established. The matter was to be elucidated in the next
few years, thanks to the histological studies of Maurice
Lev in Chicago and Jean Lenègre in Paris.[47, 48]

In 1960 in Buffalo, Greatbatch, an engineer, and William
Chardack, a cardiac surgeon, adapted Hunter's electrode
to transvenous insertion into the right ventricle.[49, 50] In
1969, lithium batteries that could last ten times longer
than conventional mercury batteries were made available
through the work of Manuel Villafana, in Minneapolis.
Villafana had just left Medtronic to start CPI.[51] He would
eventually sell CPI to Lilly and form ATS to develop the
St. Jude mechanical heart valve. The still-in-use St. Jude
became the mechanical valve most widely used in the
world. CPI, now in the hands of Lilly in Minneapolis,
would eventually put out the implantable cardioverter-
defibrillators—invented by Michel Mirowski—following
the purchase of Medrad, their original makers in
Baltimore.[52]

Valvular Heart Surgery

In 1914, some eleven years before Souttar's first
mitral commissurotomy, Théodore Tuffier, in France,
performed the first opening of an aortic stenosis by
"dilating" the aortic valve of a child with the finger
pressing the aortic wall against the aortic orifice.[53] Some
years later, again before Souttar's exploit, Elliott Cutler,
at Peter Bent Brigham Hospital in Boston, used an
instrument perfected by Claude S. Beck, his resident,
to punch out a hole through the anterior leaflet of the
mitral valve via the left ventricular apex in an attempt to
relieve mitral stenosis.[54] The first patient survived four
and a half years with some degree of mitral insufficiency
but the next six patients succumbed within a week to
severe mitral regurgitation, prompting Cutler to abandon

the procedure. A review of the literature by Beck in 1929 revealed that only three patients out of the twelve reported had survived the operation and two of them had little or no insufficiency, i.e., little or no relief of the stenosis.[55] (Bailey used a similar technique for aortic stenosis, again with significant and poorly tolerated valvular regurgitation. Later, he was the first to treat aortic stenosis successfully in 1951,[56] this time with the use of mechanical dilators inserted into the ascending aorta.) Harold Segall, who at the time was a young resident in Cutler's service at Brigham, had advised their second mitral stenosis patient to undergo the proposed operation. To Segall's chagrin, she did not survive the operation. Years later, however, he would redeem himself. Indeed, the well-known Montreal cardiologist, consulted on that epochal occasion, was to recommend surgery to Gagnon's first mitral commissurotomy at Notre-Dame Hospital in 1950.

For severe aortic stenosis, transapical dilators—used also for mitral stenosis—were to prove of great help before CPB. Lewis's technique of inflow occlusion helped Swan and others to treat scores of young adults with congenital aortic stenosis. Severe calcific stenosis requiring long débridement or valvular replacement had to await cardiopulmonary bypass and, ultimately, valvular prostheses. Mitral insufficiency also awaited similar technological developments. Aortic insufficiency, on the other hand, was tackled successfully much before such breakthroughs. On September 11, 1952, Charles Hufnagel, former trainee of Gross in Boston and now at Georgetown University in Washington, implanted a ball valve in the descending aorta to treat (although incompletely) severe aortic regurgitation.[56] Three years later, Murray in Toronto inserted a segment of human ascending aorta—containing its valvular component—

also in the descending aorta of the recipient to relieve aortic insufficiency.[57]

Open aortic commissurotomy was first performed by Swan in Denver in November 1955. Sir Russell Brock, also using Lewis's inflow occlusion technique, did the second one in London in February 1956.[58] Five days later, Lillehei would perform the first one with CPB.[59] On this occasion, Lillehei used retrograde perfusion of the coronary sinus. Myocardial protection through perfusion of the coronary sinus is an old technique therefore, going back to 1956! Lillehei was also the first to repair mitral insufficiency with CPB, that same year. Henry T. Bahnson, at Johns Hopkins, replaced an aortic valve leaflet with a Dacron cusp in 1960, and Dwight C. McGoon, at the Mayo Clinic, would replace all three leaflets with the same material in 1962.[60, 61] With time, these leaflets tended to shrink and calcify and lead to regurgitation or stenosis.

Similar attempts at replacement of the mitral valve using contraptions that imitated valve shapes and functions were also short-lived. In 1960, Nina Braunwald and Andrew Morrow successfully used a mitral prosthesis made of two flaps of Dacron anchored to the left ventricular wall through chordae.[62] A subsequent meeting on valvular prostheses held in Chicago in September 1960 concluded that prostheses imitating natural valves should be abandoned.[63] A few days later on September 21, Albert Starr, at the University of Oregon, replaced the mitral valve in a fifty-two-year-old man with a ball valve prosthesis.[64] The silastic ball tended to swell and crack through water absorption (the ball variance phenomenon) leading to entrapment or fracture of the ball. The manufacturer later replaced the silastic ball with a metallic ball. Dwight Harken used a double-cage ball prosthesis for the first aortic valve replacement.[65] The

Starr-Edwards aortic ball valve model soon came on the market and supplanted the Harken prosthesis.

In 1965, Jean-Paul Binet, in Paris, used free aortic porcine leaflets to replace an aortic valve in man.[66] Subsequently, Alain Carpentier, working with Carlos Duran and Charles Dubost, also used porcine aortic valves preserved in gluteraldehyde to replace mitral or aortic valves.[67] The leaflets were mounted on three struts serving as commissures and suspenders. Flexible struts, introduced later by Morrow[68] in 1971, helped to decrease stress on the leaflets. Barratt-Boyes used aortic homografts[69] with better long-term results than porcine leaflets—problems of procurement and availability at the time of operation notwithstanding. Donald Ross would soon attempt to circumvent this difficulty by using the patient's own pulmonary valve to replace the aortic valve.[70] Neither technique (Barratt-Boyes's nor Ross's) were used at the Montreal Heart Institute (MHI), but Paul Cartier, at the Heart Institute in Quebec City, did make extensive use of the Barratt-Boyes technique.

Current Surgical Trends in Valvular Heart Disease

In the past fifteen years, treatment of valvular heart disease has changed, not so much in the choice of prostheses which have not varied appreciably but in the approach itself. Mitral repair is common nowadays for mitral insufficiency as well as for mixed stenosis and regurgitation. At the MHI in 2002, for instance, repairs outnumbered replacements, 106 to 98. Incisions are shorter, sternotomy is either shortened or avoided. For pure mitral stenosis, surgical commissurotomy has almost become a thing of the past. Indeed, in 2002, almost all of our patients (sixty-two in all) presenting with pure mitral stenosis had their valve dilated in the cardiac catheterization laboratory. Pulmonary stenosis and pure aortic stenosis of infants and young adults have followed suit. Other congenital lesions such as PDA, ASD and even coarctation of the aorta have come under the care of invasive cardiologists.

Operative mortality has dropped markedly over the years. For valvular replacement, overall surgical mortality—for single or multiple, first time or reoperation—has decreased to under 10 percent in the nineties and to 5 percent in the past five years. The valve clinic set up by Lepage in the early seventies and currently run by Michel Pellerin has been following more than six thousand patients.

Surgery of the Aorta

Modern surgical treatment of aneurysm of the ascending aorta had to await development of cardiopulmonary bypass. Cooley and DeBakey were the firsts to report surgical correction of a fusiform aneurysm of the ascending aorta in 1956.[71] Often such dilatations are associated with aortic valve regurgitation and, not infrequently, with acute or chronic dissection of the aorta. A specific treatment may be required for each of these associated lesions. DeBakey was the first to tackle dissecting aneurysm of the aorta in 1955, even before institution of CPB. Ten years later, he described a classification of dissections still in use today.[72] Techniques of repair have varied somewhat since: for patients who present with dissection or dilatation in association with valvular insufficiency, some favor preservation of the aortic valve[73] at all cost while others, like Bentall, opt to replace the valve and the ascending aorta with a prosthesis that includes a (usually mechanical) valve and requires reimplantation of the coronary arteries.[74]

Cardiac Transplantation

In 1905, in Chicago, Alexis Carrel and Charles Guthrie, using their original arterial suturing technique, implanted in a dog's neck a nonauxiliary heart, that is, a heterotopic heart that takes no part in the circulatory function.[75] Carrel was to receive the Nobel Prize for his work in 1912. Half a century later, in Moscow, Vladimir Demikhov obtained a fifteen-hour survival with implantation in the dog's chest of an auxiliary heart,[76] all this, astonishingly, without the help of CPB! At Stanford University, in 1960, Richard Lower and Norman Shumway, using CPB, were the first to transplant a heart orthotopically in the dog (total replacement in the chest of the dog organ).[77] The technique that Shumway devised was the one Christiaan Barnard would use in the human on December 3, 1967, in South Africa.[78]

In 1965, Shumway obtained a survival of 250 days in the animal with the combination of azathioprine and prednisolone as immunosuppressive agents.[79] One year earlier, in Mississippi, James Hardy had used a chimpanze's heart in a human (the potential donor's heart not becoming available until profound deterioration of the recipient had taken place) but the organ proved too small or too weak to take over circulation upon cessation of CPB.[80] At any rate, such a xenograft was doomed to fail as was to become evident later on.

Following Barnard's success in late 1967, a host of centers and individuals began transplanting human hearts, most for end-stage coronary artery disease. Thus in 1968, forty-eight centers in seventeen countries reported a total of 108 transplantations with a low success rate, even in the short term.[81] Indeed, when Denton Cooley presented his series—the largest in the world—to the Society of Thoracic Surgeons in January 1969 (Cooley had performed the first heart transplant in America on May 2, 1968, Shumway having failed in an earlier attempt in January), seventy-one of the first hundred patients had died, half of them before the eighth postoperative day![82, 83] By 1970, most centers had put a halt to their transplantation program with a few exceptions, among them: Stanford, Capetown, Richmond, Houston and Paris. Shortly afterwards, however, the Stanford group developed the percutaneous technique of endocardial biopsy for the early detection of rejection.[84] When Shumway's team reported better control of rejection with Cyclosporin A in 1983, several investigators resumed their program or joined the fray.[85]

Coronary Artery Surgery

Direct myocardial revascularization began in the late sixties in two separate cities of the American Midwest, only a few weeks apart. René Favaloro, a young resident at the Cleveland Clinic in the early sixties, was the first in 1967 to report bypassing a right coronary artery with a segment of saphenous vein[86] sutured onto the ascending aorta (he initially had replaced segments of the right coronary artery end-to-end with a piece of vein). In the meantime, in Milwaukee, in early 1968, Dudley Johnson and Derward Lepley, a former Wangensteen trainee, reported using the saphenous vein as a bypass conduit between the aorta and the coronary arteries.[87] The technique, overshadowed somewhat by heart transplantation at the time, slowly spread to other centers.

Indirect myocardial revascularization had also had inauspicious beginnings some fifteen years earlier. After lengthy trials in the lab, Arthur Vineberg began implanting the internal mammary artery into a myocardial tunnel in 1950.[88] Proof of the efficacy of this technique awaited development of selective coronary arteriography by Mason Sones, in Cleveland a decade later. Sones actually discovered his method by accident in 1958, as his catheter slipped into the right coronary artery during an aortogram. The full 40 ml of contrast provided him with a "perfect" outline of the vessel. Sones, who abhorred writing papers, would report the technique only four years later[89] after nearly a thousand studies.

Bigelow and his group are given credit for the first demonstration, through selective catheterization of the mammary artery, of a patent Vineberg implant. Sones obtained similar proof of function of the arterial implant also in January 1961,[89] in a patient operated upon by Vineberg himself. A few weeks later, Vineberg and Gialloreto from the Montreal Heart Institute, probably unaware of the Toronto experience (the Toronto group was the first to perform mammary implantations following Vineberg's lead), brought five of their patients to the Cleveland center in early 1961 for postoperative angiographic evaluation by Sones. In the interim, Donald Effler, who had come to Montreal to observe Vineberg operate, began using this technique in large numbers of patients which helped "legitimize" Vineberg's claims, especially with Sones's postoperative studies. It is only fitting that the Cleveland group would be the one to develop the more direct form of revascularization. However, Garrett, working with DeBakey in Houston, was the first to perform an aortocoronary bypass graft with the saphenous vein in 1964,[90] These two had planned an endarterectomy for a left main coronary artery stenosis but had to revert to a vein graft to the left anterior descending artery in order to sever the patient from CPB. The case along with late angiographic demonstration of graft patency was only reported nine years later. Robert Goetz, from New York, was the first to bypass a coronary artery with the internal mammary artery[91] in 1960, thus anticipating the two surgeons most often credited with this première, Vasili I. Kolessov, from Russia,[92] and George Green, of New York,[93] by four and eight years respectively.

Surgery for Cardiac Arrhythmia

In 1930, Wolf, Parkinson and White described a peculiar form of arrhythmia in a group of eleven patients whose EKG showed a short PR interval, a large QRS with a slanted ascending limb or delta wave.[94] The syndrome—which would bear their names—stemmed in these patients from abnormal pathways between the auricles and the ventricles. At Duke University, John Boineau, Andrew Wallace and Will Sealy studied the phenomenon. Sealy had noted the occasional occurrence of ventricular tachycardia (VT) or fibrillation (VF) during OHS when deep hypothermia was utilized.[95] These investigators began recording the arrhythmias using epicardial electrodes and, in so doing, "mapped" the heart. Soon they were able to identify the abnormal pathways in the operating room through the mapping studies. In 1968, Sealy made a lower incision outside the wall of the right auricle in a thirty-two-year-old patient with the WPW syndrome.[96] The delta wave promptly disappeared. Later, John Gallagher, also at Duke, succeeded in localizing these pathways through percutaneously introduced catheters,[97] an advance that would ultimately lead in the early eighties to their interruption in the cath lab.[98, 99] Meanwhile, in the late seventies, James Cox and Sealy used better mapping techniques to remove left ventricular areas of endocardial (postinfarct) scars responsible for the arrhythmia. In Paris, Guiraudon (to work later in London, Ontario) performed an encircling ventriculotomy[100] in similar circumstances with good results. This somewhat aggressive technique did not prove superior to simple resection which, when conducted under mapping conditions, could terminate VT in 75 percent of cases.[101] In the early eighties, Cox, now at Washington University in St. Louis, developed a surgical technique to interrupt atrial reentry tachycardias[102] which he later would perfect and apply to patients with common atrial fibrillation (AF).

Technology moved rapidly in this field as treatment shifted from one moment to the next. On one hand, thrombolytic agents, introduced in the early eighties to prevent impending myocardial infarction or to limit its size, led to a considerable drop in the incidence of VT. At the same time, on the other hand, post infarct VT became the primary target of implantable defibrillators and, as such, rejoined the surgical horizon, at least for a while. Later during the same decade, surgery lost considerable ground when, in the management of the WPW syndrome, it was replaced by percutaneous ablation of the abnormal pathways through radio-frequency. It nearly became a thing of the past the day implantation of cardioverters-defribrillators began being carried out in the electrophysiological (EP) lab. Very little remained for the surgeon to do indeed in the field of arrhythmia except for complications (infections or extrusion of leads or battery units). Other avenues were to open however, more specifically in the treatment of AF where today surgery still appears to hold the lead—through the Maze (Cox) or the Corridor (Guiraudon) techniques.[103, 104] Indeed, Cox reported the highest success rate of the Maze procedure in AF and flutter. The procedure, nowadays, is (usually) reserved for patients who need concomitant mitral repair or replacement or myocardial revascularization.[104] No isolated Maze procedure has been performed at the MHI but scores of them have been done in association with other interventions. Conversely, percutaneous ablation of AF through a Mazelike procedure has not yielded results comparable to its surgical counterpart. It has been abandoned for most part as it requires widespread fulguration of the atrial endocardium. Fulguration limited to the orifice of the pulmonary veins (also used now during surgery), on the other hand, is associated with fewer complications. It is reserved for patients with intractable symptoms and offers better results in patients with paroxysmal AF.[105]

Cardiac Converters-defibrillators

Following the development of open-heart surgery in the fifties, treatment of AV block evolved rapidly with implantation of the first pacemaker in 1959. History did not repeat itself later in the case of VT or VF although the effects of these arrhythmias upon individuals were perhaps more deleterious. Indeed, for fully documented and symptomatic ventricular arrhythmias, a whole range of drugs, most with serious side effects, were used to treat VT/VF while the real and effective solution to the problem—brought forward by a young Polish expatriate—was not heeded. Indeed, Michel Mirowski published on the experimental use of an implantable device, akin to a pacemaker, that could detect and terminate VT or VF through an electrical jolt to the heart. The paper which appeared in the somewhat peripheral *Annals of Internal Medicine*[106] was entitled "An approach to the prevention of sudden cardiac death" and came on the heels of the first truly effective treatment—coronary bypass grafting—of ischemic heart disease, the condition responsible for most cases of VT/VF. Although the topic could not have been more current at the time, it failed to attract or impress Ingelfinger, the editor of the powerful *New England Journal of Medicine* or his peers, and the manuscript was rejected.[107] Ten years later, the first clinical defibrillator was implanted at Hopkins under Mirowski's supervision and, this time, the New England periodical accepted publication of the report on the historic event.[108] Several subsequent studies were required before the idea and the superiority of the device—over drug therapy—were acknowledged. The widespread use of defibrillators has helped to facilitate their implantation—now by cardiologists in the EP lab—and to diminish their cost. Today, the apparatus saves as many lives as the first pacemakers did earlier in the sixties for patients with heart block. Mirowski's contribution was to be recognized a few years later in what were to be the last of his life. He died prematurely in 1990 from multiple myeloma.[109] The pacemaker, as seen earlier, may have had several fathers. The defibrillator had only one: Michel Mirowski.

Cardioversion

In 1962, Bernard Lown, in Boston, described the "modern" technique of cardioversion of AF.[110] In February 1963, surgeons at the MHI began using this technique. Dwight McGoon happened to visit the institute a few weeks later and bore testimony to its efficacy upon his return to Rochester. He may even have initiated the procedure at Mayo, for the technique was not well known. Indeed, Lown, in a second paper a year later, reported using cardioversion in only fifty patients.[111] In contrast, defibrillation for VT or VF which Claude Beck had described first (in 1947) was widely used by then.[112] Defibrillation was initially done through the direct application of paddles on the heart but had become indirect or transthoracic by the time cardioversion, also applied through paddles on the chest, was described.

Before Lown's paper, several investigators including the Toronto group (Callaghan, Bigelow and their engineers, Jack Hopps and Orest Roy) had been working on direct current defibrillators. Leon Katz, who also was working on this topic, was in constant contact with his friends in Toronto. Ultimately, Katz and the MHI settled for the Toronto device in the operating room. But, in the midfifties, Katz, working with Gagnon and Liang, had come up with a "defibrillator" (or as should be more aptly named a "cardioverter") synchronized to the QRS complex. Sometime between 1955 and 1960, Gagnon used the device successfully in several patients with AF.[113] Neither he, Katz nor Liang reported their experience however. Although Lown was to be given credit for the "novelty," it would appear that several groups like the one at the Institute had experience with some form of cardioversion for AF before 1962. Be that as it may, true surgical interventions for arrhythmia were to await several years, here and elsewhere.

Notes:

1.   A. S. Lyons and R. J. Petrucelli, *Medicine, an Illustrated History* (New York: HN Abrams Publishers, 1987), p. 529.

2.   S. Paget, *The Surgery of the Chest* (Bristol: John Wright & Co., 1896), p.121.

3.   R. E. Gross and J. P. Hubbard, "The surgical treatment of patent ductus arteriosus," *JAMA* (1939), 112: 729-31.

4.   A. Blalock and H. B. Taussig, "The surgical treatment of malformations of the heart in which there is pulmonary stenosis or atresia," *JAMA* (1945), 128: 189-202.

5.   D. E. Harken et al., "Surgical treatment of mitral stenosis," *N Engl J Med* (1948), 239: 801-9.

6.   R. C. Brock, "Pulmonary valvulotomy for the relief of congenital pulmonary stenosis," *Brit Med J* (June 1948), 12: 1121-26.

7.   C. P. Bailey et al., "Commissurotomy for aortic stenosis," *J Int Coll Surg* (1953), 20: 393-402.

8.   E. D. Gagnon, "Commissurotomy in mitral stenosis," *Can Med Ass J* (1950), 63: 537-40.

9.   W. G. Bigelow, *Cold Hearts: The Story of Hypothermia and the Pacemaker* (Toronto, Canada: McClelland and Stewart, 1984).

10.   C. Dubost, G. Oteifa, and P. Blondeau, "Le problème technique de la commissurotomie mitrale: résultats obtenus par dilatation instrumentale de la sténose," *Mem Acad Chir* (1954), 80: 321-32.

11.   S. Westaby, *Landmarks in Cardiac Surgery* (Oxford: ISIS Medical Media, 1997), p. 180.

12.   C. Dennis et al., "Development of a pump oxygenator to replace the heart and lungs: an apparatus applicable to human patients and application to one case," *Ann Surg* (1951), 134: 709-21.

13.   J. H. Gibbon Jr., "Artificial maintenance of circulation during experimental occlusion of pulmonary artery," *Arch Surg* (1937), 34: 1105-31.

14.   S. Westaby, Opus cited, Ref #11, p. 92.

15.   C. W. Lillehei, "Historical development of cardiopulmonary bypass," In *Cardiopulmonary Bypass: Principles and Practice*, G. P. Gravlee, R. F. Davis, and J. R. Utley, eds. (Williams and Wilkins, 1993).

16.   N. E. Shumway, "C. Walton and F. John," *Ann Thorac Surg* (1999), 68: S34-36.

17.   R. E. Gross et al., "A method for surgical closure of interauricular septal defects," *Surg Gyn Obstet* (1953), 96: 1-23.

18.   J. W. Kirklin, F. H. Ellis, and B. G. Barratt-Boyes, "Technique for repair of atrial septal defect using the atrial well," *Surg Gynecol Obstet* (1956), 102.

19. W. G. Bigelow, J. C. Callaghan, and J. A. Hopps, "General hypothermia for experimental intracardiac surgery," *Ann Surg* (1950), 132: 531-39.

20. F. J. Lewis and M. Taufic, "Closure of atrial septal defects with the aid of Hypothermia: experimental accomplishments and the report of one successful case," *Surgery* (1953), 33: 52-59.

21. H. Swan, I. Zeavin, and S. G. Blount Jr., "Surgery by direct vision in the open heart during hypothermia," *JAMA* (1953), 153: 1081-85.

22. J. H. Gibbon Jr., "Application of a mechanical heart and lung apparatus to cardiac surgery," *Minn Med* (1954), 37: 171-85.

23. J. W. Kirklin, "Open-heart surgery at the Mayo Clinic—the 25th anniversary," *Mayo Clinic Proc* (1980), 50: 339.

24. A. T. Andreasen and F. Watson, "Experimental cardiovascular surgery," *Brit J Surg* (1952), 39: 548-51.

25. M. Cohen and C. W. Lillehei, "A quantitative study of the azygos factor during caval occlusion in the dog," *Surg Gynecol Obstet* (1954), 98: 225-32.

26. C. W. Lillehei et al., "The direct vision intracardiac correction of congenital anomalies by controlled cross circulation," *Surgery* (1955), 38: 11-29.

27. H. E. Warden et al., "Controlled cross circulation for open intracardiac surgery," *J Thorac Cardiovasc Surg* (1954), 28: 331.

28. R. A. DeWall et al., "Total body perfusion for open cardiotomy utilizing the bubble Oxygenator: Physiologic response in man," *J Thorac Cardiovasc Surg* (1956), 32: 591-603.

29. J. W. Kirklin et al., "Intracardiac surgery with the aid of a mechanical pump-oxygenator system (Gibbon type): report of eight cases," *Proc Staff Meet Mayo Clin* (1955), 30: 201-6.

30.   C. Crafoord, B. Norberg, and A. Senning, "Clinical
       studies in extracorporeal circulation with a heart-lung
       machine," *Acta Chir Scand* (1957), 112: 220-45.
31.   W. C. Sealy, I. W. Brown, and W. G. Young, "A report
       on the use of both extracorporeal circulation and
       hypothermia for open-heart surgery," *Ann Surg*
       (1958), 147: 603-12.
32.   F. S. Cross and E. B. Kay, "Direct vision repair of
       intracardiac defects utilizing a rotating disc reservoir-
       oxygenator," *Surg Gynecol Obstet* (1957), 104.
33.   A. C. Cooley, "Recollections of early development
       and later trends in cardiac surgery," *J Thorac
       Cardiovasc Surg* (1989), 98: 817-22.
34.   D. A. Cooley, A. C. Beal, and P. Grondin, "Open-
       heart operations with disposable oxygenators,
       5 percent dextrose prime and normothermia,"
       Surgery (1962), 52: 713.
35.   C. W. Lillehei et al., "Direct vision in intracardiac
       surgery in man using a simple disposable artificial
       oxygenator," *Dis Chest* (1956), 29: 1.
36.   W. T. Mustard and J. A. Thomson, "Clinical
       experience with the artificial heart-lung
       preparation," *J Can Med Assoc* (1957), 76: 265-69.
37.   G. S. Campbell, N. W. Crisp Jr., and E. B. Brown,
       "Total cardiac bypass in humans utilizing a pump
       and heterologous lung oxygenator (dog lungs),"
       Surgery (1956), 40: 364.
38.   H. E. Warden et al., "Direct vision intracardiac
       surgery by means of a reservoir of 'arterialized
       venous' blood: Description of a simple method and
       report of the first clinical case," *J Thorac Cardiovasc
       Surg* (1955), 30: 649-57.
39.   V. L. Gott et al., "Control of complete heart block
       by use of an artificial pacemaker and a myocardial
       electrode," *Circ Res* (1958), 6: 410-15.

40. P. M. Zoll et al., "External electric stimulation of the heart in cardiac arrest," *Arch Int Med* (1955), 96.

41. J. C. Callaghan and W. G. Bigelow, "An electrical artificial pacemaker for standstill of the heart," *Ann Surg* (1951), 134: 8-15.

42. A. Senning, in discussion of *J Thorac Surg* (1959), 38: 639.

43. S. W. Hunter et al., "A bipolar myocardial electrode for complete heart block," *Lancet* (1959), 79: 506.

44. A. S. Hyman, "Resuscitation of the stopped heart by intracardiac therapy," *Arch Int Med* (1930), 46: 553-62.

45. H. G. Mond, J. G. Sloman, and R. H. Edwards, "The first pacemaker," *PACE* (1982), 5: 278-82.

46. K. Jeffrey, "The invention and reinvention of cardiac pacing," *Cardiology Clinics* (1992), 10: 561-71.

47. M. Lev and P. N. Unger, "The pathology of the conduction system in acquired heart disease," *Arch Pathol* (1955), 60: 502-9.

48. J. Lenègre, "Etiology and pathology of bilateral bundle branch block in relation to complete heart block," *Prog Cardiovasc Dis* (1964), 6: 409-44.

49. W. M. Chardack, A. A. Gage, and W. Greatbatch, "A transistorized self-contained implantable pacemaker for the long term correction of complete heart block," *Surgery* (1960), 48: 643-50.

50. W. Greatbatch et al., "The solid state lithium battery: A new improved implantable cardiac pacemaker," *IEEE Trans Biomed Eng* (1971), 18: 313-23.

51. V. Parsonnet and M. Manhardt, "Permanent pacing of the heart 1952-1976," *Amer J Cardiol* (1977), 39: 250-54.

52. R. G. Hauser and M. S. Heilman, "The industrialization of the AICD," *PACE* (1991), 14: 905-9.

53. T. Tuffier, "État actuel de la chirurgie intrathoracique," *Trans Int Congr Med* (London: 1913, 1914), sect 7, *Surgery*, part 2, p. 279.

54. E. C. Cutler and S. A. Levine, "Cardiotomy and valvulotomy for mitral stenosis: Experimental observations and clinical notes concerning an operated case with recovery," *Boston Med Surg J* (1923), 188: 1023.

55. E. C. Cutler and C. S. Beck, "The present status of the surgical procedure in chronic valvular disease of the heart," *Arch Surg* (1929), 18: 403-19.

56. C. A. Hufnagel et al., "Surgical correction of aortic insufficiency," *Surgery* (1954), 35: 673.

57. G. Murray, W. Rocheleau, and W. Lougheed, "Homologous aortic-valve-segment transplants as surgical treatment for aortic and mitral insufficiency," *Angiology* (1956), 7: 466.

58. S. Westaby, Opus cited, Ref # 11, p. 149.

59. C. W. Lillehei et al., "The direct vision correction of cardiac aortic stenosis by means of a pump oxygenator and retrograde coronary sinus perfusion," *Diseases of the Chest* (1956), 30: 123.

60. H. T. Bahnson et al., "Cusp replacement and coronary perfusion in open operation on the aortic valve," *Ann Surg* (1960), 152: 494.

61. D. C. McGoon and E. A. Moffit, "Total prosthetic reconstruction of the aortic Valve," *J Thorac Cardiovasc Surg* (1963), 46: 162.

62. N. S. Braunwald, T. Cooper, and A. G. Morrow, "Complete replacement of the mitral valve: successful clinical application of a flexible polyurethane prosthesis," *J Thorac Cardiovasc Surg* (1960), 40: 1-10.

63. E. A. Lifrak and A. Starr, "Historic aspects of cardiac valve replacement, in *Cardiac Valve Prostheses* (NY: Appleton-Century-Crofts, 1979), p.28.

64. A. Starr and M. L. Edwards, "Mitral valve replacement: clinical experience with a ball-valve prosthesis," *Ann Surg* (1961), 154: 726.

65. D. E. Harken et al., "Partial and complete prosthesis in aortic insufficiency," *J Thorac Cardiovasc Surg* (1960), 40: 744.

66. J. P. Binet et al., "Heterologous aortic valve transplantation," *Lancet* (1965), 2: 1275.

67. A. Carpentier et al., "Biological factors affecting long-term results of valvular heterografts," *J Thorac Cardiovasc Surg* (1969), 58: 467-77.

68. R. L. Reiss et al., "The flexible stent: A new concept in the fabrication of tissue valve," *J Thorac Cardiovasc Surg* (1971), 62: 683.

69. B. G. Barratt-Boyes, "Homograft aortic valve replacement in aortic incompetency and stenosis," *Thorax* (1964), 19: 131.

70. D. N. Ross, "Homotransplantation of the aortic valve in the sub coronary Position," *J Thorac Cardiovasc Surg* (1964), 47: 713.

71. D. A. Cooley and M. E. DeBakey, "Resection of entire ascending aorta in fusiform aneurysm using cardiac bypass," *JAMA* (1956), 162: 1158.

72. M. E. DeBakey et al., "Surgical management of dissecting aneurysms of the aorta," *J Thorac Cardiovasc Surg* (1965), 49: 130-49.

73. T. E. David and C. M. Feindel, "An aortic valve-sparing operation for patients with aortic incompetence and aneurysm of the ascending aorta," *J Thorac Cardiovasc Surg* (1992), 103: 617-22.

74. H. Bentall and A. de Bono, "A technique for complete replacement of the ascending aorta," *Thorax* (1968), 23: 338.

75. A. Carrel and C. C. Guthrie, "The transplantation of veins and organs," *Am Med* (1905), 10: 1101-2.

76. V. P. Demikhov, *Experimental Transplantation of Vital Organs* (New York: Consultants Bureau, 1962).

77. R. R. Lower and N. E. Shumway, "Studies in orthotopic homotransplantations of the canine heart," *Surg Forum* (1960), 11: 18.

78. C. N. Barnard, "A human cardiac transplant: an interim report of a successful operation performed at Groote Schurr Hospital, Capetown," *S Afr Med J* (1967), 41: 1271-74.

79. R. R. Lower, E. Dong Jr., and N. E. Shumway, "Long-term survival of cardiac homograft," *Surgery* (1965), 58: 110-19.

80. J. D. Hardy et al., "Heart transplantation in man," *JAMA* (1964), 188: 114-122.

81. S. L. Lansman, M. A. Ergin, and R. B. Griepp, "History of cardiac transplantation," in *Heart and Heart-Lung Transplantation*, J. Walwork, ed. (WB Saunders, 1989).

82. J. C. Callaghan, in comment of Cooley, Ref #83.

83. D. A. Cooley et al., "Organ transplantation for advanced cardiopulmonary disease," *Ann Thorac Surg* (1969), 8: 30-46.

84. P. K. Caves et al., "Serial transvenous biopsy of the transplanted human heart," *Lancet* (1974), 1: 821-26.

85. P. E. Oyer et al., "Cyclosporin A in cardiac allograft: a preliminary experience," *Transpl Proceed* (1983), 15: 1247-52.

86. R. G. Favaloro, "Saphenous vein autograft replacement of severe segmental coronary occlusion: Operative technique," *Ann Thorac Surg* (1968), 5: 334-39.

87. W. D. Johnson et al., "Extended treatment of severe coronary artery disease: a total surgical approach," *Ann Surg* (1969), 170: 460.

88.   A. M. Vineberg and G. Miller, "Internal mammary coronary anastomoses in the surgical treatment of coronary artery insufficiency," *Can Med Ass J* (1951), 64: 204.

89.   F. M. Sones Jr. and E. K. Shirey, "Cine coronary arteriography," *Mod Concepts Cardiovasc Dis* (1962), 31: 735-38.

90.   H. E. Garrett, E. W. Dennis, and M. E. DeBakey, "Aorto coronary bypass with saphenous vein graft: Seven-year follow-up," *JAMA* (1973), 223: 792.

91.   R. H. Goetz et al., "Internal mammary-coronary artery anastomosis: A nonsuture method employing tentalum ring," *J Thorac Cardiovasc Surg* (1961), 41: 378-86.

92.   V. I. Kolessov, "Mammary artery-coronary artery anastomosis as method of treatment for angina pectoris," *J Thorac Cardiovasc Surg* (1967), 45: 535-44.

93.   G. E. Green, S. H. Stertzer, and E. H. Repport, "Coronary arterial bypass grafts," *Ann Thorac Surg* (1968), 5: 443-50.

94.   L. Wolff, J. Parkinson, and P. D. White, "Bundle branch block with short P-R interval on healthy young people prone to paroxysmal tachycardia," *Am Heart J* (1930), 5: 685.

95.   W. C. Sealy, "The Wolff-Parkinson-White syndrome and the beginnings of direct arrhythmia surgery," *Ann Thorac Surg* (1984), 38: 176-80.

96.   W. C. Sealy et al., "Surgical treatment of WPW syndrome," *Ann Thorac Surg* (1969), 9: 1-10.

97.   J. L. Cox, J. T. Gallagher, and M. E. Cain, "Experience with 118 consecutive patients undergoing operation for the WPW syndrome," *J Thorac Cardiovasc Surg* (1985), 90: 490-501.

98.   F. Morady and M. M. Scheinman, "Transvenous catheter ablation of a posteroseptal accessory

pathway in a patient with the Wolf-Parkinson-White syndrome," *N Engl J Med* (1984), 310: 705-7.

99.   W. M. Jackman et al., "Catheter ablation of accessory atrioventricular pathways (WPW syndrome) by radiofrequency current," *N Engl J Med* (1991), 324: 1605-11.

100. G. Guiraudon et al., "Encircling endocardial ventriculotomy: A new surgical treatment for life-threatening ventricular tachycardia resistant to medical treatment following myocardial infarction," *Ann Thorac Surg* (1978), 26: 438-44.

101. M. E. Josephson, A. H. Harken, and L. N. Horowitz, "Long-term results of endocardial resection for sustained ventricular tachycardia in coronary disease patients," *Am Heart J* (1982), 104: 51-57.

102. J. L. Cox, R. B. Schuessler, and J. P. Boineau, "The surgical treatment of atrial Fibrillation," *J Thorac Cardiovasc Surg* (1991), 101: 402-5.

103. A. M. T. Defauw et al., "Surgical therapy of paroxysmal atrial fibrillation with the 'corridor' technique," *Ann Thorac Surg* (1992), 53: 564-71.

104. N. Ad and J. L. Cox, "Combined mitral valve surgery and the Maze III procedure," seminars in *Thorac Cardiovasc Surg* (2002), 14: 206-9.

105. S. Nattel et al., "New approaches to atrial fibrillation management: a critical review of a rapidly evolving field," *Drugs* (2002), 62 (16): 2377-97.

106. M. Mirowski et al., "Standby automatic defibrillator: an approach to prevention of sudden coronary death," *Arch Int Med* (1970), 126: 158-61.

107. J. A. Kastor, "Michel Mirowski and the automatic implantable Defibrillator," *Am J Cardiol* (1989), 63: 1121-26.

108. M. Mirowski et al., "Termination of malignant ventricular arrhythmias with an implantable

automatic defibrillator in human beings," *N Engl J Med* (1980), 303: 322-24.

109. J. A. Kastor, "Michel Mirowski: a man with a mission," *PACE* (2001), 14: 865.

110. B. Lown, R. Amarasingham, and G. Neuman, "New method for terminating cardiac arrhythmias: Use of synchronized capacitator discharge," *JAMA* (1962), 182: 548.

111. B. Lown et al., "'Cardioversion' of atrial fibrillation: A report on the treatment of 65 episodes in 50 patients," *N Engl J Med* (1963), 269: 325.

112. C. S. Beck, W. H. Pritchard, and H. S. Feil, "Ventricular fibrillation of long duration abolished by electrical shock," *JAMA* (1947), 135: 985.

113. L. Katz, "Personal communication" (June 2003).

CHAPTER 2

EARLY DAYS IN TORONTO:
THINNED BLOOD, MONKEY LUNGS,
AND THE COLD HEART

*Reprinted with permission from *Journal of Cardiac Surgery* (2004), 19: 275-78

Shafie Fazel, William G. Williams, and Bernard S. Goldman

In reviewing the history of cardiac surgery, the reader cannot help but be overwhelmed with admiration for those pioneering surgeons and scientists whose courageous innovations, untiring work and difficult early clinical experiences finally made the heart a surgically accessible organ. The collaboration among engineers, physiologists, chemists and surgeons serves as a model for medical progress. In this article, we will review the contributions to the field of open-heart surgery that came from the University of Toronto in the very early days of this elusive goal. Although much remained within the experimental stage, the accomplishments described, nonetheless, exemplify the unique and untiring imagination of those involved at that time.

This paper will review the major advances that were made in the 1930s in purifying a commercially available and safe extract of heparin, anticoagulation being the "key to open-heart surgery,"[1] as well as the experimental and clinical work in the late 1940s and early 1950s by two pioneering Canadian cardiac surgeons: Dr. William T. Mustard and extracorporeal circulation at the Hospital for Sick Children, and Dr. Wilfred G. Bigelow and hypothermia at the Toronto General Hospital.

The Heparin Story

Heparin was discovered by Jay McLean in 1916[2] while working at "a sink and attached drain board with a shelf over the sink in a large student laboratory" supervised by the famous physiologist Dr. William Henry Howell at the Johns Hopkins University in Baltimore.[3] Dr. Howell's laboratory however was unable to extract a clinically safe form of heparin for human use. That accomplishment came many years later, to the experienced team of Dr. Charles Best at the University of Toronto. Dr. Best, a co-discoverer of insulin while still a medical student (with Dr. Fredrick G. Banting), graduated with high honours from the University of Toronto Medical School in 1925. In 1929, at the age of twenty-nine, this bright young physician-scientist was appointed professor and head of the department of physiology. Soon after this appointment, he assembled a team to undertake the study of heparin. Dr. Best writes: "I had made a comprehensive study of the literature and it became apparent that very little work was indeed being done in this field. No anticoagulant was safe for clinical work and none was being used."[4] He set out the directives that guided the research: (1) to find a readily available source of heparin and (2) to purify the extract so that it was potent and suitable for safe use in humans.

He hired Dr. David Scott, already working on purifying insulin at the Connaught Laboratories in Toronto, and as well, a young organic chemist named Dr. Arthur Charles.

Their research started in 1929, and after a painstaking eight years was completed in 1937, with the final production of a pure commercial form of heparin that could be administered safely to human patients. Dr. Albert Fisher, who collaborated on certain aspects of the heparin investigations, outlined the reasons why the research took so long: "No sooner had Charles and Scott obtained an active extract from the inexpensive bulk beef liver than liver became a popular pet food which drove the price out of range. With some misgivings, Charles and Scott turned to extraction of beef lungs that were plentiful in the abattoir. Later the pet food industry struck once again—beef lungs were needed for pet food and again the price increased. With a sense of desperation, the team turned to intestines."[5] To this day, heparin is extracted and purified from bovine lungs and porcine intestines with minor modifications to the original Best protocol. In 1933, Dr. Gordon Murray, a vascular surgeon at the Toronto General Hospital who had realized the potential for an anticoagulant in vascular surgery, joined Dr. Best's team on the advice of Professor W. E. Gallie, chairman of the university department of surgery, with the directive to take bench side experiments to the bedside. By 1935, Best, Murray and colleagues had produced a form of heparin that was safe for human use. On April 16, 1935, Murray administered heparin for the first time to a patient with deep venous thrombosis at Toronto General Hospital.[6] Dr. Murray's pioneering work clearly documented the effectiveness of heparin in reducing the incidence of pulmonary embolism from venous thrombosis as well in repairing damaged or severed arteries. [7] Dr. Murray later went on to become a highly imaginative and controversial pioneer in early cardiac operations in Toronto. In the early 1950s when open-heart surgery was becoming increasingly possible, heparin was recognized as a safe and proven anticoagulant, necessary for preventing thrombus within artificial surfaces.

Monkey Lungs

William T. Mustard received his medical degree from
the University of Toronto in 1937. After finishing three
one-year internships at the Toronto General Hospital, the
Hospital for Sick Children and the New York Orthopedic
Hospital, he enrolled in the prestigious Gallie course in
postgraduate surgery at Toronto General Hospital. During
the years 1941-1945, Mustard was the commanding field
officer of a surgical unit in the Canadian army overseas.
Following WWII, he returned to Toronto to complete
surgical training in orthopedic surgery, and through 1948-
1964, he was staff and then chief of orthopedic surgery
at the Hospital for Sick Children. During this period, his
interest in heart surgery grew steadily. However, apart
from one month of training with Dr. Alfred Blalock
at the Johns Hopkins University, he did not receive
any other formal training in cardiovascular surgery.
Nonetheless, he established the first pediatric cardiac
surgery unit in Canada at the Hospital for Sick Children
where he served as the chief of cardiovascular surgery
from 1964 until his retirement in 1976.[8] The senior
author of this paper (BSG) had the unique pleasure of
working with Dr. Mustard as a cardiac surgical resident
in 1969 performing intraatrial baffles for transposition
and total correction of tetralogy in the morning while
attending to *talipes equino varus* (clubfoot) and other
children's orthopedic deformities in the afternoon! His
best-known contribution to pediatric heart surgery was
the Mustard intraatrial baffle for transposition of the
great arteries, an operation widely adopted by cardiac
surgeons around the world. His work on establishing an
effective extracorporeal circuit is less well known. The
efforts of basic science and clinical research in heart-
lung support were at the forefront of cardiovascular
interest at that time. Reviewing Dr. Mustard's work attests

to his courage and foresight to develop some form of cardiopulmonary support to extend the dominion of the surgeon to include the interior of the heart.

The extracorporeal heart-lung machine required two components: (1) the perfusion pump and (2) the oxygenator. The Cowan pump,[9] which was designed and built at the Banting and Best Department of Medical Research in Toronto, comprised two vertical units with two bulbs in each (figure 2:1). Venous blood was pumped by the two parallel bulbs in one vertical unit through artificial valves and into the oxygenator. This blood was then pumped through a duplicate apparatus back into the subject. Compression and expansion of the bulbs was effected by the sliding action of thrust plates that could rotate at a rate of sixty rounds per minute. Flow could be adjusted independently in each circuit to provide any flow rate between zero and 3.75 L/min.

After poor results in dog experiments utilizing various artificial oxygenators, Drs. Mustard and A. Lawrence Chute (later chief of pediatrics) focused their attention on donor dog lungs to establish cardiac bypass. The first survival in a canine cardiac bypass operation was in 1949.[10] The heart was bypassed for seventeen minutes using a lung that had been removed 2.5 hours previously. The procedure involved the removal of the right lower lobe of a donor dog lung after full heparinization. The lobar bronchus and pulmonary artery were then cannulated and placed in a glass jar. The oxygenated blood would then drip to the bottom of the jar and would be pumped back to the subject. In the experimental recipient dog, the femoral veins were cannulated and the superior vena cava was cannulated indirectly through the azygos vein. The arterial cannula was placed in the right subclavian or femoral arteries with flow directed towards the aortic root. With bicaval occlusion the dog would be placed on total cardiopulmonary bypass. Numerous experimental operations were performed through the right atrium and right ventricle. These included removal of the inter-atrial septum, repairing artificial septal defects, removal of portions of the mitral valve and cardiotomies of the right and left ventricles. In a report of the first thirteen cardiotomies, two dogs suffered massive air embolism with resultant death and one other dog had prolonged hypotension. The other ten animals were sacrificed three to six months after the operation. The longest perfusion time was forty-two minutes.[11]

With these relatively successful experimental operations, work was undertaken for the first human heart operation. Initial investigations revealed adequate oxygenation of human blood when passed through aerated monkey lungs. The more specific effects on blood elements and the inflammatory/immune responses were largely unknown at that time. It was felt, based on the animal experiments, that monkey-lung oxygenation would be sufficiently safe to attempt intracardiac repair in otherwise hopeless children, such as those with transposition of the great arteries. It is of note that concepts of myocardial protection at that time were still unknown.

An attempt at an arterial switch operation with extracorporeal cardiopulmonary bypass using monkey-lung oxygenation was undertaken in seven cases.[12] The average cardiopulmonary bypass time was 110 minutes. The procedure was abandoned in two cases because of gross mismatch of the pulmonary artery and aorta—in one case because clamping of the right coronary artery resulted in brachycardia and hypertension, and in another case because of edema of the monkey lung. In the other three cases in which an arterial switch was performed to completion, two patients died with ventricular fibrillation and one patient died when the heart failed to resume an effective beat. Dr. Mustard concluded that the application of this extracorporeal circulation could potentially be undertaken in somewhat less hopeless cases.

Thus, in a report published in 1957, Mustard outlined his experience with monkey-lung oxygenation in another twenty-one human cases, excluding transposition of the great arteries and tricuspid atresia, these cases dating back to 1951.[13] Of the twenty-one patients, only three were alive and well at the time of publication. The other eighteen had passed away at the time of operation or shortly thereafter. With better operative survival being reported in the literature from multiple centers using bubble and membrane oxygenators, Dr. Mustard set aside the monkey-lung oxygenation experiments.

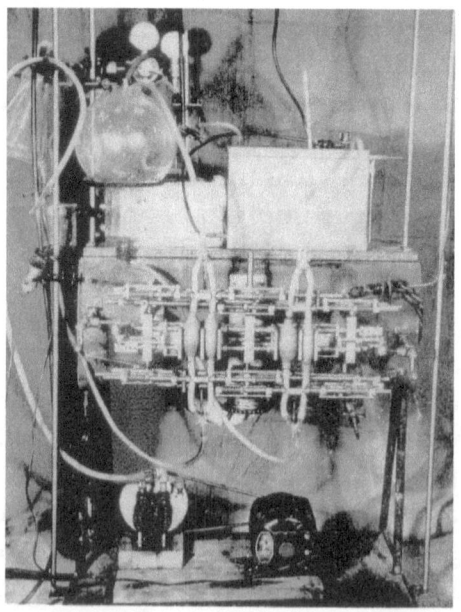

Fig 2:1 The physiologic perfusion pump designed by C. R. Cowan (Monkey-Lung Apparatus)

Hypothermia

From gangrenous toes to open-heart surgery, Dr. Bigelow's story emphasizes the crucial importance of imagination and tenacity that frequently enables progress. "My interest in hypothermia was aroused in 1941 when, as a resident surgeon at the Toronto General Hospital, I was in charge of a young man from the Canadian north woods with frostbite in his fingers that had progressed to gangrene," writes Dr. Wilfred G. Bigelow.[14] Prompted by his mentor, Dr. Gallie, Dr. Bigelow began life-long research into hypothermia that eventually allowed cardiac surgeons to open the beating but empty heart.

The observation in frostbite and its delayed evident tissue damage convinced Dr. Bigelow that tissue metabolism must be decreased thereby protecting the organ, in spite of opposing reports in dog experiments. While serving in the Canadian army during 1941-1945, he persuaded the British war office to build a cooling cabinet to help preserve a wounded limb with damaged circulation. On his later return from the war, with his manifest interest in vascular surgery, Gallie had the foresight to send the young surgeon to Johns Hopkins Hospital to train for a year with Dr. Alfred Blalock, at that time pioneering the famous "blue baby" operations. It was during his stay there that his good friend and colleague Dr. "Bill" Mustard visited Johns Hopkins. Bigelow later returned to Toronto General Hospital as a staff vascular surgeon.

At Johns Hopkins, Bigelow had come across a dynamic and intellectually charged atmosphere created by such luminaries as Drs. Blalock, Helen Taussig, Richard Bing and the technically gifted laboratory technician Vivien Thomas. Dr. Bigelow wrote: "There was an aura about the place. Here was fresh knowledge, new concepts,

new surgery, brilliant trainees, and a great teacher. This
was the birth of cardiac surgery." Dr. Bigelow awoke one
night while at Johns Hopkins with a simple solution to
surgical inaccessibility of the heart, one that did not
require pumps and tubes: "Cool the whole body, reduce
the oxygen requirements, interrupt the circulation and
open the heart."[15]

Upon his return to Toronto, Dr. Bigelow set up his
research laboratory in the Banting Institute. In 1948,
the team reported for the first time that hypothermia,
once shivering and increased muscle tone caused by the
cold temperature was pharmacologically eliminated,
did in fact reduce the oxygen requirements of living
dogs. Animals kept at 19°C for four hours did not show
evidence of oxygen deficits.[16] With this experimental
background, the team embarked on testing its original
hypothesis, namely that by cooling the animal and
decreasing tissue metabolism, the surgeon could stop
the circulation for a few minutes and open the heart
safely. In 1949, the team did just that: the dog was cooled
by cooling blankets to 22°C and the chest opened. The
circulation was then interrupted by placing clamps across
the superior and inferior vena cavae. The heart beat
itself empty, a right atriotomy was performed and the
inside of a beating heart finally visualized. Dr. Bigelow
captures the moment in his memoirs: "What a thrill to
look inside a beating heart! What a dynamic, powerful
organ—even the valve rings are contracting vigorously.
One is suddenly aware that a heartbeat is a complex
and beautifully coordinated manoeuvre."[17] The dog
lived having had its circulation interrupted for fifteen
minutes. However, the initial series showed a mortality
rate of approximately 50 percent in dogs. In 1950, Dr.
Bigelow presented these results to the American Surgical
Association in Colorado Springs.[18]

In the ensuing two years, the Toronto team perfected its approach to cooling, rewarming and the management of myocardial irritability. By 1952, having achieved 100 percent survival in monkeys with twenty minutes of circulatory arrest at 18°C,[19] the team was ready to perform its first operation on human subjects. Unfortunately, Dr. Bigelow was unable to obtain an appropriate patient referral. In 1953, Dr. F. John Lewis of Minneapolis reported the first successful closure of an atrial septal defect using the hypothermia technique developed by Bigelow and colleagues.[20] Drs. Henry Swan[21] and Charles P. Bailey[22] further validated the usefulness of this technique in open-heart procedures. Hypothermia for open-heart surgery was finally used successfully in Toronto in 1954. Thereafter an entire generation of surgical residents sought the key to artificial induction of hibernation in Bigelow's laboratory by studying groundhogs during winter sleep with unsuccessful results.

Conclusion

These reflections illustrate the melding of three key elements of mechanical assist: anticoagulation, oxygenation and body temperature control using hypothermia as needed. The origin of these separate factors within a single university is of interest and emphasizes the importance of multidisciplinary collaborative research and clinical investigation. In this modern era, cardiac surgeons perform open-heart surgery routinely and safely using extracorporeal circuits with efficient disposable membrane oxygenators. There is still concern, however, about trauma to blood elements, activation of inflammatory and immune responses and the detrimental effects of prolonged organ perfusion: thus the trend towards off-pump beating heart surgery for coronary revascularization. Heart disease remains the most frequent cause of death in the Western world. These reminiscences of the early pioneers illustrate the constant need for innovation both in surgical technique, laboratory investigation and the development of new technologies. As the domain and capabilities of the cardiac surgeon expands, these elements which are now so refined after such primitive beginnings will yet require new enthusiasm and direction. The courageous work of our predecessors does much to inspire a new generation with ongoing challenges.

Acknowledgement: The authors wish to thank Dr. W. Bigelow for his contribution.

Notes:

1.   W. G. Bigelow, *Mysterious Heparin, the Key to Open Heart Surgery* (Scarborough: McGraw Hill-Ryerson Ltd., 1990).
2.   J. McLean, "The thromboplastic action of cephalin," *Am J Physiol* (1916), 41: 250-57.
3.   W. G. Bigelow, Opus cited, Ref. # 1.
4.   C. H. Best, "Preparations of heparin and its use in the first clinical case," *Circulation* (1959), 19: 79-86.
5.   W. G. Bigelow, Opus cited, Ref. #1.
6.   D. W. G. Murray, L. B. Jaques et al., "Heparin," *Surgery* (1937), 2: 163-87.
7.   D. W. G. Murray, "Heparin and thrombosis and major blood vessel surgery," *Surg Gynecol and Obstet* (1941), 721: 341-44.
8.   M. Dunlop, *Bill Mustard, Surgical Pioneer* (Toronto: Dundurn Press, 1989).
9.   C. R. Cowan, "Physiological perfusion pump," *J Appl Physiol* (1952), 4: 695-97.

10. W. T. Mustard and A. L. Chute, "Experimental intracardiac surgery with extracorporeal circulation," *Surgery* (1951), 30: 684-88.

11. W. T. Mustard et al., "Further observations on experimental extracorporeal circulation," *Surgery* (1952), 32: 803-10.

12. W. T. Mustard et al., "A surgical approach to the transposition of the great vessels with extracorporeal circuit," *Surgery* (1954), 36: 39-51.

13. W. T. Mustard and J. A. Thomson, "Clinical experience with the artificial heart lung preparation," *Can Med Assoc J* (1957), 76: 265-68.

14. W. G. Bigelow, *Cold Hearts, the Story of Hypothermia and the Pacemaker in Heart Surgery* (Toronto: McClelland and Stewart Ltd., 1984).

15. Ibid.

16. W. G. Bigelow, "Oxygen transport and utilization in dogs at low body temperatures," *Am J Physiol* (1950), 160: 125.

17. Bigelow, Opus cited, Ref. #14.

18. W. G. Bigelow and J. C. Callaghan, "General hypothermia for intracardiac Surgery," *Ann Surg* (1950), 132: 531.

19. W. G. Bigelow and J. E. McBirnie, "Further experiences with hypothermia for intracardiac Surgery," *Ann Surg* (1953), 137: 361.

20. F. J. Lewis and M. Taufic, "Closure of atrial septal defect with the aid of hypothermia. Experimental accomplishments," *Surgery* (1953), 33: 52.

21. H. Swan et al., "Surgery by direct vision in the open heart during hypothermia," *J Am Med Assoc* (1953), 153: 1081.

22. C. P. Bailey et al., "Cardiac surgery under hypothermia," *J Thorac Surg* (1954), 77: 73.

CHAPTER 3

CARDIAC SURGERY IN ONTARIO
Memoirs, Anecdotes, Biography and History

REMINISCENCES

Ronald J. Baird, Bernard Goldman and
Raymond O. Heimbecker

Ronald J. Baird

[Editor's note:
Ron Baird was born in 1930 at the Toronto Western
Hospital where he would later become head of
cardiovascular surgery. He was first aware of "open-
heart surgery" as a medical student and vividly recalls
watching Canada's first "cardiovascular" surgeon Gordon
Murray as a final year student in 1954. In that same year
at a party to celebrate the end of final exams, his clinic
group watched a television program in black and white
on a tiny screen in which C. Walt Lillehei described the
first closure of a ventricular septal defect using his bold
technique of cross circulation from mother to child.
Ron's fascination would lead to a productive and equally
fascinating career. As a surgical resident, he elected to
work with Dr. Wilfred G. Bigelow on his investigation of
the mechanism of hibernation in the basement of the
Banting Institute, where so many surgical residents toiled
both before and after. He was witness to historical events

during training: Gordon Murray's use of a homograft aortic valve in the descending thoracic aorta in 1955, the introduction of prosthetic vascular material in 1957, and the transition from closed heart and primitive open-heart surgery with hypothermia to modern open-heart procedures with a heart-lung pump, as senior resident in 1958-59 at the Toronto General Hospital (TGH) and 1959-60 at the Hospital for Sick Children.

Ron was the first new surgeon invited to join the staff at TGH as a specifically designated "cardiovascular" surgeon. He returned from a year as a Graham Travelling Fellow in Russia, Sweden, France, England and the USA with an interest in valve repair. Bill Bigelow gave him the opportunity of performing all aortic valve replacements at TGH, initially with the individual "Kay" valve leaflets and then in 1962 with the Starr-Edwards ball valve prosthesis.

It was serendipity that placed Ron in Cleveland in May 1961 at the time Mason Sones first visualized the effectiveness of the mammary artery implant (the Vineberg operation). Both patients at the Cleveland Clinic that day had received their operations in Canada, one by Vineberg in Montreal and the other by Bigelow in Toronto. This prompted his continued interest in the various mammary artery operations and the insights they provided on myocardial dynamics and the physiology of vascular conduits.

In July 1964, Baird left TGH to join Donald Wilson at Toronto Western Hospital (TWH) where he remained for thirteen years. He pursued a vigorous and innovative career in both the experimental laboratory and cardiovascular surgery. He was an early proponent of atrioventricular cardiac pacing with leads implanted by thoracotomy, for intraaortic balloon pump assist and left ventricular assist. One of his most important contributions was to the understanding of implanted internal mammary artery patency in the myocardium for which he was awarded the Royal College Medal in Surgery in 1969. Ron Baird was appointed division head at TWH in 1972 and moved back to Toronto General Hospital as head of cardiovascular surgery at TGH. He was later named university chair for cardiovascular surgery in 1977.

Baird was quite widely recognized for his vascular surgical contributions. Baird probably had the largest vascular surgery practice and training program in all of Canada and introduced many procedures, e.g., extra peritoneal bypass from the ascending aorta to the femoral arteries. He was honoured by numerous societies, faced many uphill political battles at TGH as vascular surgery gradually separated from the cardiac program, as hospital resources were being strained by the dramatic growth of coronary bypass and as the Toronto Western and Toronto General hospitals merged.

He lived through and contributed to a remarkable era in the history of surgery and particularly in the origins of cardiac and vascular surgery in Toronto, Canada, and indeed the world. Ron has had a longstanding interest in surgical history and has written extensively on the life of Gordon Murray, the discovery of heparin and Canadian contributions to vascular surgery as well as a history of the University of Toronto teaching hospitals. The following section is excerpted from his writings.]

Cardiac Surgery in Toronto—A Memoir

Cardiac surgery in Canada began with Dr. Gordon Murray at Toronto General Hospital (TGH). Murray was born in 1894 near Paris, Ontario. He was a brilliant technician, stubborn iconoclast and courageous innovator. He "sensed" clinical need long before his peers and attempted many procedures long before enabling technology. This often placed him in conflict with the surgical establishment of the time. He was a pioneer of vascular surgery, having described a snare for peripheral arterial emboli, introduced the clinical use of heparin, invented a renal dialysis device before Kolff and ultimately operated on virtually every arterial system in the body as far back as the 1930s; indeed he pioneered the use of vein segments for arterial replacement, e.g., in the carotid artery. During the mid-1930s he described a "cardioscope," which, when pressed against endocardium, allowed him to visualize some interior structures. He introduced saphenous vein segments as a sling to reduce mitral insufficiency (similar now to posterior ring annuloplasty). Following Gross's ligation of a patent ductus in 1938, Murray soon had a Canadian monopoly on the procedure, followed then by coarctation repair and, after a short visit to Baltimore, the Blalock-Taussig shunt. These operations were essentially "vascular" procedures and Gordon Murray had by far the world's greatest experience in vascular surgery as a result of his clinical experience with heparin. Patients flocked to him from many countries and in the Canadian press he was revered as the "blue baby" doctor.

In 1947, he reported to the American Surgical Association on his bold and partially successful closure of atrial and ventricular septal defects using fascia lata sutures passed in and out of the beating heart. Before that same group in 1948, he reported on resection of ventricular aneurysm and experimental coronary bypass. Alfred Blalock, then the most famous surgeon in America, commented, "Cardiac surgery had entered a new era."

However, Murray was now in his fifties and his period of innovative surgery was almost over. In 1949, and the early 1950s, he reported on his results for both mitral valvotomy and internal mammary artery implants. He was invited to Brazil and Australia to visit, teach and operate, and is given credit for pioneering heart surgery in those regions. Murray never had the aid of hypothermia, cross-circulation, or cardiopulmonary bypass. Nonetheless, his most famous contribution to heart surgery came at the age of sixty-one when he became the first surgeon to transplant a human heart valve.

No doubt, Murray had read the clinical reports of Charles Hufnagel, who had begun canine experiments in 1952, wherein he implanted a silastic ball valve in the descending aorta to partially relieve aortic valve insufficiency, with clinical application in 1954. Fixation of the rigid lucite cage in the aorta was difficult and there were no long-term survivors. I recall, as an intern on Ward C, watching a patient bleed to death rapidly when a Hufnagel valve dehisced.

Murray experimented with a homograft aortic valve in his private laboratory near the Wellesley Hospital. In October 1955, while I was still working in Dr. Bill Bigelow's laboratory, he performed the first clinical operation (described later in this book by Ray Heimbecker). The operation was kept secret and Toronto cardiac surgeons first learned of the procedure from Murray's report in the October 1956 issue of *Angiology*, a rather obscure journal printed in Italy. The patient's pre and postoperative workup had been quietly done at Toronto Western Hospital. The secrecy surrounding this case, and its obscure publication without the exact date of surgery, reflect Murray's increasing concerns with recognition and priority, and his continuing suspicion of his colleagues.

The operation itself was a spectacular success and the valve was still functioning well nineteen years later.* As the resident at TGH in 1958-59, I assisted Bigelow, Donald Wilson and Raymond Heimbecker in the five or six of these procedures that they performed, and I, as a staff surgeon myself, performed two in 1960-61. The operation attracted international interest only when cardiologists Alfred Kerwin and Susan Lenkei reported with Wilson on the initial patient's condition six years later in the April 1962 issue of the prestigious *New England Journal of Medicine*. It is in this article that the actual date of the first operation is revealed.

Although Murray's bold operation was a great surgical contribution, his timing and luck were running out, for in 1962, Albert Starr introduced the subcoronary ball valve, which provided complete correction of aortic insufficiency. Barratt-Boyes in New Zealand implanted an aortic homograft in the subcoronary position in 1964 and did give appropriate credit to Murray who was then in his seventies. Gordon Murray's latter years were marked by controversy, paranoia, hostility, and

---

*   The editor recalls replacing the aortic valce of a patient with a Murray descending thoracic homograft implanted some eighteen years earlier: on thoracic aortic angiography the homograft was shriveled and incompetent. Nonetheless, the patient survived the aortic valve replacement depite massive cardiomegaly. Murray was indeed controversial; I recently performed coronary bypass on a patient with a sternotomy incision for apparent "blue baby" surgery performed by Murray in the 1950s with newspaper accounts of the successful procedure. Strangely, there was no evidence the pericardium had ever been opened or the heart sutured in any way.

ultimately embarrassment due to his reported successful applications of horse serum immune cancer therapy, and spinal cord resection for paraplegia. (Yet Murray had again been ahead of his time and the concepts were in fact valid.)

In 1946 following service in World War II, William T. "Bill" Mustard returned to the Hospital for Sick Children as an orthopedic surgeon. Since John Keith had just started Canada's first pediatric cardiology service there, and did not wish to work with Gordon Murray, Mustard was sent to observe Alfred Blalock in Baltimore. For the next decade, he continued as both an orthopedic and a cardiac surgeon. Only in 1959, when I was his resident, was he asked to choose only one specialty. There was a slow but steady shift of referrals from Gordon Murray at TGH. In 1953, Dr. Mustard, assisted by Bigelow, introduced hypothermia for the closure of ASDs to Canada.

Wilfred G. "Bill" Bigelow also returned in 1946 to TGH to perform general surgery. Bigelow was born in 1913 in Brandon, Manitoba, and graduated from University of Toronto Medical School in 1938. He was the son of Dr. W. A. Bigelow, a general practitioner and surgeon, a charter member of the American College of Surgeons and founder of the first private clinic in Canada. Bigelow spent the war years in a field transfusion unit and then the sixth Canadian casualty clearing station throughout Europe. He had trained under Gallie between 1938 and 1941. Bigelow's interest on the effects of cold apparently arose from his need as a resident to amputate a man's frostbitten fingers. Concerned by the lack of research on frostbite he was challenged by Professor Gallie to investigate this further. Dr. W. E. Gallie, the surgeon in chief, persuaded him to spend a year with Richard Bing and Alfred Blalock at Johns Hopkins

Hospital in 1947. On his return in 1948, he worked on Ward C under Murray and began his imaginative and productive laboratory investigations at the Banting Institute. His first interest was in blood sludging in the microcirculation, and in 1950 he began his seminal work on hypothermia. Bigelow is recognized primarily for introducing hypothermia and as well, the cardiac pacemaker (with John Callaghan and Jack Hopps). The concept of stimulating the heart electrically arose from the need to resuscitate hypothermic dogs with cold induced bradycardia. Throughout the 1950s, he was only one of two or three surgeons in the world to adopt the Vineberg procedure. His extensive clinical practice and follow-up studies proved the operation's effectiveness as documented by Sones and his presentation at the AATS in 1962 resulted in general acceptance of the Vineberg procedure. Bigelow often said that he was primarily motivated to support Vineberg as a fellow Canadian.

His landmark presentation on hypothermia research and its role in cardiac surgery was presented to the American Surgical Association in 1950. F. John Lewis of Minneapolis attended that meeting, heard the paper, and returned home to perform the world's first successful ASD in 1952 with this new technique. Bigelow performed his first clinical procedure under hypothermia at TGH in 1953 and published his first few cases from both Toronto General and Sick Children's the following year. In a 1973 interview with Gerald Ranier, Bigelow stated that he performed high-risk mitral commissurotomies with the patient orthopneic and the chest cavity irrigated with cold solution to body temperature 30°C. He is credited with removing the second atrial myxoma and the first to be resected under hypothermia. Total body hypothermia for cardiac surgery was used worldwide for almost a decade.

Bigelow was given undivided credit for this important breakthrough. Murray resigned as head of Ward C, where cardiac surgery was performed at TGH, in 1953 and Bill Bigelow was then made head of his own unit at the age of forty. Bigelow admitted that he never really thought a heart-lung pump would work due to blood sludging and too many gadgets with potential breakdown. He truly believed that some extract could be obtained from hibernating groundhogs to facilitate total body cooling in a more physiologic manner. This accounted for almost fifteen years of fundamental research on hibernation in the basement of the Banting Institute by a series of cardiac surgical fellows and reflected Bigelow's tenacity and dogged perseverance in his beliefs.

During the 1950s the most common cardiac operation performed was the closed mitral valvotomy introduced by both Bailey and Harken in the late 1940s. I believe the procedure was first performed in Canada by Gordon Murray in 1950, although Bill Bigelow in *Cold Hearts* states that he did his first in 1949, two weeks after Edouard Gagnon in Montreal. Bigelow and Don Wilson soon had large personal series. Closed valvotomy (using finger fracture, intraatrial scalpel, or the Dubost or Tubbs-Logan dilators) was slowly replaced by open valvotomy during the 1960s. I performed the last closed mitral valvotomy at Toronto General in 1981 on a woman who simultaneously went into labour and pulmonary edema—thankfully, both mother and child did well. Bill Bigelow introduced Bailey's aortic valve dilator to Toronto in 1953. Indeed he shared a single dilator with Gagnon, mailing it back and forth from Toronto to Montreal as needed. I was good at this procedure and performed quite a few during my chief residency in 1958-59. This closed approach to the aortic valve was superceded by direct vision repairs in late 1969.

While still a resident, I wrote articles on this operation for both the *Canadian Medical Association Journal* and the *Journal of Thoracic and Cardiovascular Surgery*; indeed these were my first publications on cardiac surgery.

The first operation in Toronto using cardiopulmonary bypass was performed by Bill Bigelow in January 1958, and perhaps only eight or nine patients had received operations with "the pump" by the time I became chief resident on Ward C that July. Pump surgery was reserved for ostium primum ASDs, VSDs, tetralogy and valvular insufficiency. It was during this residency that a one-room ICU was opened, room 629 on the sixth floor of the Private Patient's Pavillion at TGH, the first cardiac surgical ICU in Canada. Only one or two patients per week could be operated upon by open-heart techniques with cardiopulmonary bypass. The first oxygenator at TGH was the rotating disk, designed by Viking Bjork; its cleaning and reassembly required at least one day between operations. Around this time Donald Wilson made plans to open a cardiac surgical unit at Toronto Western Hospital, and Clare Baker, in his own independent manner, returned from training in Holland to begin heart surgery at St. Michael's Hospital a few years later.

A separate cardiovascular surgery unit then opened at TGH in the spring of 1958 and I joined it in July. This was the first such unit in Canada, was state of the art, and occupied the eighth and ninth floors of the Private Patient's Pavillion. There were two large ORs, a small room for pacemakers and vascular procedures and an adjoining new eight-bed CVICU. The staff then consisted of Bill Bigelow, James Key, Ray Heimbecker, and myself. In 1961 we were joined by Wolf Sapirstein. Wolf went to St. Mike's in 1962 and later to Harrisburg, Pennsylvania, in 1964. In July 1964, I left TGH to join Don Wilson at Toronto Western Hospital. Al Trimble soon joined the TGH group with a remarkably productive early career in valve reconstruction and correction of adult congenital problems. During my four years at TGH cardiopulmonary bypass was greatly simplified by the introduction of disposable bubble oxygenators and the Starr Edwards ball valve, which both revolutionized heart surgery.

Before the silastic ball valve became available in 1963, Bill Bigelow had arranged for most patients with aortic insufficiency to be referred to me because I had good success with bicuspidization and teflon-urethane cusp extensions. Myocardial protection at that time was by continuous intracoronary cold blood perfusion. Ray Heimbecker developed a technique of using an aortic homograft to replace the mitral valve, and in March 1962, I assisted him in the first such clinical replacement. Although early annuloplasty techniques on the mitral valve soon gave way to the mechanical ball valve, many such repairs were tried in this era. The short-term results were good but the valve ring tended to dilate with time. In 1964, I formed a complete annuloplasty ring from a Dacron graft and achieved good long-term results. In 1963 Bill Mustard had his first success with the intraatrial pericardial baffle operation for TGA. This operation was quickly accepted internationally and assured his fame thereafter. He retired at the early age of sixty-two in 1976.

I had been at TWH for three years when the procedures that would transform the volume and nature of cardiac surgery were reported: Christiaan Barnard, in Cape Town, South Africa, accomplished the first heart transplant, and Rene Favaloro, at Cleveland Clinic, performed the first aortocoronary saphenous vein bypass. These procedures captured the world's attention. Pierre Grondin, at the Montreal Heart Institute, started the first Canadian series of heart transplants in the spring of 1968 with excellent early results. We performed the first Toronto transplant at TWH on October 6, 1968.[**] The following month Clare Baker and J. K. Y. Yao performed transplants at St. Michael's Hospital. The Toronto transplant program was only modestly successful, primarily at St. Mike's and was certainly fraught with inter-hospital competition and acrimony. At TGH, there was virtually no cardiologic or immunologic enthusiasm or support. In any event, rejection and inadequate immunosuppressive therapy soon halted any further such procedures. Ray Heimbecker, by then at the University Hospital in London, Ontario, and Keith McKenzie are credited with reviving heart transplantation in Canada after their careful experimental and clinical use of cyclosporine. Tirone David and Chris Feindel started transplantation again in Toronto in 1983 at TWH and later at the Toronto General when the two clinical services merged in 1989. Wilbert J. Keon had great success with a clinical transplant program at the University of Ottawa Heart Institute, but in general, heart transplantation has never flourished in Canada. due to both a lack of available donors and improving success with other therapies for heart failure.

Coronary artery bypass, however, is a very different story. After Dudley Johnson's excellent clinical results presented to the AATS in April 1969, there was considerable enthusiasm on the part of both surgeons and cardiologists. The first coronary bypass in Canada

---

[**]   The editor brought the donor heart in a police car from TGH.

was performed by Paul Field in Sudbury, Ontario, in May 1969. Toronto surgeons soon had increasingly large series, myself at TGH and Al Trimble and Bernie Goldman at TGH. The clinical volume of coronary bypass patients grew so rapidly that most cardiac surgeons had to abandon vascular surgery and there was much discussion and controversy over the allocation of scarce hospital resources to cardiac versus other surgical specialties. This debate raged most notably at Toronto General Hospital and contributed in part to the opening of a cardiac surgical unit at Sunnybrook Hospital (University of Toronto Clinic) in late 1989. While I was university head and chief at TGH, there was increasing recognition of the clinical research productivity of Richard Weisel and the clinical innovations of Tirone David in valve repair. Tirone David became head of cardiac surgery in 1987 and created a superb international reputation for himself and Toronto in the years that followed.]

During my tenure as university chair the Toronto Residency Program attracted numerous residents and fellows from around the world and especially the United States. Bill Bigelow had established the first complete inter-hospital university training program for cardiac surgeons in 1956. He chaired the University of Toronto Cardiovascular Residency from 1960-1977, and after my tenure (1977-1987), Tomas Salerno (1987-1992), William G. Williams (1992-1997), and Richard Weisel (1998-present) were all subsequently appointed.

The attractiveness of our program to American residents changed with the controversial decisions of the American Board of Thoracic Surgery regarding accreditation. There were numerous difficult decisions at that time, the most notable to me being the agreement in 1981 to form a separate division of vascular surgery at TGH and the university, both headed by my former resident Wayne Johnson. I had always enjoyed the combination of vascular and cardiac surgery but year by year the services inevitably moved farther apart and it was more difficult to find time and space for vascular operations. It was happenstance not design that allowed my vascular interest to become more and more focused on the thoracic aorta. Thus in 1982 I introduced the technique of hypothermic total circulatory arrest for repair of aneurysms of the arch and descending thoracic aorta to Canada. During the 1980s I was pleased to be elected president of the Canadian Society of Cardiovascular and Thoracic Surgeons, to be the first Canadian invited to give an honoured guest lecture before the Japanese Society of Thoracic Surgeons (having trained over a dozen young surgeons from Japan), the first Canadian to be elected president of the International Society for Cardiovascular Surgery and elected to honorary membership of numerous other vascular and surgical societies. In the meantime, Tirone David had taken over as head of the merged units at Toronto General; Tom Salerno was appointed university chair, replaced by Bill Williams in 1992, and finally in 1994, I closed my TGH office and decided to "semi-retire," content with my life and my career.

I was privileged to have lived through a remarkable era. Who is the prophet who can foretell the future? In my professional lifetime, cardiovascular surgery had grown from a new and struggling discipline, to one so large it had to be separated into separate specialties, cardiac and vascular. From 1991 onwards, over two thousand patients each year have had cardiac operations and almost a thousand have had vascular operations at TGH. This was inconceivable when I began practice as a cardiovascular surgeon in 1960.

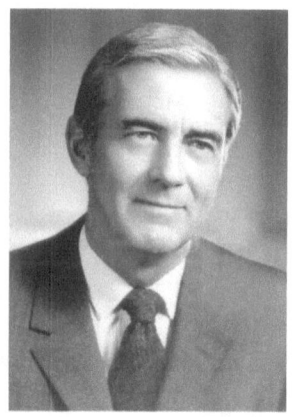

Fig. 3:1a
Wilfred G. Bigelow

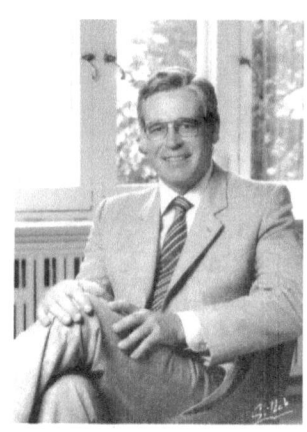

Fig. 3:1b
Ronald J. Baird

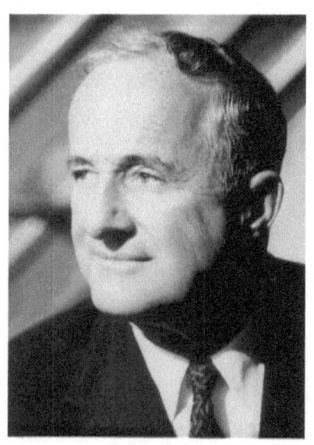

Fig. 3:1c
Raymond O. Heimbecker

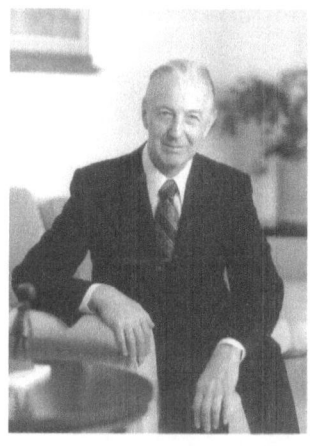

Fig. 3:1d
James A. Key

Raymond O. Heimbecker

[Editor's note:
Ray Heimbecker was born in Calgary and received his MD at the University of Toronto in 1947. He trained in Toronto with Wilfred Bigelow, Richard Bing and Alfred Blalock at Johns Hopkins, and Sir Russell Brock in London, England. He was a protégé of Dr. Gordon Murray. Ray was known as a superb researcher, a brilliant and innovative surgeon, a tinkerer with machines and devices, sailor, glider pilot, and all-round raconteur. He really has had three careers—at Toronto General Hospital from 1955, as professor and founding chief of cardiovascular surgery at the new University Hospital in London, Ontario, in 1974, and as the local doctor for island residents, fishermen and tourists in the Bahamas. The following reminiscences are typical Heimbecker stories.]

A Medical Milestone—Canada's First Adult Open-heart Operation

The year was 1949, and my new chief, the famous Alfred Blalock of Johns Hopkins Hospital in Baltimore, had asked me to review with him the status of heart-lung machines as a surgical tool. It was a stifling hot day there in Baltimore and certainly no air-conditioning in 1949. His first words were "Mary, please bring us each a Coke." What a wonderful, humble, and unassuming man was Blalock. Many had worked in this field over the years, including Charles Lindbergh, and Blalock was kind enough to show me the Lindbergh heart-lung apparatus, which he had kept in storage for many years. After a wonderfully informal discussion, the two of us agreed quite clearly that this was a "pie in the sky" situation with absolutely too many barriers to make it a feasible tool at that time. However, by 1956, my chief in Toronto, Wilfred Bigelow, had asked me to review the problem once again for the heart-lung machine was now somewhat more developed. Would it ever be possible to use for open-heart surgery? Most of all, would it ever become a practical day-to-day tool for the cardiac surgeon? Many centres were using general body hypothermia with circulatory arrest for brief periods of up to five or six minutes, the technique which Bigelow had pioneered. William Mustard of Toronto had used a monkey lung as an oxygenator to correct tetralogy of Fallot. Above all, the legendary John Gibbon of Philadelphia had performed a successful operation with his amazing and complex heart-lung apparatus, which he had developed over many years of research.

A Glimmer of Optimism

My answer to Bigelow was yes. This controversial apparatus, if developed and fine-tuned, would become a useful tool and indeed might revolutionize the surgical world. For the next twenty-four months, I proceeded first to reorganize my animal laboratory in the Banting Institute at the University of Toronto so that I could do weekly heart-lung machine experiments with various homemade and artificial lungs, different blood pumps, many primitive types of blood filters and connectors, arterial and venous cannulae and precise heat exchangers. All had to be carefully designed to be atraumatic to blood components, especially the fragile erythrocytes and platelets. Moreover precise temperature control was vital. I was fortunate to have a home workshop where I could make prototypes of these components in metal and plastic. My designs were then manufactured by Canadian Pipe and Steel Fabricators, 160 Dutchess Street, Toronto, and by Hartz Surgical Supplies, Toronto.

The commercial device was developed by myself with Dr. W. E. Young and Dan Sanford assisting.

Home Workshop a Must

None of the instrument companies were the least bit interested in this field for they felt there was "no future out there." Friends and colleagues were even more outspoken, "Ray, you're wasting your time," "Ray, get out of your ivory tower," "Ray, it can never become a safe practical apparatus," "Ray, there is no future in open-heart surgery, you will surely starve." One surgical fellow (Dr. Mitchell Tanz) wrote an article on "The Thousand Things That Go Wrong with the Heart-Lung Machine Experiments." My greatest support came from my wonderful and tolerant wife and family, for I was spending all of those overtime hours in the dingy windowless lab in the subbasement of the Banting Institute. At the same time, my routine work in student and postgraduate teaching and clinical surgery continued day by day. Great things were happening at other centres, especially Houston, Minneapolis, and the Mayo Clinic. How exciting to be on the cutting edge with them.

Exciting Progress

By January 1957, we had performed over a hundred animal experiments. A simple bubble oxygenator had won out over vertical screens, primitive membrane lungs, and even monkey lungs. Our favourite blood pump was the one that had been originally designed to atraumatically pump beer (the Sigma motor). Arterial blood filters were still problematic. We found most designs to be very traumatic, especially to platelets and fibrinogen—so they often did more harm than good and perhaps hindered the progress of heart-lung machine development.

January 12, 1958

The operating room was electric that day—indeed the whole hospital became electric. Wilfred Bigelow, James Key, Don Wilson and myself were preparing for a huge step forward. A wonderful dedicated man, Dr. Barry Fairley, had spent many late hours with me in the Banting lab and was the chief anaesthetist. Our patient, E.J., was a twenty-five-year-old woman from Northern Ontario suffering from a large atrial septal defect. The cardiologist, Bill Greenwood, had found the intracardiac shunt to be massive and pulmonary hypertension developing so that surgery was imperative to avoid the complications of chronic pulmonary hypertension, arrhythmia, and heart failure. It was difficult to keep our plans secret in the hospital. Personnel everywhere were talking about it "being too early," "was it too risky at this time?" "was the heart-lung machine an invention of the devil?" "could this be done by hypothermia instead?" Of course, we had all performed many brief open-heart operations with general body cooling and circulatory arrest as the standard procedure, but with a five-minute time limit.

The local Red Cross was able to provide twenty units of fresh blood less than twenty-four hours old. This was the essential ingredient for any open-heart surgery in that year of 1958, otherwise surgery would have had to be postponed indefinitely or even cancelled. An intensive care unit did not exist. We surgeons would take turns all night, every night, to help the dedicated nurses so that the new and somewhat overwhelming problems they encountered with postoperative heart surgery patients could be managed. Early recognition and rapid effective treatment was extremely important whether it be for acidosis, arrhythmia, or persistent blood loss.

A Brilliantly Successful Operation

Much to our delight the operation proceeded beautifully. The pump run was no longer than about twenty-five minutes and the defect was closed without a patch for the tissues were very lax. I also had to supervise the operation of the heart-lung machine, for I was in fact the chief perfusionist! All of us were very new in this field and I was the one who had had two years of constant exposure to all the minor problems that could develop during every pump run. So I would scrub and unscrub throughout the procedure. It was thrilling to see inside the living human heart and to leisurely examine the internal structures in a living state.

The patient left the operating room in excellent condition and had a very smooth postoperative course, without arrhythmia, without coagulopathy, or undue blood loss. She was discharged home on the tenth day much to the delight of all, but especially the excitement and delight of the entire hospital, and of course her loyal and supportive family.

Follow-up

Postoperatively over the years, Bill Greenwood followed E.J. with great care and I was delighted to get periodic reports, usually in the form of yearly Christmas cards, which she faithfully sent from Northern Ontario. What a wonderful beginning to a whole new era of medical care and what an exciting experience! Perhaps the four of us were really on the right track. Maybe in the near future we would be able to replace or repair heart valves, repair coronary artery disease, and even totally correct many forms of congenital disease. Perhaps the "pump" was not "a pie in the sky" or an "invention of the devil" after all.

The World's First Homograft Heart Valve Replacement

1955 was the year of my Royal College of Surgeons Examinations. I was now a full-fledged university teacher and my role model Gordon Murray had become a colleague. He and I had discussed many times the flood of patients who became cardiac invalids because of the ravages of rheumatic fever and damage to the heart valves. There had been some recent improvements in medical therapy but heart valve damage was still the underlying culprit for chronic heart failure. Murray was now approaching retirement. He was a slim, vigorous, and quick-witted man, popular with students and nurses. His fertile mind and quick wit invariably stimulated me to consider new approaches and we often discussed the concept of transplanting a healthy heart valve into a disabled patient.

Animal experiments in his laboratory had already shown that other tissues such as blood vessels could be transplanted without rejection, but the heart valves are exquisitely complex and there was concern, not only of rejection, but also durability. It was our premise that valve leaflets were different from organs such as the kidney that underwent rejection because of the inherent blood supply and inevitable immune response. Valve leaflets did not have a true blood supply, being bathed only with tissue fluid, and we both undertook experiments to transplant leaflets, one animal to another. This was difficult experimental surgery because the current heart-lung machines were too primitive and this prevented us from working inside the heart for accurate placement of the transplanted valve in the appropriate location.

Our perseverance finally paid off. We found that heart valves could indeed survive transplantation without rejection. Patient J.P. from Northern Ontario had been known to have a leaking aortic valve for several years, but gradually suffered such cardiac enlargement and failure that at the age of twenty-five he was an invalid. He and his doctors had heard about our experimental work but felt that it was too early to even consider surgery without information on how long the transplanted delicate tissue could survive and function. There was concern about blood clot on the valve leaflets and embolism, which had been noted with plastic valves and valve leaflets. However, by November 1955 it was clear that our laboratory leaflets were surviving and without the dreaded complications of blood clotting. J.P. had deteriorated and was eager to accept the dangers of an entirely new heart operation.

Excitement was at a high pitch in operating room C that day. I had harvested the heart valve under sterile technique from the hospital morgue twenty-four hours before and had placed it in a sterile container with penicillin and refrigerated it overnight. To avoid publicity the operation was booked simply as a left lateral thoracotomy, but in spite of the secrecy there were more than enough visitors in the gallery and looking over our shoulders.

Dissection of the aorta was considered relatively new and dangerous, especially in a seriously ill patient with gross cardiomegaly. Nonetheless the aorta was finally dissected and clamped gradually to avoid sudden strain on the ailing left ventricle. The aorta was then divided and the aortic valve then transplanted in place and forty minutes later the clamps were gradually released. The transplanted leaflets began to open and close with each heartbeat which we could confirm by palpation, and as well, note that the left ventricular contraction was less vigorous and slower. A few days later J.P. was back with his jubilant family. Selective angiography at thirteen years demonstrated normal valve function without calcification or distortion of the leaflets. The adjacent aortic sleeve was calcified as would be expected. The patient underwent a total correction of the native aortic valve twenty years later at another centre.

Intracardiac Valve Replacement

Many writers are simply not aware of the Canadian origins of the principal of valve homograft and porcine heterograft for heart valve replacement, techniques now widely accepted and used universally. My own interest in valve replacement began at Johns Hopkins when Dr. Blalock and I created gradually progressive valve insufficiency in experimental animals. Beginning in 1955, working with Dr. Gordon Murray, my colleagues and I carried out a series of successful clinical aortic valve transplantations into the thoracic aorta for the partial correction of aortic insufficiency and further optimism came from a similar series performed by Dr. Don Wilson in Toronto. In 1961, Dr. Bryan Barratt-Boyes of New Zealand visited the Banting Institute laboratory showing great interest in the procedures and clinical results and returned to New Zealand to continue similar work. By 1962, we in Toronto were able to conduct a very satisfying seven-year follow-up of patients who had received such transplants in 1955.

Armed with these results and assisted by Ron Baird, I was able to implant the first intracardiac aortic valve homograft for the total correction of valvular heart disease at Toronto General Hospital on March 27, 1962. Barratt-Boyes and Donald Ross conducted similar homograft valve implants some months later. Ross reported his successful implantation performed July 24, 1962. By 1986, Ross confirmed that our twenty-year follow-up was the longest of its kind for homograft or any tissue valve implant. On March 23, 1962, we were able to accomplish the first successful open-heart replacement of the human mitral valve.

A Historical Essay On Heart Transplantation

"Neil, here is another rejection letter from our research applications." The year was 1979, and Calvin Stiller, Neil McKenzie and I, at University Hospital in London, Ontario, had just finished a pilot study on the mysterious properties of a new drug Cyclosporin A.

Twelve years before, in 1967, Christiaan Barnard had electrified the world by performing the first world's heart transplant. True, it was a piggyback type of transplant and also true that Norman Shumway at Stanford University was the real pioneer with many years of heart research transplantation behind him. Barnard, on the other hand, had considerable courage but very little background research experience.

Before long centres around the world were following the lead. Don Wilson and Ron Baird at the Toronto Western Hospital successfully performed the first heart transplant in Toronto, in 1968. Clare Baker and Jim Yao of St. Michael's Hospital in Toronto had several successes including a man who became quite famous for long-term survival in good health for many years. Tony Dobell at McGill and Pierre Grondin at the Montreal Heart Institute also had many immediate successes. However as the world experience became tabulated it was quite clear that the operation was not successful on the one hand due to rejection and on the other to the toxic effects of immunosuppressive drugs available at that time. No research funding was therefore possible.

Stiller, McKenzie and I were terribly dejected when all the granting bodies informed us that there was "no future" in heart transplantation research. The Ontario Heart Foundation, which had been so supportive of my work for twenty years or more gave us a simple no. The Medical Research of Council, also supportive, said, "No funding possible in this hopeless field of research." We knew this was negative thinking, for Roy Calne of Cambridge had shown that Cyclosporin A (Sandoz Pharmaceuticals), a fungal metabolite, had a beneficial effect in laboratory and clinical kidney transplantation. His friend John Borel of Switzerland had developed this drug as a new antibiotic, only to find out that it was a rather poor antibiotic, but that it might have some immunosuppressive properties

Research Funding?

Why not check out our own funds before we became completely demoralized? For the three of us were all on "hard income ceilings" in which our surplus of funds from clinical earnings were placed in a special account. We were delighted to learn that we had accumulated an overage (i.e., surplus) of some $150,000 in this fund. With special permission from Douglas Bocking, dean of the faculty of medicine, University of Western Ontario, we were able to continue our exciting laboratory research for another two years using our own hard earned research funds. We clearly established all the pharmacological properties of Cyclosporin A, its dosage, toxicity, side effects and potency and especially nephrotoxicity. It was clearly a fantastic drug that produced selective immunosuppression of implanted foreign tissue but without the generalized immunosuppression that had occurred with all earlier drugs such as azathioprine (Imuran).

Exciting Research

By 1981, there was much excitement in our laboratory at University Hospital, London, Ontario, for our transplanted animals were doing so well. It was time to forge ahead in a field that the medical world had deemed hopeless.

G.M. was a fifty-year-old male who had suffered severe heart failure, not responding to optimal medical care, a true cardiac invalid with a hopeless bed-to-bathroom existence. On April 18, 1981, we excised his enlarged heart (cardiomyopathy with only mild coronary disease) and replaced it with a heart of an accident victim. The new wonder drug Cyclosporin A made the postoperative course so much smoother and manageable because his own immune system was still functioning rather well and he was able to avoid the common complications of pneumonia, kidney infection, etc. Words of encouragement came from a few medical centres but there was also alarm and criticism. "What are you people doing over there, Ray? You know that cardiac transplantation is a bad operation without future." Norman Shumway had been especially delighted for they had done Cyclosporin A heart transplantation shortly before us. We were glad to be in touch with each other day by day during this exciting period. Our research and organ preservation and transport had also been a big step forward based on the cardioplegia methods generally used during that period. Since few in North America were performing heart transplants, donor organs were frequently available to us everywhere in most major cities. We were able to bring them in from many American centres miles away and even from our own West Coast city of Vancouver, British Columbia.

Endomyocardial Biopsy

Serial postoperative myocardial biopsies were a tremendous step forward in the monitoring of cardiac rejection. Bill Kostiuk of cardiology, Malcolm Silver and Cameron Wallace of pathology were vital in such histologic monitoring. We were now able to anticipate and diagnose early rejection with great accuracy and sensitivity while all other methods of monitoring had clearly proven to be almost useless. The right ventricular specimens were obtained via a cardiac catheter "nibbler" and were obtained with great ease and no morbidity.

University Hospital Becomes a Multiorgan Transplant Centre

We were then able to carry out our first "en bloc" heart and lung transplantation in 1982, following the impressive techniques of Bruce Reitz of Stanford. What a blessing for patients with terminal cystic fibrosis or other advanced pulmonary disease. *Kidney transplantation* clearly benefited from the improved organ storage and especially with the addition of Cyclosporin A to postoperative therapy (Jack Sharpe). *Liver transplantation* had been a difficult field before Cyclosporin A, but our colleague Bill Wall was quick to appreciate this exciting breakthrough. In short order he was obtaining spectacular results with worldwide recognition. Our hospital of only five hundred beds was becoming rapidly known as a major multitransplant centre. Our excellent results were recognized throughout the world. It was almost two years before any other Canadian centre had mobilized its facilities and expertise to undertake such transplant work. These were exciting times for all of us at University Hospital in London, Ontario. What would have transpired if our own hard-earned but surplus funds from clinical earnings had not been there to make our dreams a reality?

[Editor's note:
To summarize Ray Heimbecker's important research highlights: 1951, development of a continuous dye dilution recording with Richard Bing at Johns Hopkins; 1955, descending thoracic aortic valve transplantation with Gordon Murray; development of extracorporeal circulation resulting in the first adult open-heart operation in Canada 1958; world's first intracardiac heart valve transplantation March 1962 with Ron Baird; studies of ventricular modeling and resection for arrhythmia and low cardiac output 1967; routine open-heart surgery without blood with R. Barr 1974; cyclosporin research and Canada's first heart transplant with cyclosporin April 1981.]

TORONTO GENERAL HOSPITAL

Tirone E. David and Bernard Goldman

The cardiac surgical program currently at Toronto General Hospital (TGH) is the one the largest in Canada since its merger with Toronto Western Hospital in 1989. The two programs were consolidated at the TGH site of the University Health Network. Tirone David, then head at TWH, was invited to lead the merged programs after Ronald Baird's tenure at TGH and as chair of the university program was completed. Just over two thousand open-heart operations are performed each year. The clinical outcomes remain second to none according to the Cardiac Care Network of Ontario and the Society of Thoracic Surgeons database. The program enjoys an international reputation and continues to be sought by doctors from around the globe who wish to take additional training in cardiac surgery. Six international fellows are trained each year.

During the past two decades, a major academic focus has been on cardiac transplantation, left ventricular assist device and other forms of surgical treatment for end-stage congestive hearts failure under the stewardship of Dr. Vivek Rao.

Dr. Lynda Mickleborough along with Dr. Eugene Downar had developed a unique program of surgical ablation of ventricular dysrhythmias but with the introduction of implantable defibrillators the need for this service diminished, and some of that technology was transferred to surgery for atrial dysrhythmias. The Maze procedure was introduced in 1994 and has become a common operation. Lynda's accomplishments in high-risk surgery for patients with severe LV dysfunction were beautifully presented by her as a twenty-year follow-up at the AATS meeting in Boston, Massachusetts, in 2003 marking the end of her clinical practice.

Another very successful program on heart valve surgery has been spearheaded by Drs. Christopher Feindel and Tirone David. Numerous new operative techniques such as reconstruction of the mitral annulus, reconstruction of the base of the heart, replacement of chordae tendineae with expanded polytetrafluoroethylene sutures, aortic valve repair, aortic valve sparing operations, stentless aortic valves, new approaches for the Ross procedures, and mitral valve repair for ischemic mitral regurgitation were developed. These have been among the most significant and landmark contributions to the understanding of valve function and the innovative procedures that evolved have become milestones in the history of cardiac surgery. Dr. David has been acknowledged and honoured as one of the finest cardiac surgeons in this country and world. He served as President of the prestigious American Association for Thoracic Surgery in 2004/5 after serving 5 years as its Secretary. Dr. David was elected to the rank of university professor, the University of Toronto's highest honour bestowed

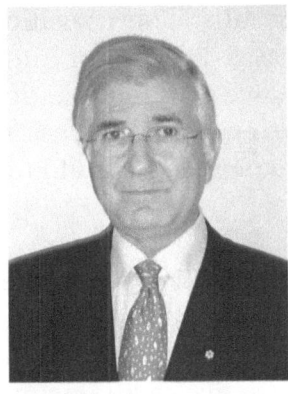
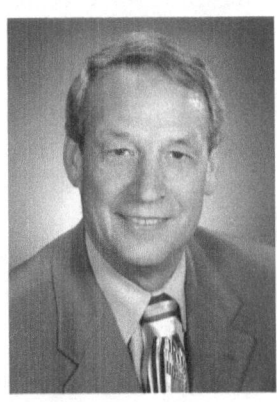

Fig. 3:2a Tirone E. David   Fig. 3:2b Richard D. Weisel

Dr. David brought Drs. Chris Feindel and Irving H. Lipton with him from Toronto Western Hospital to the new merged unit along with other members of the nursing and perfusion team in 1989. Lipton had been recruited to the TWH in the early 1970's from the University of Sherbrooke, Quebec, where he had been instrumental in creating a new open-heart unit with Dr. Claude Labrosse. Lipton spent 20 years at TWH and TGH and earned a solid reputation as a clinician and teacher in cardiac, vascular, and pacemaker/ICD programs before retirement.

At the time of the merger, Dr. Donald Wilson was not only Surgeon-in-Chief at the Toronto Western, but also Professor of Surgery at the University of Toronto and not directly involved in the clinical aspects of the merger. Alan S. Trimble had left Toronto General Hospital early in his career for medical reasons. He had been Bill Bigelow's "wunderkind" and had returned to TGH in the mid 1960's after a fellowship year away. He was a brilliant technician and prolific publisher with numerous important papers in his first years of practice. He tackled the most difficult cases, e.g., the adult redo tetralogy, the end-stage multi-valvular rheumatic patients, etc., at a time when few surgeons had good results. The transition to delicate coronary artery surgery was difficult for him and he ultimately withdrew from practice working as a surgical assistant until late in life. However his contributions to the Toronto General Hospital experience should not be neglected nor forgotten.

Dr. William G. Williams developed the largest program on congenital heart surgery in the adult in North America. He also has the single largest surgical experience in treating patients with hypertrophic obstructive cardiomyopathy, using the original septal myectomy technique introduced by W. G. Bigelow many years earlier. Dr. Williams retired from clinical practice in 2006 but remains active in managing the multi-center congenital heart surgery database.

Dr. Richard Weisel contributed immensely to our understanding of myocardial protection and myocardial cell culture and has established the foundations for a program entirely dedicated to myocardial regeneration. Weisel has been one of the most important surgeon-scientists in Canadian heart surgery and mentor to an entire generation of trainees who have moved to academic positions throughout North America. Weisel was born in the United States and completed his medical school at Marquette University in 1969. After surgical residency in Boston, at Boston University Medical Centre, he came to Toronto for CVT training in 1976, joining the TGH staff in 1978. He retired from clinical practice early on this millennium but remains very active as a basic sciences investigator.

Dr. Hugh Scully is known for his excellence in redo valve surgery and his leadership in university and professional associations. He has been a major contributor in medical economics and government relations. He has been president of the Canadian Medical Association and Canadian Cardiovascular Society as well as pursuing his interest in the medical care of Formula One racing on an international scale. Dr. Scully retired from clinical practice in December 2008.

More recent staff members include: R. J. Cusimano, a superb technician, innovative and courageous in his practice; Anthony Ralph Edwards, a well-liked and respected clinician with a major interest in coronary bypass; Terrence Yau, with a major interest in coronary bypass surgery and the application of anastomotic connectors; and Stephanie Brister, an important teacher and excellent surgeon. Michael Borger returned after fellowship in Leipzig with Friedrich Mohr, and began a program in minimally invasive valve surgery. Dr. Borger returned to Leipzig after practicing in Toronto for 3 years.

Toronto General Hospital has been the cornerstone of Toronto cardiac surgery and carries on as the major player in terms of clinical volumes, fellow and resident training, and research productivity.

ST. MICHAEL'S HOSPITAL

Clare Baker, Lee Errett, and Bernard S. Goldman

Interns, residents, and medical students have always enjoyed their time at St. Michael's Hospital due to an eclectic mix of "downtown and uptown" patients, considerable clinical volume, and diversity with excellent teaching. Yet no cardiac surgical resident was ever allocated to St. Michael's during his/her formal training in the university program until Tomas Salerno was appointed head and university chair for cardiovascular surgery. There was a degree of antipathy mixed with considerable respect, between Bill Bigelow at Toronto General Hospital and Clare Baker at St. Michael's. Bigelow was of course responsible for resident training. This prevented many residents from exposure to and the benefit of working with Baker and later his associate J. K. Y. Yao.

Clare Baker attended medical school at the University of Saskatchewan in the accelerated program during World War II. His junior internship was spent at Toronto General Hospital. It was impossible to secure a surgical residency in Toronto after the war due to these positions being held for medical officers recruited by the military. Baker was able ultimately to find a position through the influence of a Dutch Nobel laureate, father of a colleague in Toronto. After a residency in the Prince Albert Sanitorium, he obtained three years general surgical training in The Hague and later thoracic surgery in Utrecht under Drs. Klinkenberg and Gerard Brom. He returned to Canada as a fellow at St. Michael's in 1951-52; his experience and facility with lung resection caused some difficulties with Drs. Robert Janes and Fred Kergin, prominent leaders and noted chest surgeons at

Toronto General Hospital (where thoracoplasty was still being performed for tuberculosis).

Baker then spent a year at Johns Hopkins Hospital in Baltimore working with Henry Bahnson and Alfred Blalock prior to joining the staff at St. Michael's. This introduction to the U.S. crucible of cardiac investigation and surgery led to his career as a heart surgeon. Indeed, on return to St. Michael's, he arranged for space in the OR to develop a cardiac catheterization laboratory, performing transthoracic and transatrial hemodynamic studies himself with the aid of a hospital engineer.

Baker was a dynamic and talented surgeon performing general, thoracic, vascular and the usual closed heart operations until an open-heart program could be started with the purchase of a Mayo-Gibbon pump oxygenator in 1958. Of interest, he and Bahnson had visited Corning, New York, where a rudimentary pump was being developed at the glass works there. With the decline of the Canadian aerospace initiative (the Avro Arrow) he tried to utilize their hydraulic engineering expertise to develop an Avro pump, but predictably the University of Toronto refused co-sponsorship, which was required. Baker attributed this reluctance to the ongoing tensions from his past experiences with lung surgery.

Clare Baker had a unique relationship with the colourful chief coroner of Ontario, Dr. Smirlie Lawson, a fraternity brother, who instructed all pathologists on call to notify Baker prior to any postmortem examinations. Baker carried a sterile instrument bundle in his car trunk so as to harvest aorta and femoral arteries, which were then freeze-dried or utilized fresh after irrigation with plasma/ antibiotic solutions, long before the advent of prosthetic vascular grafts. Throughout his career, Baker had to work independent of the university program but was supported by the sisters who ran the hospital. Indeed, he brought dogs from the Banting Institute to St. Michael's in order to train anaesthetists and nurses in open-heart surgery with perfusion using a "Rube Goldberg" assembled pump and later a Pemco device. No dogs survived of course and the project was halted rather abruptly when a dead canine was returned and left outside the Banting Institute doors on a hot summer Friday evening after the Banting staff had left. Thus a canine experimental laboratory was developed at St. Michael's Hospital without reliance on university facilities. Wolf Sapirstein joined Baker for a few years after a fellowship at TGH but went to Harrisburg, Pennsylvania, to develop a private practice. Sapirstein ultimately became responsible for Medical Devices at the United States Food and Drug Administration. John Hart came up from the United States and Jimmy Yao joined Baker for the rest of his career until Baker's retirement in May 1990. John Hart retired in the past few years and Jimmy Yao continues to work part-time at St. Michael's and in the Philippines.

Under Clare Baker's direction, cardiac surgery at St. Michael's thrived despite any direct involvement with the formal U of T training program. Residents and fellows came from elsewhere, or from other programs, to St. Michael's because of the large and diverse volume and the opportunity to develop their own skills with an excellent teacher. Baker became widely known for his success with open-heart surgery in Jehovah's Witnesses and indeed performed major operations on 147 such patients with only a single death after double valve replacement. He performed over two hundred open mitral operations without a single mortality. St. Michael's performed five heart transplants with one perioperative death and indeed recorded the second longest survivor in

the world (Perrin Johnston, seven years survival) despite
a demonstrable lack of enthusiasm for this venture from
Dr. Bigelow and a direct order from the then professor
of surgery, William Drucker, not to proceed with the
transplant.

Tomas Salerno and Samuel Lichtenstein were recruited
to St. Michael's in 1984 and 1986 respectively. Salerno
is one of the most colourful cardiac surgeons in North
America with an interesting, provocative, and productive
career described elsewhere in this book. He developed
a thriving research laboratory, became a "Pied Piper"
and mentor to a generation of young cardiac surgeon-
scientists and was appointed chairman of the university
division of cardiovascular surgery in 1987. Not only did
this bring St. Michael's into a much better research
position, but also brought CV residents eager to train
at that institution. The university professor of surgery
at that time, Dr. Bernard Langer, invested heavily in the
academic and training potential at St. Michael's.

As partners, Salerno and Lichtenstein were truly "the odd
couple," Tomas being extroverted and Sam somewhat
more self-effacing. However, together they evolved
the concept of continuous normothermic myocardial
protection with oxygenated warm blood cardioplegia.
This created a stir within a city and university whose
history was based on hypothermia and attracted
worldwide attention with international visitors, clinical
demonstrations, and seminal publications.

Clinical and research success at St. Michael's at that
time was so intense that patient management became
somewhat chaotic and ultimately a patient died after
CABG surgery, having had his operation cancelled on
numerous occasions (1988). This resulted in intense

media and public focus and the Ministry of Health and Provincial Government subsequently established an inquiry into the practice of cardiovascular surgery at St. Michael's and indeed throughout Ontario. While this almost destroyed St. Michael's reputation at the time, it ultimately benefited the cardiovascular and patient community in Ontario by the establishment of the Cardiac Care Network of Ontario. This established uniform definitions of clinical urgency, appropriate waiting times and the placement of nurse coordinators in each full service hospital. (This development is described elsewhere in the book.) Salerno later took up the position as chief of cardiac surgery at Buffalo General Hospital and Lichtenstein as head of St. Paul's Hospital in Vancouver, ultimately being appointed university chair for the University of British Columbia Cardiovascular Training Program.

Lee Errett, a graduate of McGill University, left a staff position at Montreal General for practice in New Haven, Connecticut, and a teaching position at Yale University. Errett was recruited as head at St. Michael's Hospital in 1994. He redeveloped and reestablished the cardiac surgical clinical and research program at St. Michael's and was able to fund numerous innovations with the generous support of an old friend and mentor. The Terrence Donnelly Cardiovascular Residents' Research Day has become a national institution. The team at St. Michael's is uniquely composed of non-Torontonians: David Latter, trained at McGill and Stanford University; Daniel Bonneau, trained in Toronto and later head of cardiac surgery at University of Sherbrooke, Quebec; and Yves Leclerc, trained in Montreal, Birmingham, Alabama, and Toronto and ultimately appointed head of cardiac surgery at the prestigious Montreal Heart Institute. They have developed an excellent reputation in

clinical practice and resident training and are respected
as full members of the university program. Indeed David
Latter is director of the Cardiac Surgical Residency
Program—the ultimate vindication of Clare Baker's
pioneering efforts.

Recent additions to the surgical staff include Subohd
Vermah, a well respected lipid metabolism researcher,
who is well funded and on the Editorial Board of
Circulation, as well as having a growing surgical practice.
Mark Peterson returned from a Fellowship with Ed
Dietrich at the Arizona Heart Institute to focus on
endovascular aortic surgery.

St. Michael's continues to stimulate residents and the
larger cardiovascular world with the annual Landmark
Lecture Series and the Terrence Donnelly Residents'
Day.

SUNNYBROOK HEALTH SCIENCES CENTRE

Stephen Fremes and Bernard S. Goldman

Wilfred G. Bigelow performed the first closed mitral valvotomies in Toronto and second in Canada at Sunnybrook Hospital in the early 1950s. Sunnybrook was then a Veteran's Hospital in the north suburbs of the city. He was later granted permission to perform this operation at the Toronto General Hospital. He and James A. Key continued to perform closed procedures for many years at Sunnybrook.

A cardiac catheterization laboratory was opened by Drs. Art Chisholm and Sam Shane in July 1969. Only four procedures were done by the time Sal Naqvi joined them in November of that year. Jim Key consulted on all cases requiring heart surgery and these patients were then brought to the Toronto General Hospital. In 1980, Bernard Goldman was named the cardiac surgical consultant, as successor to Key, ultimately bringing over three hundred cases per year "downtown" to TGH.

The Department of Veterans' Affairs transferred Sunnybrook to the University of Toronto, becoming Sunnybrook Health Sciences Centre and University of Toronto Clinic in 1966. Despite the hopes and plans of Drs. Chisholm, Key, and Al Harrison (then chief of surgery), a formal open-heart surgical program would not develop at Sunnybrook for many years. Indeed, nineteen years would pass from the initial application. The original suggestion of a cardiac surgical team at Sunnybrook was made in 1970 after a presentation by Drs. Al Harrison and Art Chisholm to Dean John Hamilton, then vice provost of Health Sciences at the University of Toronto. The proposal was part of a planned new medical school at York University. Sunnybrook's CV plan was accepted in concept for a full forty-eight hours! Not only did the York University Medical School plan falter, but the University of Toronto (presumably Bill Bigelow) wanted Sunnybrook Hospital "to mature" and generate at least a hundred open-heart cases per year (for TGH naturally). Nonetheless a "promise" was extracted that Sunnybrook would indeed be the next open-heart unit.

The waiting list crisis of the late 1980s with its intense media focus and significant political pressure resulted in a ministry and university decision to create a fourth heart surgical program in Toronto. Drs Ron Baigrie, then chief of cardiology at Sunnybrook, and Goldman at Toronto General had been delegated to find a means to facilitate urgent referrals: "Metro Triage" resulted. Ultimately, with the help of Dr. David Naylor, later dean of medicine and subsequently president of the University of Toronto, the Cardiac Care Network of Ontario and the open-heart program at Sunnybrook both evolved. The first case was performed on November 27, 1989; 167 patients then underwent successful surgery before a mortality, thereby establishing the new team as safe and successful.

Initially there were numerous university and local political problems to surmount; the intent of the "downtown" surgeons was that Sunnybrook simply become a "coronary mill" to ease the waiting lists while the cancer, orthopaedic and trauma surgeons on site were less than enthusiastic about the potential for excess resource utilization by a new cardiac team. However, Goldman, Stephen Fremes and George Christakis (initially a fellow) were determined that the Sunnybrook program should be part of the University of Toronto Cardiovascular and Thoracic Surgery Residency Program, that it provide a full service, and that it become a major academic centre. Both Fremes and Christakis had been research fellows under Richard Weisel at TGH, who groomed them as clinician scientists. Sunnybrook surgeons have contributed significantly in clinical research relating to myocardial preservation, aortic valve surgery, left ventricular dynamics, arterial conduits, and demographic and outcome studies.

Sunnybrook has had both the pleasure and honour for some members of our surgical staff to populate other excellent centres. Labib Abouzar left for Hamilton Civic Hospital and McMaster University, Gopal Bhatnagar and Charles Cutrara opened the new Trillium Heart Centre, and Mark Pelletier was recruited to Stanford University Medical Center in Palo Alto, California, after which he became the divisional head in Saint John, New Brunswick.

Sunnybrook was the host site for much of the training and resource personnel for Trillium Heart Centre: indeed two cardiac anaesthetists, nurse managers and OR assistants left for Trillium, which initially caused some difficulties with our own OR and ICU staffing. Later, the opening of the new cardiac surgical unit at Southlake Regional Centre in Newmarket added to our volume woes already precipitated by the SARS incident. Nonetheless, we were pleased to see a reunion at Southlake of three former residents in the Toronto program during Tom Salerno's tenure as university chair, Drs. Byung Moon, Charles Peniston, and Richard Bauset.

After Goldman became Surgeon-in-Chief, Stephen Fremes was made Head of Cardiac Surgery and later Head of the combined units of Cardiac and Vascular Surgery. Gideon Cohen, a Toronto trainee and PhD student of Richard Weisel, returned to Sunnybrook after a fellowship at Cleveland Clinic. He has demonstrated an interest in minimally invasive valve procedures, mitral valve repair and arrhythmia surgery. Fuad Moussa joined the staff as an Associate, having trained with Tomas Salerno in Miami. Moussa has focused on off pump coronary bypass as well as thoracic surgery.

The vascular section of the Sunnybrook Division has been expanded and re-invigorated. Current members of the vascular section of the combined division include longstanding Sunnybrook surgeons Robert Maggisano and Daryl Kucey, and the recent recruit Andrew Dueck who specializes in catheter-based vascular procedures. Dueck spent valuable time with Dietrich at Arizona Heart Institute. Joe Papia will be joining the combined division with a cross-appointment in Critical Care Medicine in May 2009, following completion of an advanced EVAR fellowship in the Cleveland Clinic. Both contribute greatly to the Clinical Centre of Excellence for Endovascular Aortic Surgery developed by Maggisano and Kucey.

Sunnybrook continues to thrive in both clinical and academic realms with specific interests in arterial conduits, valve function, intraoperative coronary bypass graft imaging, and outcome determinants. Drs. Christakis and Cohen have contributed seminal clinical trials of functional effects of various aortic valvular prostheses, while Dr. Fremes' landmark studies on the radial artery bypass have been significant and widely quoted.

A very exciting development has been the creation of the Bernard Goldman Chair in Cardiovascular Surgery, which will help foster research in the Division. To ensure future academic success at Sunnybrook, there is a now a search for a new clinician scientist in cardiac surgery.

REFLECTIONS ON BILL MUSTARD AND THE EARLY DAYS AT HOSPITAL FOR SICK CHILDREN, TORONTO

George A. Trusler

[Editor's note:
I had the pleasure of working with Bill Mustard and George Trusler for almost two years during my own residency and it was delightful to share lunch with George Trusler and Bill Williams in Toronto on June 11, 2004. What follows is partly taken from Trusler's personal recollection, the Fourth Keon Lecture, which he delivered on the tenth anniversary of the University of Ottawa Heart Institute and a summary prepared by Bill Williams of the major contributions from Sick Children's over the years.]

With some nostalgia, I recollect Bill Mustard, in the fall of 1949, working in the old Sick Children's Elizabeth Street Hospital, a Victorian institution opened in 1892. I was doing a rotating internship then at the TGH and one of the options was two months at HSC, the first month in the out-patient "Dresser's Room" and the second month on the combined John Keith-Bill Mustard service. Mustard's patients were a mix of orthopedic, general, and cardiac surgery. Cardiac had only started about two years earlier with one operating day per week, mainly doing patent ductus, coarctation, and Blalock shunts.

Let me digress and relate Bill Mustard's history: of Scottish ancestry, William Thornton Mustard was born on August 8, 1914, in Clinton, Ontario, the third of four boys and a girl. Both parents were teachers. As a young boy, in addition to the usual games and sports, he cultivated some unusual interests such as raising pigeons and collecting butterflies and was said to be exceptionally bright, reading widely. He attended UTS, perhaps the most academic high school in Toronto, but his main interest there seemed to be football. He was short, strong, coordinated, and ambitious and became captain of the 130 lb. football team. An indication of some of his personality traits and interests that he himself later admitted was his tendency to avoid the mundane chore of dishwashing by entertaining his siblings with stories of his day's activities—while they did the work.

He entered the University of Toronto at the early age of sixteen and chose the Faculty of Medicine because his second eldest brother was already there. He literally coasted through medical school, applying his energies to theatrical skit nights where his wit and sense of humour allowed him to write and play in most of the productions. He was a leader and always loved centre stage: active in sports, chiefly football, where he was quarterback and captain of the second varsity team. In summers as a camp counselor his athletic ability led to a high degree of excellence in water sports, swimming, diving, and paddling. He acknowledged, as he left university in 1937, that although he did fairly well academically he had come nowhere close to his potential. It was later in postgraduate training that he started to take his career seriously. In 1937, he did a standard junior rotating internship at the TGH, and in 1938 a year of surgery at HSC. In September 1939, his father perished in the sinking of the passenger ship *Athenia*. There was little money in the family and Bill Mustard took several months off his internship to earn enough to help his youngest brother through university. Dr. A. B. Lemesurier, chief surgeon at HSC, took an interest in Bill and slanted some of his training toward orthopedics. He then spent six months at the New

York Orthopedic Hospital and was later back at Ward C of TGH with Gordon Murray, with some subsequent training in neurosurgery with K. G. MacKenzie. His sense of humour was ever present and many stories are told of his antics in the interns' quarters.

In 1941, he enlisted in the Royal Canadian Army Medical Corps and was sent to England where he was asked to form a field surgical unit. He subsequently took mobile field surgical unit 7 into Europe on D day plus two, going all through the European campaign, operating at front line level. It is here that he first showed the brilliance, boldness, and enterprise, which was to mark his career. From his experience with Gordon Murray, who was pioneering the use of heparin, he had a unique supply of vitellium tubes, heparin, and arterial sutures. At the front line unit, he inserted the vitellium tubes and administered heparin to soldiers with severely damaged leg arteries in an attempt to save their limbs. This was probably the first time a prosthetic material was used in the human cardiovascular system and he was awarded an MBE. Unfortunately, he was ahead of his time, and of eighteen soldiers so treated only one leg survived, this in a soldier who had the tube replaced with a vein graft two days later back at base hospital.

Wherever he was, he could be relied on for wit and humour, some of it outlandish and some at others' expense. Bill Bigelow relates a story of a gala Christmas party in the officers' mess at Aldershot, United Kingdom, where Mustard took centre stage by swallowing goldfish until requested (ordered?) to leave. Bigelow said that Mustard could never resist the temptation to poke fun at the pompous, which might include all officialdom. Bigelow and Mustard were close friends throughout their careers and Bigelow with his own great sense of humour and showmanship was often the perfect straight man for a Mustard act.

Following the war in Europe, Mustard returned and completed his surgical training with a residency at HSC followed by a year's fellowship at the NY Orthopedic Hospital. He returned in 1947 on staff at HSC in both general and orthopedic surgery. Meanwhile Dr. John Keith, after his service in the navy, started a congenital heart service at HSC and asked Dr. Lemesurier to assign a surgeon. Thus was Bill Mustard appointed and sent to Baltimore for a month to watch Dr. Blalock. At the time, Bill Bigelow was working there, and later Ray Heimbecker worked with Richard Bing also at Hopkins. When Mustard returned to Toronto, he added cardiac surgery to his pediatric surgical responsibilities.

At that time, cardiac surgery was rather limited. Coarctation repairs were usually performed between six and twelve years of age and the surgery could be hazardous: there were no specialized clamps, Kelly clamps either damaged the arterial wall or slid off with predictable results. Patent ducti were all ligated and usually in childhood, two years and older. Blalock shunts were performed nearly always on tetralogy patients mostly two to four years of age. At this point Mustard had performed forty-seven Blalock shunts, which I reviewed (heady stuff for a junior intern), and my naïve but correct conclusion at that time was that better follow-up was needed. Mustard would later devise his own version of the special Blalock clamps which worked very well.

During the first ten years of his practice, Mustard accomplished much. In 1948, one year after starting, he did the first total blood replacement of an infant with

Rh incompatibility. He became well known in pediatric surgical circles, particularly in the surgical section of the Academy of Pediatrics. He was frequently asked to speak or even entertain and one-armed push-ups were a specialty that he would demonstrate at any time or place. Frequently irreverent, his antics were enjoyed by most but not all, but at least they were renowned. On several occasions in the middle of a formal function, he took the spotlight by diving into the fountain or pool, or crawling under the head table. Nonetheless, all agreed he was a gifted and slick orthopedic surgeon with a huge volume of patients. Postpolio patients formed a large group and he developed an operation, the ileo psoas transfer, for treatment of weak hip abductors. This operation became known internationally as the Mustard operation.

During my twelve-month rotating residency in 1953-54, I spent two months on the Mustard service. In 1951, the new children's hospital (the sixth) had opened on University Avenue providing improved facilities for the advances soon to come. Cardiac volumes had increased and now included vascular rings, Blalock-Hanlon shunts, Brock procedures for pulmonary stenosis or atresia, Potts shunts for tricuspid and/or pulmonary atresia. Clamps had improved but the ORs in those days, like the rest of the hospital, had no air-conditioning. As well, the steam sterilizers were adjacent and contributed to the heat. During a very hot spell in summer, temperatures in the OR would soar to over 90°F and this was particularly difficult for cyanotic children—Mustard would sometimes arrange to have a fan blow over buckets of ice in order to provide some cool air. Mustard achieved some prominence in these early days with a number of firsts: the first to ligate a ductus in an infant in failure and the first to repair a coarctation in infancy, both of which now seem routine. Early on, and independently, he envisioned the potential for a heart-lung pump and he worked on this in the laboratory. Open-heart surgery was just about to begin. Bigelow had done the early experimental work on hypothermia but had no clinical cases. F. John Lewis had closed an ASD with hypothermia in 1953. Bill Mustard had had some problems with the Blalock-Hanlon procedure so he and Bigelow attempted this, using hypothermia, on an infant with TGA but unfortunately was unsuccessful. This was probably the first use of hypothermia at HSC and perhaps in Toronto. Bubble oxygenator experiments were unreliable because antifoaming agents were not yet available. Mustard subsequently used monkey lungs as an oxygenator before Gibbon's pump oxygenator had been used clinically. Mustard attempted arterial repair of TGA in seven small sick children without success, but again he was ahead of his time with this courageous and imaginative enterprise. The monkey lungs were only good for fifteen to twenty minutes before they became edematous. The pump, designed by Campbell Cowan, is described elsewhere in this book.

By modern standards, conditions at HSC in the early 1950s were fairly primitive. Blood pressure was taken by cuff, oximetry was just starting, and there was no intraoperative ECG monitoring since the hospital had a single cumbersome large ECG machine kept on cardiology. Children were kept in the recovery room for four hours after surgery and then transferred to the ward. Despite the simplicity of monitoring and the primitive nature of the Cowan pump and monkey-lung oxygenator, the cases that Mustard performed were among the first extracorporeal circulation procedures done in the world. Mustard continued to apply this modality to the occasional patient with tetralogy of Fallot or VSD. I believe it was in 1953 that he had his first surviving patient, the first in Canada surviving a congenital repair on cardiopulmonary bypass. In a 1957 paper, Mustard described a total of twenty-one cases in addition to the previous seven with TGA, with three survivors—a nine-month-old with tetralogy operated on in May 1955 and two—and four-month-old infants, both with VSDs repaired in 1956. The tetralogy was the first surviving heart-lung pump case in this country. Bigelow had earlier performed several successful open-heart cases using only hypothermia. In early 1957, Mustard changed to a bubble oxygenator similar to the DeWall-Lillehei model.

In most cities in the 1950s pediatric surgeons did pretty well all types of surgery without subspecialization. At HSC, Dr. Alfred Farmer, the newly appointed chief of surgery, decided to change this practice and in 1957 Mustard was asked to choose between orthopedics and cardiac surgery, choosing the latter. (Nonetheless, a host of residents including Goldman, Keon, Williams, and others, would work with Mustard on orthopedic cases in the afternoon after the cardiac caseload for the day was completed, for many years.) As I completed my training in 1956, I was asked to join the staff at HSC to help Mustard with the fledgling cardiac surgery program. I took a six-month traveling fellowship and returned for a one-year chief residency before entering practice in June 1958. In the traveling fellowship, my focus was divided between general pediatric and cardiac surgery but the major purpose was to collect as much information and detail as possible on heart-lung pumps and relay this back by letters to Mustard every few weeks. I visited eighteen different surgical centres in the United States and Mexico. In July 1957, I returned to HSC and this year marked a significant change for cardiac surgery. We began performing one pump case per week despite the new and in some ways relatively crude perfusion technology. In addition our knowledge of congenital anatomy and repair techniques were just being developed. Heart monitoring had advanced so there was now arterial pressure, ECG and some oximetry although the old van Slyke apparatus required at least a half hour for oxygen saturation. We did not fully understand the anatomy of the Bundle of His, and heart block was common after VSD repair (about 15 percent). Cardiac pacemakers had just become available but they were large, bulky and external. If heart block was persistent the patient would not survive since epicardial leads invariably led to infection. Later Sick Children's would apply external radio frequency energy through a specially designed jacket that the child would wear over the implanted pacemaker and induction coil.

Postoperative care in 1957 was still problematic. We soon realized that after cardiopulmonary bypass, every organ system was liable to malfunction and that postoperative care for children on a regular ward was cumbersome, inadequate and unsafe. Thus as volume increased a portion of the recovery room was set aside, particularly after a major donation from Colonel Sam McLaughlin and a dedicated ICU and staff were developed by Dr. Al Conn of anaesthesia. The volume of cardiac surgery continued to increase steadily. Instruments and surgical techniques were improving; patent ductus and some coarctations were being repaired in infancy as were some Blalock shunts. For many years, indeed throughout the 1960s, atrial septal defect, aortic and pulmonary stenosis were all corrected with surface hypothermia and inflow occlusion, although it was obvious that more time was required for some of the more complex repairs.

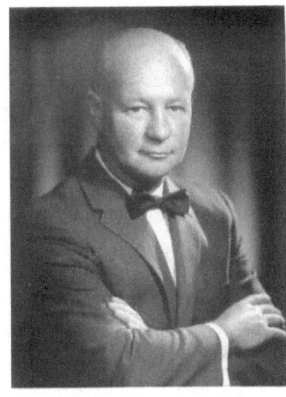 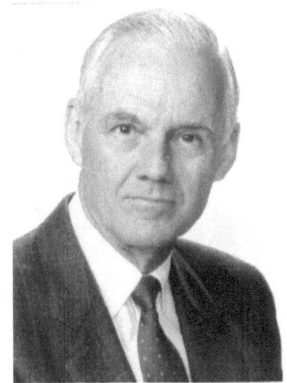

Fig. 3:3a William T. Mustard   Fig. 3:3b George Trusler

Bill Mustard, HSC, and TGA are a story important to relate. TGA is a fairly common complex congenital malformation making up about 5 percent of congenital heart disease and without treatment 90 percent of infants die in their first year. Many procedures had been devised, e.g., the Blalock-Hanlon shunt in 1948, Mustard's 1952 attempt at arterial switch, Tom Baffes's 1957 graft from the IVC to LA (a difficult and complicated procedure), and Senning's complete venous repair in 1959, also ingenious but complicated. Mustard had attempted both the Baffes and Senning procedures but without success. Despite his brilliance and ability, Bill Mustard was not a detail man and these procedures, which were meticulous and somewhat tedious, did not appeal to him for he was impatient. In 1963, he conceived a repair for TGA whereby he removed atrial septum and replaced it with a baffle of pericardium, which would divert the pulmonary venous return to the tricuspid valve and the caval venous return to the mitral valve. He performed this procedure in the animal laboratory numerous times and it seemed perfectly feasible. In May 1963, he did his first baffle operation on a two-year-old girl who survived and the case was published in 1964. In the spring of that year,

he presented five patients at the annual AATS meeting
in Montreal and the operation was greeted with much
enthusiasm, being relatively simple, easily reproducible,
with good early results. For the next thirteen years
Mustard lived with increasing fame and Sick Children's
enjoyed a wonderful reputation with patients coming
from all over the globe. He built a five-foot-high inflatable
see-through plastic model of the atrial chambers of the
heart with the Mustard baffle in place and he would take
residents and visitors on a walk through the model in
his own inimitable style, usually making everyone more
confused than ever and he would finally pronounce
the whole procedure "baffling." There has been some
speculation as to how Mustard first conceived the
operation. Whitmer Firor, his resident at the time (and
later cardiac surgeon and aerospace physiologist in
Saskatoon), thought that it related to several instances
where a caval vein had inadvertently been rerouted into
the wrong atrium—if it can be done inadvertently, then
why not on purpose, thought Mustard.

Bill Mustard's successes could not have been achieved
without great support from many others in the hospital
community, in particular the Division of Cardiology led
by Dr. John Keith, later Richard Rowe, and subsequently
Robert Freedom. All were natural leaders and superb
cardiologists, who fostered an atmosphere where the
interests of the child were foremost and importantly they
were strong supporters of innovative surgical procedures.
While no one surgeon ever achieved the renown and
reputation of Bill Mustard, it is fair to state throughout
this period of intense growth and change Canada was
blessed with a number of excellent pediatric cardiac
surgeons. The first who deserves mention is Gordon
Murray who while essentially an adult surgeon, did some
early pediatric surgery at the TGH. He was an outstanding

surgeon and a superb technician and probably did the first Blalock operation in Canada, going on to perform a whole series of these with excellent results. Phil Ashmore pointed out that even way back then Murray recognized the virtue of nursing all children in the same unit. The true pediatric cardiac surgeons in Canada include: David Ross Murphy, Tony Dobell, and Paul Stanley (all of Montreal); Colin Ferguson (Winnipeg); Phil Ashmore (Vancouver); David Alton Murphy (Halifax); and George Trusler and Bill Williams (Toronto). All of these surgeons in their separate communities established or helped to establish open-heart units for children and provided excellence in pediatric cardiac surgery. Ashmore has pointed out that the results of congenital heart surgery are best when done by a small group of individuals with a concentrated high volume, persons who are able and prepared to dedicate most of their time to that subspecialty. Perhaps thanks to a certain historical bias towards children's hospitals, Canada learned the lessons early in comparison to many centres in the United States. All of the surgeons mentioned contributed excellent material and published papers of excellent quality and achieved international recognition. Furthermore, they trained a generation of young surgeons who now serve Canada well.

Let me finish these thoughts with a few more remarks on Bill Mustard. While very athletic in earlier years, Mustard played hard along the way but failed to maintain his physical capacities. Perhaps the discipline of continuing physical fitness was not as popular in his generation and he was extremely busy both in his professional life and with a large family of seven children. In his last few years of practice, he was physically slower and less comfortable with surgery and he retired in 1976 at age sixty-two. Retirement was not easy for such a talented, ambitious, and busy soul. Ultimately, he went into florid pulmonary edema at his cottage in Muskoka but was fortunately resuscitated by a visiting Israeli surgeon (Dr. Dani Goor) there to do an interview. He was ultimately transferred to TGH with the clinical picture of severe calcific aortic stenosis with coronary artery disease. But when Bill Bigelow and Bernie Goldman visited him in the CCU to discuss angiography and surgery he adamantly refused. He passed away in 1987 at age seventy-four, and on October 21, 1991, the Toronto Historical Board dedicated a plaque on the northwest corner of the new Sick Children's Hospital grounds honouring William Thornton Mustard. At the dedication ceremony Bill Bigelow stated, "William Mustard was a legend in his time. He will be remembered as an impressive, buoyant personality whose surgical career featured imagination and creativity. He may be the last of a breed who combined being a character with excellence in surgery."

It was a great treat and a privilege for me to be associated with Bill Mustard for all of those years as resident, fellow, colleague and partner, to share not only in his brilliance, creativity and irreverence, as well as participating in the training of so many superb pediatric heart surgeons across Canada and abroad.

THE HOSPITAL FOR SICK CHILDREN IN TORONTO

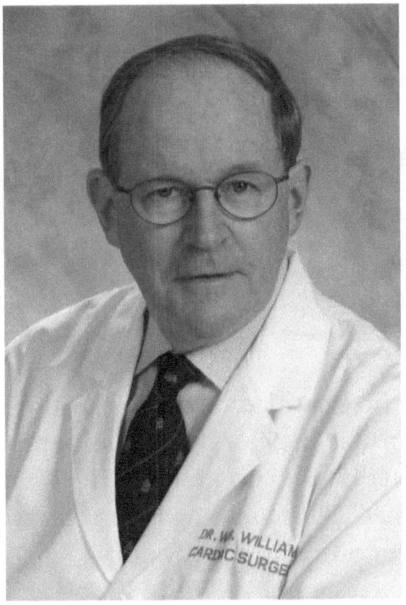

Fig. 3:4 William G. Williams

The Beginning of Heart Surgery

The outlook for children with heart disease was poor in the era prior to operative intervention. Dr. Robert Gross of Boston performed the first operation for congenital heart disease, a patent ductus ligation, in 1939. In that era, studies of the natural history of congenital heart disease provided a foundation upon which physicians and surgeons could build and also to judge the effects of their developing interventional techniques.

William T. Mustard was appointed to the faculty of the Hospital for Sick Children (HSC) and the University of Toronto in 1947 as a pediatric general surgeon with an interest in orthopedic surgery.

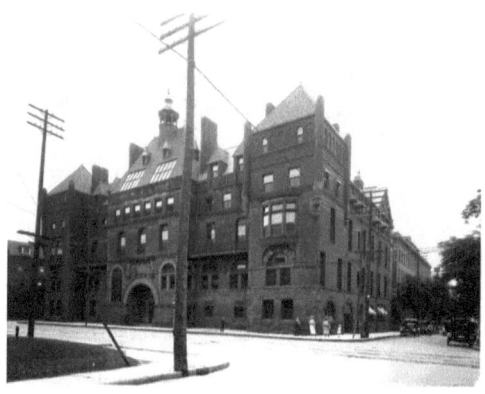

Fig. 3:5 The first cardiac operation at the Hospital for Sick Children was in 1947. The photograph shows the College Street building occupied by the Hospital for Sick Children in 1947. This building is currently the Canadian Blood Services office and laboratory.

There was no cardiac surgery program at that time but the division of cardiology was well established. Cardiology had a busy clinical service organized by Dr. John Keith. Keith's service formed the basis for publication of his internationally recognized textbook of pediatric cardiology in 1958.[1]

Mustard's interest in the potential of surgical treatment for children with cardiovascular disease came from his experience in treating vascular injuries as an army surgeon during the Second World War.[2, 3] He described the process that led to limb gangrene as follows:

> *Whether the ischemia progresses to recovery or not depends upon the volume of blood the limb receives, the pressure at which it is delivered, the length of time the ischemic state has existed, and the metabolic demands of the limb itself.*

Mustard repaired major arterial transections of limbs from war wounds by inserting interposition glass tubes. He used heparin to prevent clotting. Gordon Murray of Toronto had developed both the use of heparin and the interposition tubes in 1940, but Mustard was the first to use the tubes in man. The tubes were an emergency measure that would allow evacuation of the soldier and subsequent elective replacement of the damaged artery with an interposition autologous venous graft. He reported his results in eighteen soldiers, including six who underwent the second stage artery repair. He summarized his results as:

Disappointing but not discouraging.

Mustard's careful observation of his clinical experience, systematic approach to understanding a problem, and careful analysis and description of his results were the foundation for an outstanding career in academic surgery and as a pioneer in pediatric cardiac surgery.

The first cardiac operation at HSC was a patent ductus ligation in 1947.[4] Operations for coarctation of the aorta, palliation of tetralogy of Fallot, pulmonary stenosis and five other cardiac anomalies soon followed. By 1954, he had accumulated experience in 480 infants and children. Survival after patent ductus repair was excellent with only two deaths among 176 children.[5] However, the outlook for many other children was less favourable with an operative mortality rate of 37 percent. It was much higher in the infant group. Mustard was critical of centres that reported selected groups of patients:

> *If one did not operate upon tetralogy of Fallot before three years of age the mortality figures would be much better for the surgeon but not for the patients, since a number would be dead before operation was undertaken.*

His early reports established a precedent for honesty in reporting. The noncompetitive system of centralized health care in Ontario ensured patient referrals so that "manipulation" of results as an enticement to patient referrals was unnecessary.

All of the surgery for children with tetralogy of Fallot during that era was palliative. He stated that surgical repair of the infundibular and pulmonary valve stenosis should be delayed until such time as the ventricular septal defect could be closed, a feat that Lillehei performed in 1953 to begin the era of open-heart surgery.

Beginnings of Cardiopulmonary Bypass

The experience referenced above was accumulated prior to the first open-heart operations. Development of a "heart-lung" machine was being investigated in many centres. Mustard and A. Lawrence Chute (Chute was subsequently appointed chief of pediatrics and then dean of medicine at Toronto) reported upon their experimental work in developing a heart-lung machine in 1951.[6] They used a biologic oxygenator (dog lung) because as they explained, lungs have a massive surface area for gaseous exchange, are a first-rate filter, and because the lung "carries out certain detoxification functions which are not clearly understood at this time."[7]

The pump for their heart-lung machine was also custom built and consisted of a mechanical piston that compressed the outside of a rubber bulb that was scavenged from a syphingomanometer.[8]

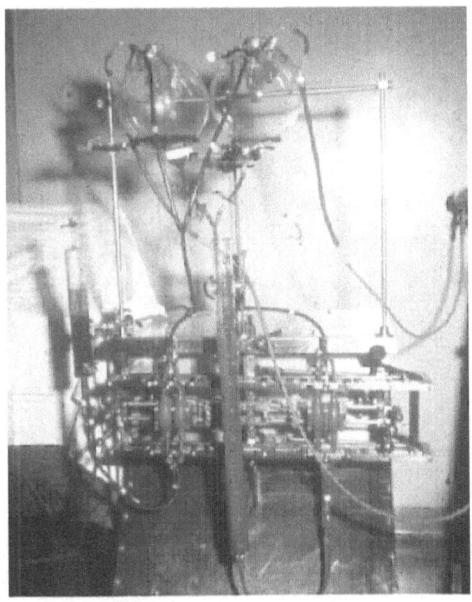

Fig. 3:6 The "monkey-lung oxygenator" and cardiac bypass pump was used in a number of children in the early 1950s. Note that the "pump" consists of a blood pressure bulb compressed by steel pistons. Blood dropping out of the left chamber of the lung is collected in a Bell jar before being pumped back into the child's arterial system.

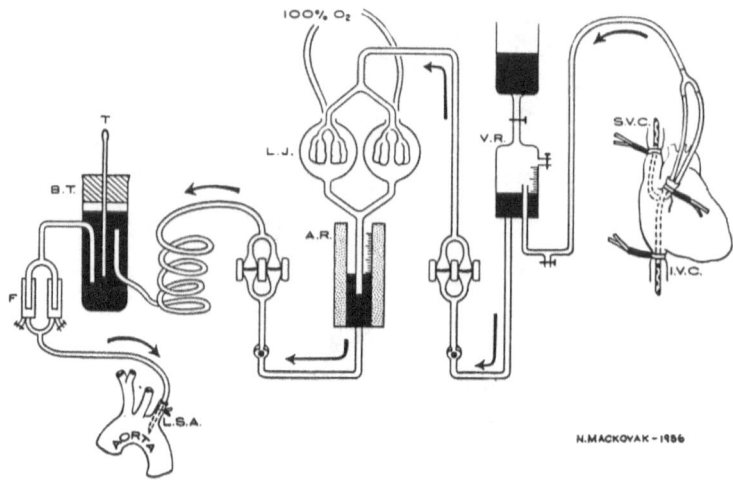

Fig. 3:7 Diagram of the heart-lung machine designed by
Mustard, Chute and Cowan, circa 1950.

They reported a series of seventy-six experimental bypass
operations in dogs with the circulation completely
supported for periods of nine to forty-seven minutes.
They also explored the safe limits of anticoagulation with
heparin, developed a bubble trap to reduce air embolism,
and examined the response of the heart to incision and
suture repair. They concluded:

> *The possibilities of applying this principle of a*
> *biologic oxygenator to human beings are now being*
> *investigated through the study of human lungs*
> *obtained at autopsy and operation, and the study of*
> *lungs of other species.*

During this work, Mustard could not make a living wage
performing only sixty-five closed heart operations per
year, so he had an active practice in general pediatric
surgery and in orthopedic surgery. He developed an
orthopedic operation in 1953 (an iliopsoas tendon

transfer) for children who were paralyzed by poliomyelitis. The tendon transfer allowed them to sit upright.[9] It was the original "Mustard operation."

The first open-heart operation at the Hospital for Sick Children was in 1951 using the monkey-lung oxygenator. The sixteen-month-old child with tetralogy of Fallot died after an attempt at relieving right ventricular outflow tract stenosis without closing the ventricular septal defect. Mustard made more than twelve subsequent attempts at open-heart surgery before his first success in 1955. In a remarkable paper in 1957, Mustard reported his entire clinical experience (but excluded infants with transposition and tricuspid atresia because they were universally fatal) using the biologic oxygenator in twenty-one children.[10] There were only three survivors. Each child's course was carefully reviewed and the reason for failure described a format he had used previously in describing his "*disappointing but not discouraging*" results with arterial war wounds. During this pioneering work with the heart-lung machine, all other aspects of clinical care for these children were being invented by necessity including cannulae, bypass tubing and connectors for the heart-lung machine, vascular clamps, methods of suture repair of the heart and vessels, clinical monitoring and intensive care facilities including methods of respiratory support, techniques of managing the coagulation system, and development of the cardiac pacemaker. A remarkable list of formidable obstacles was overcome by enormous effort and perseverance to achieve success.

Expansion of the Cardiac Surgery Service

Given the primitive state of cardiac surgery in 1958 and the limited clinical experience, it took considerable foresight to appoint a second cardiac surgeon, Dr. George Trusler.

A graduate of the University of Toronto and of the Gallie course in surgery, Trusler spent time in Dr. W. G. Bigelow's laboratory investigating hypothermia and its potential use in cardiac surgery. Dr. Trusler had a cross-appointment to the division of pediatric general surgery but by 1968 restricted his practice to cardiovascular pediatric surgery.

Trusler contributed to the ongoing development of heart surgery by designing a novel vascular clamp and venous cannulae. The team of Mustard and Trusler produced many reports of their expanding clinical experience in all aspects of cardiac surgery. Among these were many contributions to the understanding and management of neonates with pulmonary atresia / intact ventricular septum, innominate artery suspension for life-threatening tracheal compression, and palliation of transposition of the great arteries. Unique contributions include the first successful one-stage repair of interrupted aortic arch with ventricular septal defect, and a method of achieving predictable control of the pulmonary over-circulation in children with a ventricular septal defect.[11, 12] He banded the pulmonary artery to a specific circumference based upon the baby's body weight. He also varied the band circumference to adjust for varying degrees of mixing of the two circulations caused by the cardiac lesion associated with the ventricular septal defect.

Another major contribution is Trusler's description of a novel operation to repair the aortic valve in children with a ventricular septal defect and associated aortic insufficiency.[13] His method of repair was widely adopted by other surgeons around the world.

Trusler made notable contributions to the development of the cavopulmonary anastomosis for palliation of cyanotic heart disease. The operation became the precursor to the

Fontan procedure, and a valuable staging procedure in the management of children with functionally single ventricle. His contributions were recognized by the American Heart Association's invitation to give the first Glenn lecture in 1989.[14] During his career, he trained numerous residents and fellows from all parts of the world and published two hundred peer-reviewed clinical papers.

Transposition Surgery at the Hospital for Sick Children

The surgical management of neonates with complete transposition of the great arteries is intricately entwined with pediatric cardiac surgery at HSC. And the evolution to the neonatal arterial switch operation had a major impact on the management of all congenital cardiac lesion everywhere, and especially at HSC.

Keith's text illustrated that prior to the 1950s, newborns with complete transposition (TGA) would die within days or weeks. Blalock and Hanlon demonstrated that surgical enlargement of the atrial septal defect improved the short-term survival for these children by increasing the mixing of the pulmonary and systemic circulations. Beginning in the early 1950s, Mustard and Trusler performed this palliative operation and a variation (Sterling-Edwards) in a large number of newborns with TGA. These palliative operations only postponed certain early death as there was nothing further to offer these children until the atrial repair of TGA was devised by Senning (1959) and later by Mustard (1964)—see G. A. Trusler's contribution, re: development of the Mustard. The children surviving because of the septectomy operations provided a much large cohort of children amenable to the Mustard operation and facilitated its development.

In the era prior to atrial repair, many surgeons were trying to develop techniques to repair TGA by "switching" the great arteries. Mustard devised (and tried in seven infants in 1952) a switch of the great arteries that included transfer of the left coronary artery to the neo-aorta. The right coronary artery was not transferred from the neo-pulmonary artery because he thought the low pressure and saturation in the pulmonary artery would be sufficient for the low-pressure right ventricle. While this seems naïve, there were other surgeons at the time that attempted the arterial switch operation without transferring either coronary artery!

The Mustard operation changed dramatically the outlook for children born with TGA. Survival improved from the natural history of a one-year survival < 10 percent to over 90 percent survival to age twenty years. With longer follow-up of these children however, the late complications from the right ventricle supporting the systemic circulation became evident, especially among those with TGA and an associated VSD. Consequently, when Jatene reported success with the arterial switch operation in 1975, it was not a difficult decision for us to abandon the Mustard operation for children with TGA+VSD.

Because our results with the Mustard operation for isolated TGA were outstanding (<1 percent operative risk, > 93 percent ten-year survival) it was very difficult for us to change to the arterial switch operation in this cohort of neonates. At HSC we had inherited a philosophy of managing neonates by low-risk palliative operations in order to delay intracardiac repair to a later, and presumed safer age. Beginning in 1987, and after considerable discussion, we changed to the neonatal arterial switch operation for all variants of TGA. The operative risk during this early experience increased substantially, as it did also in other institutions making this transition. The "learning curve" lasted about two years before the operative mortality became low. In recent years, the switch mortality has matched the < 1 percent risk of the Mustard operation for isolated TGA, but with the important differences that the arterial switch eliminated the impact of an associated VSD, and the late result is associated with fewer complications than after Mustard's operation.

The arterial switch operation demonstrated conclusively that the neonate could successfully withstand a complex repair requiring long cardiopulmonary bypass and aortic cross-clamp times. This clinical experience and the newfound confidence with neonatal intracardiac surgery had a profound impact on the management of neonates with other cardiac lesions.

As a result of the arterial switch experience, our management of infants with tetralogy of Fallot changed from one of palliation prior to later repair to that of an early primary repair in infancy. Although our results for tetralogy had been good with the older "conservative" two-stage approach, the change to primary repair, spearheaded by Dr. Glen Van Arsdell, reduced operative risk to < 1 percent, preserved the pulmonary annulus and right ventricle in most children, and will undoubtedly improve the very late outcomes for these children, especially during their adult life.

Experience with the neonatal switch also led to improvements in the care of neonates with hypoplastic left heart syndrome, and other forms of single ventricle; lesions that are rapidly fatal without intervention.

Data Collection and Analysis at the Hospital for Sick Children

Dr. John Keith recognized early in his career that progress in caring for children with heart disease would require careful consistent recording and collation of data. In the 1930s he devised data collection sheets that were folded sheets four pages long. To make these easily identifiable in the child's hospital file he had striped black lines drawn diagonally along the right hand border of the data pages and they became known as the "Zebra" forms. There were separate four-page zebra forms for recording clinical findings, for catheterization data, for autopsy information, and for postoperative information. He also formed his own medical record room for cardiology where each child had a packet containing their demographics, copies of electrocardiograms, X-ray reports, and the various zebra sheets. The collated data formed the basis for his textbook of pediatric cardiology.

As a resident in training, Trusler reviewed Mustard's initial results with the Blalock-Taussig operation and noted that the postoperative follow-up of these children was inadequate. When he joined the faculty, Trusler established a cardex system of recording demographics for groups of children with similar operations. He also devised a "cardiac operation sheet" similar in concept to Keith's zebra forms. The surgeon filled in a cardiac operation sheet after each operation. It contained the basic demographics and separate sections of the sheet had details specific to each operation. These were filed in the division of cardiac surgery with a copy in the cardiology packet. The operation sheets were readily accessible and formed the basis of many clinical reviews.

In 1982, we developed a computerized database.* Every operation performed by the division since July 1, 1982, is recorded. The information is entered from the operation sheets that the surgeons continue to use for data collection. For every operation a concise dataset is entered including patient demographics, details of diagnosis and surgical procedure, length of stay and in-hospital outcome. As well, there are several more detailed data tables for specific diagnostic and surgical groups of special interest. Currently the database is in a relational format allowing access from the surgical data tables to current patient status and follow-up information. The data entry and maintenance, creation of built-in reports, and continuous upgrading of the database have been provided for twenty-two years by M. Gail Williams. The database now contains information on over thirteen thousand children with approximately twenty thousand records of surgical data. It is one of the largest institutional databases in congenital heart surgery. It is continually maintained and updated with each new surgical patient and current follow-up status of previously entered patients. We have developed automated preformatted reports that are an invaluable source of information for administrative purposes, quality assurance, clinical result summaries, and as a basis for initiating clinical studies. CVSDB is used by five of the eight pediatric cardiac surgery centres in Canada and two centres in other countries.

In 1998, the Congenital Heart Surgeon's Society (CHSS) moved their database centre from Birmingham Alabama to the Hospital for Sick Children. The CHSS consists

---

* CVSDB is a registered copyright. M. Gail Williams, gwillms@istar.ca

of seventy surgeons from the United States, Canada, Brazil, and Argentina who are committed to improving the care for patients with congenital heart disease. The data centre began in 1985 with a study of all newborns admitted with a diagnosis of transposition to any of the CHSS institutions. Within four years, the data centre had collected information on the care of > nine hundred newborns with transposition. Subsequent studies were added for eight other diagnostic groups of infants with congenital heart disease and form the basis for analysis and > twenty publications from the data centre that are available though our website.[**] The analytic expertise of the CHSS statistical consultants Drs. Eugene H. Blackstone and Brian W. McCrindle had been invaluable to the data centre and of considerable benefit to our HSC clinical studies.

Present and Future at the Hospital for Sick Children

The strength of any organization is the people that are the organization. The division of cardiovascular surgery at HSC has had outstanding individuals, not just within the division, but also in the allied professions of nursing, anaesthesia, intensive care, administration, and of course cardiology. The co-operative and collegial association between cardiology and cardiovascular surgery deserves particular emphasis and has been a major asset for over fifty years. Care for children with congenital heart disease could not be developed except through close collaboration between our two divisions. Beginning with the partnership of Keith and Mustard, and continuing through the leadership of Trusler and Rowe, Freedom and Williams, and currently Drs. Andrew Redington

---

[**]   http://www.CHSSdc.org

and Glen Van Arsdell, our two divisions have functioned symbiotically as a model of collegial co-operation in fostering the improvement in care for children with congenital and acquired heart disease.

The surgical practice of congenital heart disease has changed remarkably over the past five years and continues to evolve. The interventional cardiologists have made remarkable advances and provide care for many children that in previous years would have required surgery. This trend will continue. Expansion of congenital cardiac surgery has occurred at both ends of the age range. Neonatal surgery has become well established and currently > 50 percent of pediatric cardiac surgery is in infants < one year old. At the same time, the majority of people living with congenital heart disease are now adults > eighteen years. An increasing number of adults are requiring further surgery late after repair in childhood. In association with Dr. Gary Webb of the Toronto General Hospital, our division has helped develop one of the world's leading centres for the care of the adult with congenital heart disease. Adult surgery currently accounts for 20 percent of the congenital heart surgery volume.

The science of congenital heart surgery is also evolving. Our enviable long-term follow-up will become even more valuable in the future, but the emphasis is shifting from one of survival towards outcome measurements of quality of life. Clinical and laboratory studies of cardiovascular physiology and haemodynamics are yielding to the evolving science of molecular biology. Dr. John Coles has maintained peer-review research funding for > twenty years and is currently investigating novel techniques of gene manipulation. Dr. Christopher Caldarone is an internationally recognized expert in cellular apoptosis and is investigating new methods of controlling cell death and cellular remodelling of the heart. Under the leadership of Dr. Glen Van Arsdell, the division of cardiovascular surgery at HSC is extremely well positioned to continue its traditional leadership role of improving care for patients of all ages who are affected by congenital heart disease.

Of note, Christopher Caldarone, cardiac surgeon at HSC, was selected as Chairman of the University of Toronto Division of Cardiac Surgery in April 2009. With his training and initial practise in the U.S. and his considerable research interests and clinical talents he is in a wonderful position to oversee the residency program and the evolution of the university as they face the inevitable health challenges of the future.

Notes:

1. J. D. Keith, R. D. Rowe, and P. Vlad., *Heart Disease in Infancy and Childhood* (New York: MacMillan Company, 1958).
2. W. T. Mustard, "The problem of damaged artery in forward surgery," *Can Med Assoc J* (1945), 53: 128-30.
3. W. T. Mustard, "The technique of immediate restoration of vascular continuity after arterial wounds," *Annals Surg* (1946), 124: 46-59.
4. W. T. Mustard, "Suture ligation of the patent ductus arteriosus in infancy," *Can Med Assoc J* (1947), 57: 340-41.
5. W. T. Mustard, "Mortality in congenital cardiovascular surgery," *Can Med Assoc J* (1955), 72: 740-44.
6. W. T. Mustard and A. L. Chute, "Experimental intracardiac surgery with extracorporeal circulation," *Surgery* (1951), 30: 684-88.

7.   W. T. Mustard, A. L. Chute, and E. H. Simmons, "Further observations on experimental extracorporeal circulation," *Surgery* (1952), 32: 803-10.

8.   C. R. Cowan, "Physiological perfusion pump," *J Appl. Physiol* (1952), 4: 695.

9.   W. T. Mustard, "Iliopsoas transfer for weakness of the hip abductors," *J Bone and Joint Surg* (1952), 34: 647-50.

10.   W. T. Mustard and J. A. Thomson, "Clinical experience with the artificial heart-lung preparation," *Can Med J* (1957), 76: 265-69.

11.   G. A. Trusler and T. Izukawa, "Interrupted aortic arch and ventricular septal defect," *J Thorac Cardiovasc Surg* (1975), 69: 126-31.

12.   G. A. Trusler and W. T. Mustard, "A method of banding the pulmonary artery for large ventricular septal defect with and without transposition of the great arteries," *Ann Thorac Surg* (1972), 7: 324-28.

13.   G. A. Trusler et al., "Late results after repair of aortic insufficiency associated with ventricular septal defect," *J Thorac Cardiovasc Surg* (1992), 103: 276-81.

14.   G. A. Trusler et al., "The cavopulmonary shunt: Evolution of a concept," *Circulation* (1990), 82: 132-38.

Table 1: Cardiovascular Surgeons at HSC.

Name	Academic Rank	Years at HSC
William T. Mustard Order of Canada	Professor of Surgery	1947-1986
George A. Trusler Golden Jubilee Medal	Professor of Surgery	1961-1997
William G. Williams University Chair, 1992-1998	Professor of Surgery	1973-present
John G. Coles	Professor of Surgery	1984-present
Ivan M. Rebeyka Chief of Pediatric Cardiac Surgery, U of Alberta, 1997-present	Associate Professor	1987-1997
Michael Black	Assistant Professor	1995-1999
Glen Van Arsdell Chief of Pediatric Cardiac Surgery at HSC, 2002-present	Associate Professor	1996-present
Christopher A. Caldarone	Associate Professor	2003-present

Table 2: Cardiovascular Surgeons, University of Toronto

		Hospital	University Appointments
Ronald	Baird	UHN	1968/07/01-1995/07/01
Gopal	Bhatnagar	SHSC	1968/07/01-2000/10/31
William	Bigelow	UHN	1947/07/01-1979/06/30
Michael	Black	HSC	1995/07/01-1999/01/01
Daniel	Bonneau	SMH	1995/01/01
Michael	Borger	UHN-TGH	2002/11/02
Stephanie	Brister	UHN-TGH	1998/11/01
Christopher	Caldarone	HSC	2003/07/01
George	Christakis	SHSC	1990/07/01
Gideon	Cohen	SHSC	2002/07/01
John	Coles	HSC	1984/07/01
Robert J.	Cusimano	UHN-TGH	1993/07/01
Tirone	David	UHN-TGH	1978/07/01
Lee	Errett	SMH	1994/06/01
Christopher	Feindel	UHN-TGH	1985/07/01
Stephen	Fremes	SHSC	1990/01/01
Bernard	Goldman	SHSC	1968/07/01
John	Hart	SMH	1973/07/01-2002/07/01
David	Latter	SMH	1996/06/01
Yves	Leclerc	SMH	1998/07/01
Samuel	Lichtenstein	SMH	1985/07/01-1992/10/31
Irving	Lipton	UHN-TGH	1976/07/01-1996/12/31
Lynda	Mickleborough	UHN-TGH	1981/07/01-2003/07/01
Marc	Pelletier	SHSC	2001/07/01-2004/02/01
Charles	Peniston	UHN-TGH	1992/07/01-2003/07/01
Mark	Peterson	SMH	2008/07/01
Anthony	Ralph-Edwards	UHN-TGH	1992/07/01-2003/07/01
Vivek	Rao	UHN-TGH	2001/07/01
Ivan	Rebeyka	HSC	1989/07/01-1996/08/30
Tomas	Salerno	SMH	1983/06/01-1996/04/30
Hugh	Scully	UHN-TGH	1974/07/01
George	Trusler	HSC	1971/07/01-1994/12/31
Glen	Van Arsdell	HSC	1996/08/13
Subodh	Verma	SMC	2007/07/01
Richard	Weisel	UHN-TGH	1979/07/01
William	Williams	HSC	1974/07/01
Donald	Wilson	UHN-TWH	1966/07/01-1984/06/30
James	Yao	SMH	1973/07/01-1998/07/01
Terrence	Yau	UHN-TGH	1998/07/01

HEART SURGERY IN LONDON

VICTORIA HOSPITAL

Martin M. Goldbach

Heart surgery in London began in 1956 when John C. Coles returned from post-fellowship training with Lord Russell Brock to take on the responsibility of developing this new specialty. Dr. Angus McLaughlin (the Chief) trained all the future surgeons at the University of Western Ontario, designating his disciples not only to develop expertise in a specific area of surgery, but also to return to London and head that program. John Coles was chosen to develop Cardiovascular and Thoracic Surgery.

Dr. Coles recruited a cardiac anesthetist (Dr. George Butlin) from Houston, Texas and trained an orderly (Mr. Gus Fabricus) to run the complex Mayo Gibbon heart-lung machine. That orderly went on to become one of the most respected perfusionists in Canada. Dr. Coles had the pioneer spirit that was so necessary for that first generation of cardiac surgeon. Another McLaughlin graduate, Dr. Alan Lansing, joined him soon thereafter. Dr. Lansing's tenure in London was brief; he left for the United States, where he was very successful both as an excellent surgeon and for his efforts in the mechanical heart program in Louisville, Kentucky. Dr. Nicholas Gergely came to London from Hungary via Toronto and not only helped Dr. Coles, but also established himself as a thoracic and vascular surgeon. Dr. Gergely ran an active research laboratory in the 1960s, where he pursued his interests in the very new field of heart transplantation. Dr. Coles had a friendship with Dr. Albert Starr, who sent one of his fellows, Dr. Aftab Ahmed to London for further experience. Dr. Ahmed was of great assistance to Dr. Coles in moving this challenging new specialty forward. Dr. Ahmed returned to Portland, Oregon, in partnership with Dr. Starr.

Over the years Dr. Coles introduced a large number of medical students and residents to their first taste of cardiac surgery. Many have gone on to careers in cardiac or thoracic surgery. Students such as Ernie Spratt, William G. Williams, Lloyd Black, Martin Goldbach, and Mary Lee Myers all had their first exposure to cardiothoracic surgery in OR 5 at Victoria Hospital. In addition, Dr. Cole's surgical volume stimulated the development of Critical Care at Victoria Hospital. Dr. William Sibbald, a graduate of the internal medicine program in London, was asked to return from a fellowship in the United States to develop Critical Care, which he did successfully.

Over the years, many future surgeons came to London to work with Dr. Coles as fellows for one or two years. This was a win-win situation as new fellowship graduates would learn from Dr. Coles and gain surgical experience, while they brought new techniques from other centres to London. In addition, surgical residents from the McLaughlin training program were exposed to cardiothoracic surgery.

Under Dr. Coles, London became a major centre for cardiac surgery, serving all of Southwestern Ontario. Cardiology and pediatric cardiology developed in tandem with cardiac surgery. In 1978 Dr. Martin Goldbach returned to London from surgical training at the University of Toronto and post-fellowship training in pediatric cardiac surgery at the Children's Hospital Medical Center in Boston. Dr. Goldbach joined Dr. Coles as a second adult cardiac surgeon at Victoria Hospital and established the pediatric cardiac surgery program. Adult cardiac surgery was in its rapid growth phase as coronary artery bypass surgery became very popular. The pediatric program grew to over one hundred cases per year, and moved from Victoria Hospital to a new children's hospital on the Westminster Campus. Dr. Goldbach was assisted by one of the program's graduates, Dr. Stan Rosenblum, who returned to London from his thoracic and vascular surgery practice in Sarnia to offer experienced assistance. The program moved forward to a full range of complex pediatric procedures, including Tetralogy, Transposition, AV Canal, and Hypoplastic Left Heart Syndrome cases. One of our trainees, who started his career in the orthopedic surgery program, was convinced to transfer to cardiac surgery. Dr. John G. Coles completed his surgical training in Toronto, and has gone on to a distinguished career in pediatric cardiac surgery at the Hospital for Sick Children in Toronto.

Dr. Mary Lee Myers trained in cardio-thoracic surgery at the University of Western Ontario after graduating from the McLaughlin general surgery program. She completed a research fellowship with Dr. Robert Roberts in Houston Texas, and returned to Victoria Hospital in 1984 to join Drs. Coles and Goldbach. She brought a strong academic and research presence to the program as well as clinical and surgical excellence in adult cardiac surgery.

Dr. Byung Moon joined the Victoria Hospital staff in 1992 as Dr. Coles was winding down his practice. Dr. Moon brought his enthusiastic surgical expertise to London following his surgical training at the University of Toronto. He worked at Victoria Hospital for 11 years, leaving in 2003 to start the new cardiac surgery unit at Southlake Regional Health Centre.

Dr. Ray Guo joined the Victoria Hospital surgical staff in 1997 as an associate staff surgeon, following his surgical training in Beijing, China and fellowship training at Sunnybrook Health Sciences Centre and Victoria Hospital. Dr. Guo mastered the English language in a very short period of time and was appointed to the full-time staff in January, 2005. He is known for his excellence in clinical surgery and as a teacher.

As part of the restructuring program in London, cardiac surgery was consolidated at University Hospital in May 2005. The closing of Victoria Hospital as a cardiac surgery centre marked the end of an era that extended from the very beginning of open-heart surgery in the mid-1950s and treated 18,442 patients who required cardio-pulmonary bypass.

UNIVERSITY HOSPITAL

F. Neil McKenzie

University Hospital was opened in September 1972 by Dr. Wilder Penfield, the culmination of close to a decade of planning by a small group of enthusiastic citizens. The need for an academically oriented medical institution in this city was vigorously debated as was the suggestion that a second cardiac surgical unit should be opened at the new hospital. However, the new unit with its first and at that time, only cardiac surgeon, opened in January 1974 with the appointment of Dr. Raymond O. Heimbecker from TGH. Several months were spent hiring and training staff and buying equipment while in the interim performing thoracic and vascular surgery, which at that time were part of—and indeed the progenitor of—the specialty of cardiac surgery. The first open heart operation, the repair of an atrial septal defect, was performed in August 1974 by Dr. Heimbecker. He was assisted by Dr. R. Del Maestro, an intern who had just graduated from UWO and who subsequently went on to a distinguished neurosurgical career, whose knowledge of cardiac surgery was then quite modest, and Dr. N. McKenzie who had just arrived from Scotland with an even more meager fund of knowledge.

The main academic interest of the new unit at this point was blood conservation, with the use of a prototype membrane oxygenator to minimize cellular injury and autotransfusion of shed blood among other techniques. Likely the most important message was to lower the hemoglobin "trigger" for transfusion and acceptance of normovolemic anemia. In the late 1970s cyclosporine, a new and highly specific immunosuppressive agent, became available for experimental use. A detailed evaluation of a variety of forms of this new drug was performed in different experimental animals and led to the first human transplant procedure at University Hospital in April of 1981. This first patient died of coronary graft vasculopathy in 1993. The second patient, transplanted in October 1981, also for dilated cardiomyopathy, remains alive and well 26 years later. Thoracic organ transplantation has remained a strong interest of the cardiac surgical division since that time and all the cardiac surgeons have contributed significanttly to this program.

Techniques to divide aberrant electrical pathways in the heart were also being developed in the late 1970s. The appointment of Dr. Gerard Guiraudon to University Hospital in 1981 catalyzed the development of a large program in electrophysiological surgery. Just as with the transplant program, patients came from all points of the compass and for a number of years well over 100 patients per year were treated surgically by these new techniques. Quite abruptly, it seemed, the interventional electrophysiologists discovered that aberrant pathway interruption could be achieved by catheter-based techniques, and surgical volumes rapidly slowed to a trickle and then stopped entirely.

In addition to Dr. Guiraudon, appointees to the division of cardiac surgery included Dr. Alan Menkis, an Ottawa Heart Institute graduate, now Medical Director of the Cardiac Sciences Program at St. Boniface General Hospital in Winnipeg, and Dr. Richard J. Novick who had trained at McGill and Stanford universities. Following Dr. Heimbecker's retirement in 1984 they participated in the expanded clinical programs as well as transplantation.

In the 1990s attention was directed to the fields of minimally-invasive, off-pump and robotic cardiac surgery.

Dr. Douglas Boyd, also an Ottawa Heart Institute trainee, used a prototype robot for mammary artery harvesting with subsequent performance of coronary artery bypass grafting through a small thoracic incision. Continued refinement of the technology (and a lot of hard work) has enabled Dr. Bob Kiaii, our most recent graduate in 2004, to extend this work to totally robotic revascularization in selected cases.

The University Hospital Division of Cardiac Surgery officially disappeared in April of 2005 with the merger of University and Victoria Hospitals. With this formal merger the city returned to a single unit with eight surgeons now operating. Richard Novick is the Professor and Chair of Cardiac Surgery at the University of Western Ontario and Hospital Chief of Cardiac Surgery at London Health Sciences Centre.

SUDBURY MEMORIAL HOSPITAL

Avdesh Mathur

The cardiac surgical unit in Sudbury evolved as early as 1959 through the determination of Dr. George Walker— Dr. Wilfred Bigelow had suggested that Walker sponsor a cardiovascular and thoracic unit in the Ontario north, which initiated the recruitment of Dr. Paul Field. Field had been a senior fellow at the Toronto General Hospital (the editor recalls Paul Field as a superb technician, Belsey-trained in thoracic surgery). Field pioneered the open-heart surgery program in Sudbury and the cardiovascular and thoracic unit there was unique in that it was the only open-heart program in Canada located in a nonteaching centre. In 1967 Paul Field performed the first open-heart operation in Sudbury. At first, all cases were presented at TGH and Alan Trimble went up to Sudbury to assist. Later, in December 1968,* Field performed the first coronary artery bypass in Ontario, perhaps Canada. Avdesh Mathur completed formal cardiovascular and thoracic training at the University of Alberta in Edmonton, having previously been a fellow at Henry Ford Hospital in Detroit and the Hospital for Sick Children in Toronto. He initially joined the cardiac surgical unit as an assistant and progressed to staff surgeon in April 1974. Dr. Edwin O. W. Night joined the staff in 1977 and recently retired in 2002.

The cardiac surgical unit continued to evolve and it was the overall commitment, diligence, excellence, and determination of the team that brought forth a new

---

*   The exact date of this Canadian "first" keeps changing from one report to another.—Editor.

aspect when a task force commissioned by the Ministry of Health recommended in 1982 that Dr. Mathur begin elective valve surgery. Dr. Mathur was also responsible for initiating the formation of the Mended Heart Inc. chapter #154 at the Sudbury Memorial Hospital, which contributed greatly to social aspects and community liaison for the cardiac surgical program. In addition, Dr. Mathur was constantly active in fundraising towards expansion of the unit, which required considerable lobbying of media, Ministry and Cardiac Care Network of Ontario, despite the usual local and governmental barriers.

In 1983 Sudbury Memorial Hospital was designated as the regional centre for cardiovascular investigation and cardiac surgery for the northeastern region of Ontario. Its surgical excellence has been recognized many times throughout the ensuing years and in 1994, the Cardiac Care Network listed Sudbury as "The Best Cardiac Centre" in the province. In 1985 Sudbury's first eight-coronary artery-bypass graft operation was performed. In 1986 with the increasing demand for cardiac surgery the addition of more manpower became evident and Dr.Sewaaul was recruited from Ottawa. He contributed an interest in pacemaker and other cardiac rhythm device surgery. Dr. Rowan was recruited for thoracic surgery, and in 1987 due to the increase in manpower, Mathur dedicated his practice to cardiac surgery only.

In 1991 the first beating heart off pump coronary bypass surgery in Canada was performed. With the continued development of advanced technology, Sudbury expanded the indications for off-pump surgery in 1996. Mathur introduced stentless aortic valve replacement surgery, valve sparing operations, the Ross procedure, and the Maze procedure, as well as coronary bypass surgery using total arterial conduits. Since 1992, the Sudbury unit has performed almost 300 stentless aortic valve replacements and 145 mitral valve repairs. These advanced procedures increased Memorial Hospital's reputation as a centre of excellence despite remaining a nonteaching institution. Recognition of Memorial Hospital's cardiac surgical unit was achieved through presentations and publications in Canada, the USA, and internationally, but unfortunately due to lack of resources, i.e., research support, assistants, residents, etc., these publications are acknowledged to be few and far between.

As the volume of cardiac surgery continues to expand the cardiac unit pursued increased recruitment and Dr. Avinash Garg joined the team in 1995. He had additional training in cardiac transplantation, although not performed in Sudbury. At the time of writing, the cardiac surgical service consists of three full-time active surgeons. The service remains under the cardiology/cardiac surgery department and each of these services has a service head elected yearly. Members of the multidisciplinary cardiac working group have business meetings once a month and cardiac work rounds are held once a week. NOMEC (Northeastern Ontario Medical Education Corporation) residents usually spend some elective time largely in cardiology. Being an isolated, nonteaching centre, located in Northern Ontario with poor access to the larger Ontario centres, the cardiac surgical unit at Sudbury Memorial Hospital has faced many challenges over the years and continues to do so, e.g., manpower recruitment difficulties affecting anaesthesia and surgical assistants, as well as limited support services. Transportation to larger centres has also been problematic due to local weather conditions. Nonetheless, the unit continues to provide superb service.

CARDIAC SURGERY IN OTTAWA

Pierre Bédard

In the spring of 1967, late one evening in the residents' on-call room on the ninth floor of the Private Patient Pavilion at the Toronto General Hospital, the chief resident in cardiovascular surgery, Wilbert Keon, explained to his junior resident, Pierre Bédard, that he planned to return to Ottawa to build a Heart Institute that would be the equivalent of the National Institutes of Health in the US. He had a vision of creating an Institute which would specialize not only in cardiac medicine and surgery, but also in cardiac rehabilitation, prevention, education and research.

Jean-Jacques Lussier, dean of the University of Ottawa Medical School, had previously met with Keon and convinced him to develop a cardiac institute there. Unfortunately Dean Lussier did not witness the full realization of his dream as he died of a myocardial infarction in 1975.

Forty years later the University of Ottawa Heart Institute (OHI) is flourishing and is well known not only in Canada but throughout the world.

EARLY DAYS

During the 1960s cardiac surgery was being performed at three sites in Ottawa: the Ottawa General Hospital, the Civic Hospital and the National Defense Medical Centre (NDMC), a Canadian Forces facility. There were three surgeons involved: Dr. André Crépeau, Dr. Harold J. Sachs, and Dr. J. David Hooper. Under the guidance of Dean Lussier, meetings were organized to amalgamate cardiac surgery and tertiary cardiology at one site. After numerous lengthy discussions and consideration of various plans, an agreement was reached to use the Civic Hospital facilities. Following his training in Toronto, Dr Keon spent some time in Boston and then returned to Ottawa in 1969 to form the cardiac unit at the Ottawa Civic Hospital. He surrounded himself with a team of dedicated nurses and was on call 24/7 for two years.

FROM A DREAM TO REALITY

Because of budgetary restraints, it was decided following numerous meetings with various organizations including the University of Ottawa, the Civic Hospital, the Ottawa Regional Hospital Planning Council and the Provincial Ministry of Health, to develop the Heart Institute in three phases.

The Ontario Hospital Services Commission approved the construction of **Phase 1** in 1970. With capital funding of $5,000,000 from the University of Ottawa, Phase 1 of the University of Ottawa Cardiac Unit was officially opened in May 1976. It incorporated all life support services on one floor: two heart catheterization laboratories, three operating rooms, a six bed recovery room, an eight bed surgical intensive care unit and eight coronary care suites. This unit was attached to the old East Lawn Pavilion where inpatients' and outpatients' services were provided.

Plans were then made for **Phase 2,** which were approved by the Provincial Ministry of Health in June 1979. Phase 2, consisting of 136 inpatient beds and outpatient clinics, was completed in 1983, and was known as the University of Ottawa Heart Institute (OHI).

For **Phase 3** plans were developed to build a research centre adjacent to the Institute on the grounds formerly occupied by the East Lawn Pavillon. Approval was obtained from the Ministry of Health in 1987 and construction was completed in 1989.

In order to achieve his dreams, Dr. Keon surrounded himself with other key players. In 1975 he attracted Dr. Donald Beanlands to become Chief of Cardiology. Under Dr. Beanlands' guidance, the Department of Cardiology has flourished and has been in the forefront of the new developments in cardiology. In 1982 Dr Keon recruited a Cardiac Rehabilitation specialist, Dr. William Dafoe, who developed a cardiac rehabilitation and prevention program.

THE DIVISION OF CARDIAC SURGERY AT THE OHI

In addition to his vision for a Heart Institute with all its ramifications, Dr. Keon wanted the best for his division—cardiac surgery. Over the years he attracted and educated young surgeons and scientists to fulfill the various needs of his division: clinical services, education and research.

CLINICAL SERVICES

Dr. Keon recognized that cardiac surgery cannot be done without a strong team. He hired Rosemary Cooms who organized a team of dedicated cardiac nurses in the recovery room and intensive care unit. He also recruited Mary Powers who did the same on the cardiac surgical ward. As well he obtained the services of Mary Clinkett, a physiotherapist. With the help of his devoted secretary, Dorothy Surcouf, Dr

Keon was able to handle his medical work as well as his administrative duties.

Dr. Wilbert Keon graduated in Medicine from the University of Ottawa and undertook his surgical training at McGill University and Toronto. After completing a fellowship in Boston he started his clinical practice in 1969 and gradually developed a very active operating schedule. Some of his many areas of interest were emergency surgery for acute myocardial infarction and shock, assisted circulation with either contra pulsation or artificial heart, various aspects of coronary artery bypass grafting for congestive heart failure, the use of endarterectomy, and studies of various valve prostheses. In the course of his career he became Chairman of the Department of Surgery at the University of Ottawa, was appointed to the Canadian Senate, and was nominated to the Order of Canada. Dr. Keon retired from surgery in 2001.

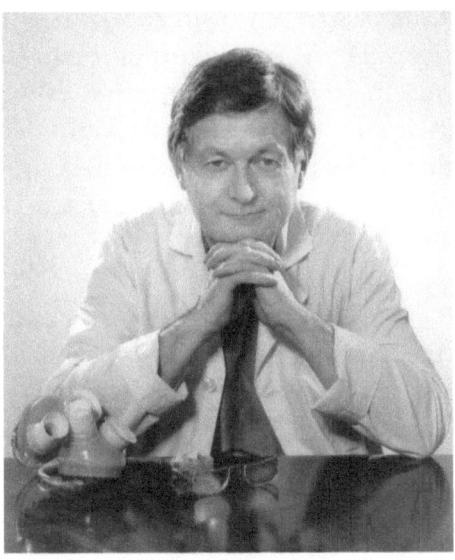

Fig. 3:8 Wilbert J. Keon © 1986 Yousuf Karsh

Dr. Pierre Bédard graduated from Laval School of Medicine in Quebec City. Following his surgical residency in Toronto, he received a McLaughlin Traveling Fellowship to pursue additional training at Toronto's Hospital for Sick Children and at the University of Alabama Medical Centre with John Kirklin. In 1971 he joined Dr Keon, who took a one-month break after having been on call continuously for two years. (Bédard could not believe that he was trusted to handle calls alone just one month after his arrival in Ottawa). Bédard developed an interest in intensive care and after attending Alain Carpentier's Club Mitral developed an interest in mitral valve reconstruction. He was a cofounder and member for over 20 years of the subcommittee on cardiovascular perfusion of the Canadian Medical Association's Conjoint Committee, which gives accreditation to allied health programs.

Dr. Yashar Akyurekli came to Ottawa in 1968 after completing his surgical training at McMaster University. He was Dr Keon's right hand surgeon, assisting him with all his operations. Dr. Akyurekli obtained his fellowship in general surgery in 1971 and became a dedicated cardiac surgeon with a special interest in arrhythmia surgery and pacemakers. He implanted the first defibrillator in Canada as well as using atomic pacemakers. Dr. Akyurekli retired in 1991.

Dr. Maurice Brais from Montreal graduated and completed his training in surgery at the University of Montréal. He spent a year as a fellow to Dr. Keon and in 1975 joined the staff of OHI. Because of his interest in congenital cardiac surgery he spent a number of months in Boston under Dr Castadina. In addition, he established a valve clinic which has been running for over 30 years and has resulted in the publication of numerous research papers by various OHI surgeons.

Dr. William Goldstein graduated from McGill University and pursued his surgical training in Ottawa and Toronto. Dr Goldstein then completed a clinical fellowship in cardiac surgery in Ottawa and joined the staff of OHI in 1978. Dr. Goldstein has a special interest in electrophysiological surgery including pacemakers.

Dr. Arvind Koshal completed his training in cardiac surgery at the OHI and then joined the Harvard Medical Centre in Boston as a Canadian Heart Foundation research fellow. Thereafter in 1980 he joined the OHI, becoming an accomplished cardiovascular surgeon. Among his various achievements he performed Canada's first implantation of a thoracic left ventricular assist device and was a member of the team that performed the first total artificial heart implant in Canada. In 1991, Dr. Koshal left the OHI to become the chief of Cardiac Surgery in Edmonton and director of the Development and External Affairs of the Mazankowski Alberta Heart Institute.

Dr. Roy Masters obtained his MD from Memorial University in Newfoundland in 1978. Following his surgical training in Ottawa and a year as a fellow at the OHI, he joined the staff in 1986. Dr. Masters has a special interest in circulatory support, devices and transplantation. He has also been closely associated with the valvular clinic and has published numerous articles.

Dr. Paul Hendry from Nova Scotia obtained his MD from the University of Ottawa and completed his Masters in Physiology. Following his surgical training in Ottawa, Dr. Hendry obtained a fellowship from the Medical Research Council of Canada, and pursued his training at Duke University in North Carolina. He joined the OHI in 1990. Dr. Hendry has a special interest in electrophysiological surgery and heart failure as well as assisted circulation devices (he has a vast experience with the use of Thoratec and Novacor assist devices) and transplantation.

Dr. Inderjit Gill did his surgical training in Ottawa and at the Cleveland Clinic. He joined the staff of the OHI in 1993 and left for Cleveland in 1998. Dr. Gill's interests were beating heart surgery and intensive care.

Dr. Fraser Rubens joined the OHI in 1995. A native of Kingston Ontario, he completed his medical training at Queen's University and then completed his surgical training in Ottawa. He undertook research training as a fellow from the Medical Research Council in the Department of Pathology at McMaster University for which he received a Master of Science degree. His main focus is on the process of thrombosis and cardiovascular devices, off-pump surgery, and pulmonary thrombo-endarterectomy. He has established an active program in the treatment of chronic pulmonary embolism from which more than 120 patients have benefited. Referrals come from all over Canada and his results have been recognized internationally.

Dr. Thierry Mesana, PhD, became the chairman of cardiac surgery at the University of Ottawa in 2001 following the retirement of Dr Keon. He received his MD degree at the University of Méditerranée, Marseille, France. Following his training, he became a full professor of cardiac surgery and chairman of thoracic and vascular surgery at the University of Marseille. He was a visiting professor at Harvard Medical School from 1996-1997. Dr. Mesana brought a vast experience in mitral and aortic valvular repair, aortic surgery, assistive devices and transplantation to the OHI. He has made significant changes in the Division of Cardiac Surgery and is directly involved in most of the Division's research projects.

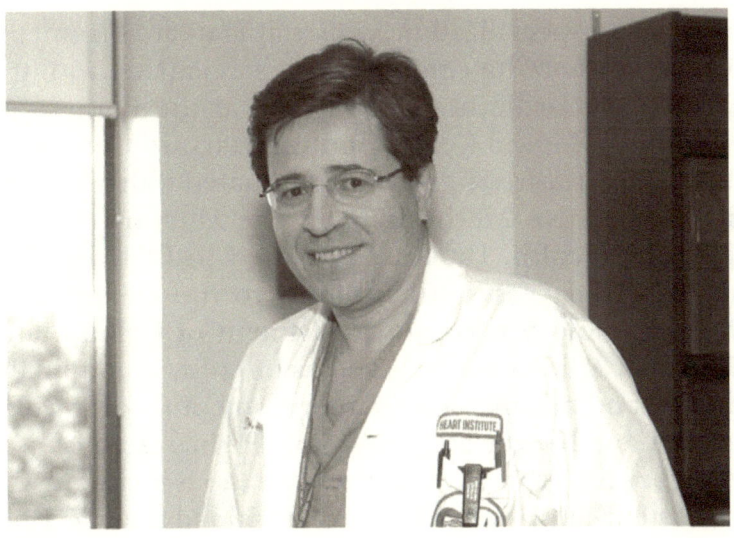

Fig. 3:9 Thierry Mesana

Dr. Gyaandeo Maharajh completed his MD degree at McGill University in 1990. He completed his training in surgery at the University of Manitoba in 1995 and received a MSc in surgery. He then undertook his cardiac surgery residency training at the OHI. Following fellowships in congenital cardiac surgery at the Hospital for Sick Children in Toronto and the University of Colorado, Denver Children's Hospital, he joined the staff of the Children's Hospital of Eastern Ontario and the OHI in 2002. He has research interests in allograft tissue degeneration and myocardial protection in a pediatric setting. He returns to Trinidad every four months to perform congenital cardiac surgery with a team of allied Canadian health professionals.

Dr. Marc Ruel, a native of Quebec City, received his medical degree at the University of Ottawa and completed his surgical training in Quebec City and Ottawa. Following his training, he received an award to pursue post-specialization studies at Harvard University in Boston where he completed his scholarship with the Division of Cardiothoracic Surgery at the Beth Israel Deaconess Medical Center and the Harvard Center for Minimally Invasive Surgery. He graduated with a Masters in Quantitative Methods from the Harvard School of Public Health. Dr. Ruel returned to OHI in 2002 and received cross-appointments to the Department of Epidemiology and the Department of Cellular and Molecular Medicine. Dr. Ruel has interests in minimally invasive and beating heart surgery, outcomes of valvular surgery, and heart transplantation. He has established a new laboratory to study innovative methods including the use of stem cells to improve coronary blood flow. Dr. Ruel has received numerous awards, most recently the Gold Medal in Surgery from the Royal College of Physicians and Surgeons of Canada.

Dr. B-Khangh Lam, originally from Montreal, received his MD from McGill University where he trained in surgery prior to completintg his cardiac surgery residency at the OHI. He then pursued his clinical research training at the Cleveland Clinic Foundation as a research fellow of the Heart and Stroke Foundation and the Canadian Institutes of Health Research where he obtained his Masters in Public Health Epidemiology with a special emphasis on advanced parametric outcomes analysis. He completed his surgical fellowships on complex pulmonary and valvular surgery, minimally invasive valve surgery, aortic surgery and atrial fibrillation surgery. Dr. Lam's research interests include novel anticoagulation strategies for patients with mechanical heart valves, valve outcomes analysis, minimal surgical approach to the treatment of atrial fibrillation and therapeutic options for the treatment of ischemic mitral regurgitation. He joined the OHI in 2003.

EDUCATION

Undergraduate Education: Third and fourth year medical students may spend one to three weeks with the Division of Cardiac Surgery as an elective or selective rotation. Under the direction of Drs. Paul Hendry, Pierre Bédard and, now, Khanh Lam, a program has been established to introduce medical students to cardiac surgical disease. Medical students spend time in the operating room learning basic surgical techniques. They are exposed to cardiac patients on the ward and in the clinics under the supervision of the resident staff and staff surgeons. Surgeons give the medical students one-on-one lectures on coronary artery disease, valvular heart disease, pacemakers, and aorta disease.

Postgraduate Education: Since 1974 the Division of Cardiac Surgery at the OHI has trained residents in cardiac surgery. Dr. Fraser Rubens is currently the director of the post-graduate training program. He was preceded by Drs. Arvind Koshal and Roy Masters. Canadian and foreign residents, mostly from the Middle East, have obtained, over the years, a high degree of success at the Royal College Fellowship exams. Residents prepare research projects under supervision, most of which are presented at international meetings and/or published in major journals. Graduates of the program are in practice in Quebec City, Montreal, Ottawa, Kingston, Sudbury, Hamilton, Mississauga, Winnipeg, Calgary, Edmonton, and Vancouver as well as in a number of centres in the United States and the Middle East.

RESEARCH

A research program was established under the guidance of Dr. Keon in the early 1970's. Both basic and clinical research projects have led to articles published in the medical literature. With the arrival of Dr Mesana, research has continued to further evolve.

Basic Research: Dr. Keon first hired **Gerry Taichman**, a post-graduate PhD student, to study the relation between coronary flow and cardiac function in acute cardiac failure, the effect of ultrasound on cardiac muscle, and various studies on the human atrial tissue. Unfortunately Dr Taichman died in 1987, ending a brilliant career. **Rosalind Labow,PhD**, director of the Taichman Laboratory, joined the staff to study the mechanism of cell—material interaction. Part of her research deals with the role of mechanical strain in monoyte-derived macrophage-mediated biodegradation of polyurethane medical devices.In the 1990's,**Tofy Mussivand, PhD**, came to the OHI from the Cleveland Clinic to study mechanical support devices and established a program to develop a totally implantable artificial heart.

Under Dr. Mesana, Dr. Marc Ruel was appointed director of cardiac surgery laboratory research at OHI. Dr Ruel established a new laboratory to study innovative methods to enhance cardiac blood flow and with **Erik Suuronen, PhD,** laid the ground work for tissue engineering research within the Department of Cardiac Surgery. Their research includes the investigation of stem and progenitor cells and their potential for promoting angiogenesis within the heart to restore blood flow to damaged tissue and improve function.

Clinical Research: Under the leadership of Dr Keon, various aspects of cardiac surgery have been studied. While coronary artery surgery was in its infancy, investigations by various members of the Division were done on coronary bypass grafts for acute myocardial infarction, cardiogenic shock, congestive heart failure and the use of coronary endarterectomy as an adjunct to coronary artery bypass grafting. In addition, results of clinical experience with the intra-aortic balloon pump assist were published.

In Dr Brais' Valve Clinic, Dr Andrew Pipe (now director of the cardiac rehabilitation and prevention centre) and then Dr Harry Lapierre have monitored valve surgery patients for the past 30 years. Outcomes for the various prosthesis used at the OHI have been published. More recently, under the guidance of Dr Ruel and Dr Lam, director of the valve clinic, a focus on an in-depth analysis have been formulated.

Shu-Tim Cheung PhD is the Chief Information Officer at the OHI. He has overseen the development of the Institute Hybrid broadband telehealth network for cardiac consultation and the randomized clinical trial on telehome care.

Dr Mesana recruited **Dr Rosendo Rodriguez, PhD** as a clinical scientist and manager of the clinical research unit of the Division of Cardiac Surgery at the OHI. His research interest is in the use of transcranial Doppler ultrasound for detecting peripheral emboli during cardiac procedures and following implantation of mechanical valves. In addition he has been investigating whether ultrasound technology is capable of differentiating between solid and air emboli.

In summary, Cardiac Surgery is flourishing in Ottawa thanks to the dedication of individuals whose efforts have achieved a high level of proficiency in patients' care, education and research. The Division of Cardiac Surgery at the OHI has attained a highly respected foundation on which to build for future achievements in the 21st century.

CHAPTER 4

THE HISTORY OF CARDIAC SURGERY IN NEWFOUNDLAND AND LABRADOR

Kevin Melvin

Cardiac surgery in this province is generally considered to have begun in 1969 with the opening of the Faculty of Medicine at the Memorial University of Newfoundland. Dr. James Beaton Littlefield, the first professor of surgery, performed cardiac procedures as did his wife, Dr. Phyllis Ray Ingram. In addition to setting up a training program in general surgery at the university, they introduced open-heart surgery at the General Hospital in St. John's. Since that time, cardiac surgical services have been continuously available in the province. The real history of the specialty in Newfoundland, however, is much longer and more colourful.

As early as 1950, Dr. Ian E. Rusted, a Newfoundland native who would later become the first dean of medicine at the Memorial University Medical School, became involved with Dr. John Kirklin and the evolving cardiac surgery program at the Mayo Clinic in Rochester, Minnesota. Having already had experience in the early development of a cardiac catheterization laboratory at the Royal Victoria Hospital in Montreal, Rusted pursued further training in cardiology at the Mayo Clinic. As a research fellow, he was engaged in studying the anatomy and function of the mitral valve at a time when surgical intervention was coming into vogue. Rusted co-authored a number of seminal articles on the subject, specifically addressing mitral stenosis and the anatomy of the fused commissures.[1, 2] These investigations coincided with Kirklin's return from a year spent at the Peter Bent Brigham Hospital with the Boston thoracic surgeon Dwight Harken. Rusted was present, at the surgeon's request, when Dr. Kirklin performed his first closed mitral valvotomy at the Mayo Clinic. Some photographs of diseased mitral valves identified as part of Rusted's research were subsequently published in Dr. Charles P. Bailey's *Surgery of the Heart* (1955),[3] an early textbook in the field.

Although Dr. Rusted was offered positions at both the Mayo Clinic and the Royal Victoria Hospital, he chose instead to assist in the development of modern medical facilities in his native province. When Rusted returned to St. John's in late 1952, he was the first formally trained internist in Newfoundland and cardiac services were in their infancy, with only two or three electrocardiographs in the entire province. In addition to establishing a busy private practice, Rusted became a medical consultant to the Newfoundland Department of Health and in 1953 director of continuing medical education at the General Hospital. Dr. Rusted's practice included a large proportion of patients suffering from both congenital and acquired heart disease, many of whom were referred for surgical intervention at mainland centres. (It was not until 1955 that the personnel and resources became available to perform closed cardiac procedures locally.) By this time a second Newfoundland-born physician, Dr. James Bagg Roberts, had completed his training as an internist in Boston and Toronto and introduced cardiology services at the General and Grace hospitals in St. John's.

Extracardiac and Closed-Heart Procedures, 1955-1969

Two general surgeons trained in cardiovascular surgery also returned to St. John's in 1955 and joined the staff of the General Hospital: Dr. John Douglas Baird had recently finished his postgraduate training in Toronto and Dr. Angus J. Neary at the Mayo Clinic. Baird's primary interest was in thoracic surgery, including closed cardiac and major vessel procedures. He performed a number of mitral splits, patent ductus ligations, and coarctation repairs during his career in Newfoundland, but did not practice open-heart surgery. Dr. Neary focused on general thoracic and pediatric surgery. His practice included patent ductus ligations, pericardectomies, aortopulmonary shunts and vascular ring releases. During his final period of training at the Mayo Clinic Neary had taken advantage of the opportunity to observe some of the first open cardiac procedures being performed by John Kirklin. Yet his surgical practice in Newfoundland was likewise confined to extracardiac and closed heart procedures.

Cardiopulmonary bypass was not introduced clinically in Newfoundland until the arrival of Drs. Littlefield and Ingram in 1969. Until that time, all patients requiring open-heart procedures had to be referred to a mainland centre. Yet Newfoundland had narrowly missed entering the open-heart era several years before this—in a most unlikely setting.

The St. Anthony Experience

St. Anthony is a community located at the very tip of the Great Northern Peninsula of the Island of Newfoundland; it is best known as the main administrative and medical centre associated with the International Grenfell Association. A modern medical facility has been maintained there since its foundation in 1901 by the British medical missionary Sir Wilfred Grenfell, who also established several smaller hospitals and nursing stations on the Labrador coast in the late 1890s. Beginning as the Grenfell Mission, this system eventually evolved into the International Grenfell Association. Headquartered in New York, the association coordinated an ambitious social program of which medical care was central. The hospital in St. Anthony provides tertiary care to a large portion of the northeast and northwest coasts of the Island and to the coast of Labrador.

Dr. Gordon Thomas arrived in St. Anthony in 1946, fresh from a year of training with Dr. Wilder Penfield at the Montreal Neurological Institute. Thomas would spend the next thirty-six years in the service of the International Grenfell Association (known after April 1981 as the Grenfell Regional Health Services.) Having developed an interest in the emerging field of cardiac surgery, Thomas spent some time in Stockholm in 1957-58, with Clarence Crafoord. His interest continued on his return to St. Anthony where, as surgeon in chief, he performed a number of closed procedures, beginning with a patent ductus and a coarctation repair in 1960. Taking special leave from his post in 1961-62, Thomas spent a year in Toronto with Dr. Wilfred Bigelow. At the same time, he encouraged a local anaesthetist to do extra training in cardiac anaesthesia in Montreal. Recognizing that open cardiac procedures were not being done in Newfoundland, Thomas set out to develop a program in St. Anthony upon his return to the province in 1962.

Thomas persuaded the IGA board to approve $10,000 to set up a dog lab and purchase special equipment, including a cardiopulmonary bypass machine. Experimental surgery was performed one morning a week and included refinement of the hypothermic techniques with which Thomas had become familiar with while working with Dr. Bigelow. These experimental procedures went well as did a number of closed mitral splits; the next step was obvious.

As Thomas would later explain in his autobiography,[4] he had become blind to the fact that his personal goals were dividing his staff. Many of the surgeon's colleagues felt that his priorities were wrong and that the hospital's resources were insufficient to support such an ambitious program. Thomas, on the other hand, felt that there was a patient need, and since the equipment and trained staff were available, the program should be pursued.

In 1965, during a visit by Dr. Ray Heimbecker, a well-known cardiac surgeon, and Dr. Ray Matthews, an anaesthetist from the cardiovascular unit of the University of Toronto, a young woman with an atrial septal defect was booked for surgery. The staff's displeasure was such that the night before the scheduled procedure the patient was injected with an anti-typhoid inoculation. The resulting fever resulted in its cancellation. Only after this incident did Dr. Thomas discover the depth of feeling amongst his staff. The proposed operation was never performed, and the program was abandoned. Given the choice of abandoning cardiac surgery or leaving St. Anthony, Thomas decided to stay and continued developing a regional hospital system. He performed a few more closed procedures, but the number of candidates for this type of surgery was small and eventually it proved more practical to refer patients to larger centres.

Establishing Provincial Cardiac Services, 1962-1969

Medical care in Newfoundland and Labrador improved significantly after it became a Canadian province in 1949. Yet both federal and provincial royal commissions on health services conducted in the early 1960s revealed that the region was still lagging behind the rest of the country, with the poorest physician-population ratio, the fewest specialists[5] and the lowest ratio of hospital beds[6] in Canada. By this time, the Newfoundland Department of Health had likewise begun to recognize the need for cardiac investigative and surgical services in the province, but perhaps because of limited resources and many competing demands, did not initiate a program in this area. Despite the lack of a coordinated official plan, however, a group of physicians trained in both pediatric and adult cardiology emerged independently to establish what would eventually become a comprehensive cardiac service for the entire province.

Dr. John F. Collins, a native of St. John's, returned to Newfoundland in 1956 after completing his medical and pediatric training in Scotland. As one of only five pediatricians in the city he soon built up a practice in neonatology and cardiology. A 1961 research fellowship from the Ontario Heart Foundation allowed Collins to spend a year at the Hospital for Sick Children in Toronto. Following his return to Newfoundland, Collins became involved in the establishment of the province's first pediatric hospital, becoming head of cardiology at the new Dr. Charles A. Janeway Child Health Centre in 1966, and chief of neonatology at the Grace Hospital in 1974. Collins also served as national chairman of the Canadian Medical Association's Child Health Committee (1965-

68) and president of the Canadian Pediatric Society for 1970-71. He subsequently went into politics, becoming the provincial minister of finance (1979-88) and then minister of health and deputy premier of Newfoundland (1988-89).

In 1962, Collins wrote a proposal to the Newfoundland Department of Health outlining the need for a local cardiac diagnostic unit and identifying the human resources already available. In addition, he developed a recruitment plan—complete with statistics on the incidence and prevalence of congenital heart disease in the province—to justify the establishment of such a facility. The same year, the health department contacted Dr. Arnold L. Johnson, director of the cardiovascular division for the joint cardio-respiratory service of the Royal Victoria and Montreal Children's hospitals, for further information and guidance in this area. Johnson's response focused on congenital heart disease in the pediatric age group and outlined criteria to be considered in the establishment of a properly equipped cardiac service, including a full time pediatric cardiologist and surgical personnel. In 1963, an attempt was made to recruit a cardiac surgeon: Dr. Gordon Thomas showed some interest in the position, but eventually decided to stay in St. Anthony. No further efforts toward recruitment were made at that time, and the majority of Dr. Johnson's recommendations were not implemented until the establishment of the Memorial medical school in 1969.

The province's cardiology resources had continued to expand, however, following the return of Dr. Gerald B. "Bud" Peckham to St. John's in 1965. As part of his postgraduate training, Peckham had spent three years as a cardiology resident and fellow at the Toronto General Hospital and a year with Dr. John Keith at Toronto's

Hospital for Sick Children. In addition, a portion of Peckham's Ontario Heart Foundation grant monies were earmarked to help establish a cardiac catheterization laboratory at the General Hospital so that upon his arrival the equipment was in place and the laboratory began to function in 1966. A considerable volume of valvular and other congenital heart problems were investigated, and those requiring surgery were referred to Drs. Wilfred Bigelow and Bernard Goldman in Toronto and to Dr. Ray Heimbecker in London, Ont.

The first implantable pacemaker was inserted in 1966 and coronary angiography was begun in 1969. But most candidates for coronary artery surgery continued to be referred out of province until the arrival of Drs. Cecil Couves and Garry Cornel in 1974.

Establishing Canada's Newest Medical School, 1961-1969[*]

The first step in the establishment of a medical school at Memorial came as early as 1961 when the university moved from the original 1925 Memorial College campus on Parade Street to its present location in a newer section of St. John's which offered plenty of room for expansion.

The same year, a federal Royal Commission on Health Services chaired by chief justice Emmett H. Hall began a

---

[*]   In September 2005, the Northern Ontario School of Medicine, a new initiative of Lakehead and Laurentian Universities, was opened with campuses in Thunder Bay and Sudbury, thus supplanting Memorial as "Canada's newest medical school."

full-scale investigation into Canada's present and future health care needs. At a November 1961 hearing held in St. John's, Newfoundland Medical Association chairman John Douglas Baird presented a submission calling for the creation of "a medical school in Newfoundland in connection with our Provincial University, or in affiliation with Dalhousie University" in addition to expanded hospital facilities including "a University Hospital . . . to meet the needs of the medical school."[7] A separate survey of medical manpower in Canada undertaken for the commission concluded that the nation's twelve existing medical schools "cannot satisfy our future needs for physicians" and that both expansion and new schools were urgently needed.[8] In its 1964 report, the Hall Commission recommended the construction of four new schools of medicine in Canada, including one in Newfoundland.[9]

By 1961, the provincial health department had also begun contemplating the possibility of a medical school in the province and, in 1963, began a series of meetings with representatives from Memorial and the Newfoundland Medical Association. In 1965, following the Hall Commission's recommendations, the Newfoundland government, and the university each launched investigations of their own into the state of health care in the province and the feasibility of establishing a medical school in St. John's.

The Memorial University's feasibility study, headed by Dr. James Arthur MacFarlane, former dean of medicine at the University of Toronto, concluded that plans for a medical faculty should be instituted as soon as possible in order to meet the province's need for more physicians. The 1966 MacFarlane commission report recommended the Health Sciences Centre model exemplified by the recent facilities established in Gainesville, Florida, and Lexington, Kentucky, which integrated medical education with teaching and research in the basic sciences as well as with clinical care. The new school should thus include a strong research program and a four-hundred-bed university teaching hospital located "on the Memorial University Campus in as close proximity as possible to the preclinical medical departments."[10] This new facility would replace the antiquated General Hospital as the province's main training and acute care centre.

In February 1965, meanwhile, the Newfoundland government had appointed Lord Walter Russell Brain, an eminent British medical educator, to undertake a Royal Commission on health care in the province. Lord Brain's findings agreed with those of the Hall and MacFarlane commissions: a new medical school was urgently needed. Like the MacFarlane commissioners, his report recommended the construction of a teaching hospital on or near the university campus, and the integration of teaching and clinical medicine with medical research. He considered it important that students and health care personnel should have an opportunity to witness or take part in clinical research, "and that research workers and teachers should meet over lunch or a cup of coffee."[11]

Following the MacFarlane commission's recommendation that the new medical school be organized as quickly as possible, Dr. Ian Rusted was appointed by Memorial in 1966 as coordinator of planning. The following year, the Faculty of Medicine was inaugurated with Rusted as the first dean and professor of medicine. As a pioneer of medical education in the province and a key player in the effort to establish a medical school at Memorial, he was well qualified for the challenges of developing an undergraduate training program, recruiting faculty members, and overseeing the planning of the Health Sciences Centre. Under his leadership, the first class of undergraduate medical students was admitted in September 1969, a year ahead of schedule. Dr. Rusted retired from the university in 1989 and was appointed dean emeritus, after going on to become vice president of Health Sciences (1974-88) and pro vice chancellor (1981-88).

Research efforts in cardiology developed at Memorial under the leadership of Dr. Albert R. "Al" Cox, who supervised a number of graduate students in this area. A cardiologist and former associate professor of medicine at the University of British Columbia, Cox was recruited in 1969 as the university's first professor and chair in medicine, with appointments at the four hospitals in St. John's. Dr. Cox served as Memorial's second dean of medicine between 1974 and 1987 and oversaw the faculty's move from its original temporary quarters to the present Health Sciences Centre. Officially opened to patients in 1978, the new facility took the university hospital concept a step further by integrating teaching, research and clinical care within a single structure.

In 1968, Dr. James Littlefield was selected by an international advisory committee as professor of surgery on the basis of his achievements at the University of Virginia. Accompanied by his wife, Dr. Phyllis Ingram, a fellow graduate of the University of Maryland medical school who became Memorial's first assistant professor of surgery, Littlefield succeeded in setting up a training program in surgery at Memorial and introducing adult and pediatric cardiac surgery at the General and Janeway hospitals. During the latter few years of his tenure in St. John's, however, Dr. Littlefield was plagued by poor health; the surgical training program grew slowly, and the cardiac service was dormant for the last year of so of his career at Memorial. By the mid-1970s, Drs. Littlefield and Ingram had returned to the United States.

The Evolution of Cardiac Services, 1974-82

In 1974, Dr. Cecil M. Couves was appointed to the chair of surgery at Memorial and a new era was ushered in, both for the university and the future of cardiac surgery in the province. A native of Saskatchewan, Couves graduated in medicine from the University of Manitoba in 1945 and went on to postgraduate training in surgery at the University of Edinburgh and the Sheffield Royal Infirmary. As a result of a chance meeting with Dr. Michael DeBakey, he proceeded to Houston where he spent two years as a fellow in cardiovascular and thoracic surgery (1954-1956) at Baylor University. He subsequently moved to Edmonton and went on to become professor of surgery at the University of Alberta. Attracted to St. John's as professor of surgery in 1974, Couves instilled an irresistible energy in the local surgical scene. With him, he brought Dr. Garry Cornel, another cardiovascular surgeon who had trained with him in Edmonton and whose area of interest was pediatric cardiac surgery.

A team, including personnel that had accompanied the two surgeons from Edmonton—complete with interventional cardiologists—was soon established in St. John's, and programs in both adult and pediatric cardiac surgery were reenergized. Visiting professors, including Dr. Wilbert Keon from Ottawa and Dr. David Mulder from Montreal, were soon to be seen in the operating rooms and lecture halls. Regular teaching rounds were established and the profile of cardiac surgery in Newfoundland was suddenly prominent. The need for expensive and inconvenient visits to mainland facilities for complex cardiac surgical procedures was a thing of the past for the residents of the province.

A man of many parts, Cec Couves contributed significantly to the cultural life of the community as a musician and originator of a choral group, as well as to its professional life as an educator. Nowhere was this more apparent than in his near obsession with continuing medical education. Teaching rounds for house staff, specialists, and general practitioners seemed never-ending and embraced all areas of medicine. A strong department of surgery became a priority at Memorial and many young surgeons were encouraged to pursue subspecialty training in areas as diverse as head and neck surgery, ophthalmology and thoracic surgery. The continued presence of many of these individuals on staff to this day is part of this man's legacy.

The new chairman quickly closed what seemed initially to be a major gulf between the local academic and private-practice communities. Dr. Couves brought the two groups together socially and professionally, and in the end, they became indistinguishable.

Basic research was encouraged and an animal laboratory was established with a full-time scientific investigator. Dr. Yves M. LeGal (who had joined the department of surgery as a graduate research assistant in 1971, completed his PhD at Memorial and was appointed assistant professor of experimental surgery in 1979) investigated the role of a left ventricular assist device (LVAD) in the treatment of experimental myocardial infarction. Out of this program grew an initiative involving a number of surgical trainees and research assistants and led to the participation of all residents in basic research throughout the duration of their surgical training.

Stricken with heart disease in 1978, Couves's last years at Memorial were dedicated solely to educational efforts. He died in 1991, officially retired but still very much active as director of continuing medical education at Kelowna General Hospital in British Columbia. By the time he retired, Dr. Couves had recruited two young cardiac surgeons to join Garry Cornel in the practice of the specialty at Memorial. Dr. Terrill E. Theman joined the team in 1978 and Dr. Victor Aldrete in 1981. Along with an expanded team of cardiologists, perfusionists, and nurses they enlarged and further developed the program to fulfill Cec's dream of providing the people of Newfoundland with a full range of cardiac services.

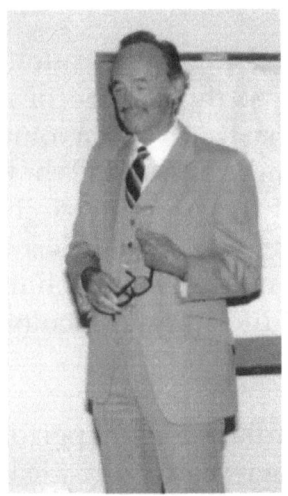

Fig. 4:1 Dr. Cecil Couves

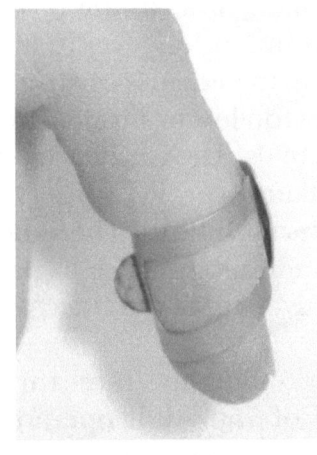

Fig. 4:2 Finger instrumentation for mitral valvotomy (Dr. Gordon Thomas)

1982 to the Present

Despite an ever-increasing demand for adult cardiac surgery, the number of procedures performed in

Newfoundland remained below two hundred per year until 1982, when efforts were made to increase the volume to a level more in keeping with the needs of the province's population. During this period there was a significant change in the surgical staff. Drs. Theman and Aldrete left, to the United States and Calgary respectively. Dr. Kevin Melvin, a native Newfoundlander, completed his cardiac surgery training in Toronto and returned home to take up practice in 1982. Dr. Amin Addetia, a graduate of the program in Edmonton, was recruited in 1984, and in response to continuing increase in volume, a third surgeon, Dr. Kam Mong, another Edmonton graduate, was recruited in 1998.

Meanwhile, a declining birth rate and out-migration of Newfoundlanders eventually led to the demise of the program in pediatric cardiac surgery. Faced with a volume of cases too low to support his team's clinical skills by the early 1990s, Dr. Cornel accepted the position of chief of pediatric cardiac surgery at the Children's Hospital of Eastern Ontario. There he developed a large clinical and academic practice as part of the surgical faculty of the University of Ottawa.

At the present time, these three cardiac surgeons perform a total of 750 adult operations per year at the Health Sciences Centre in St. John's. With the exception of heart transplantation, a full range of adult cardiac surgical services, is currently available in the province. With the departure of Garry Cornel, the pediatric component of the program was closed and pediatric cases are performed at one of the mainland centres.

With the transfer of all health services from the General Hospital to the new Health Sciences Centre complex in 1978, accommodation for the expansion of the cardiac surgery service was given priority and adequate dedicated operating space and ICU beds were allocated. Despite these provisions, competition between the cardiac unit and other services for hospital resources remained a significant problem. It was not until the consolidation of services under a new health care board in 1999 that geographically identifiable resources in the form of a new cardiac intensive care unit and a second operating room dedicated to the cardiac service were made available.

The development of a new cardiac catheterization laboratory and the subsequent addition of a second catheterization room has led to a marked increase in the volume of patients being investigated and to greater demands for cardiac surgery. While the present volume would appear to be adequate for a population of a little over a half a million, there is a long waiting list for elective surgery. The problem is multifaceted: The province has an inherently high incidence of coronary artery and cardiac valvular disease due to its aging population. In addition, the ever-increasing waiting list was not adequately addressed in past years and sufficient resources to deal with this backlog were not available. Only within the past three years has the volume of cases come close to reflecting the requirements of the population, and as recently as 2001 elective cases were sent to mainland centres because of strained local services. Additional resources have since been allocated to allow for a level of service that will eliminate excessively long waiting lists for elective operations and for an ongoing service that will keep wait times in line with those in mainland Canadian centres.

Current Developments and Future Trends

Given the province's aging population, the demand for cardiac surgery services in Newfoundland is not likely to decrease and may in the short term continue to grow. Since the problem of resource allocation has finally been addressed by the provincial government, physical facilities, nursing staff, and perfusion services are currently adequate. Yet medical personnel, particularly anaesthetists, are in short supply, and because there is no local training program in cardiac surgery and the service no longer shares general surgery residents, surgical staffing remains a problem. To address this challenge, a program for Registered Nurse First Assistants has been developed, and at present, four of these individuals provide intraoperative support for all procedures. This approach has eliminated dependence on part-time physicians as surgical assistants and has added greatly to the stability of the service.

In addition, a group of tertiary care nurse-practitioners provide perioperative support. These nurses, currently four in number, have advanced critical care training and are educated to the level of Master of Nursing. This group provides a continuity of pre-and postoperative care as well as a program of staff and patient education. This has eliminated the need for house staff and the acquisition of a number of these individuals is recommended to any centre performing cardiac surgery.

Notes:

1. I. E. Rusted et al., "Guides to the commissures in operations upon the mitral valve," *Proc Staff Meeting Mayo Clinic* (1951), 26: 297-305.

2. I. E. Rusted et al., "Studies of the mitral valve: I, Anatomic features of the normal mitral valve and associated structures," *Circulation* (1952), 6: 825-31.

3. C. P. Bailey, *Surgery of the Heart* (Philadelphia: Lea & Febidger, 1955), 497, fig. 368.

4. G. W. Thomas, *From Sled to Satellite: My Years with the Grenfell Mission* (Toronto: Irwin Publishing, 1987), esp. ch.12.

5. S. Judek, Canada, Royal Commission on Health Services, *Medical Manpower in Canada,* (Ottawa: Queen's Printer, 1964), 27-28 and tab. 103; "Provincial physician-population ratios" (1911-61), 158-59 and tab. 4-35; "Ratios of general practitioners and certified specialists to population, for provinces and Canada" (1961).

6. "Proceedings of the hearing at St. John's, Thursday, November 2, 1961," Canada, Royal Commission on Health Services, *Transcripts,* vol.6. (Toronto: Canadian Pharmaceutical Association, 1961); Submission of the Department of Health of Newfoundland, 1417 and 1545-46.

7. "Proceedings of the hearing at St. John's" (1961), Submission of the Newfoundland Medical Association, quotes at 1544 and 1546.

8. J. A. MacFarlane, chair., "Report of a survey of the feasibility of establishing a medical school in Memorial University of Newfoundland at St. John's, Newfoundland," St. John's: Memorial University of Newfoundland (Feb. 1966), quote at VIII-2.

9.   Memorial University of Newfoundland, Faculty of Medicine, *Calendar* (1970-71), 20-1; (1979-80), 17-18.

10. *MacFarlane Report* (1966), quote at VIII-2.

11. Newfoundland and Labrador, *Royal Commission on Health*, Lord Brain, commissioner, St. John's: Government of Newfoundland and Labrador (1966), 3 vols., quote at vol.1, 124.

CHAPTER 5

THE DEVELOPMENT OF CARDIAC SURGERY IN THE MARITIMES

David Murphy

As in other parts of Canada, no surgeon in the 1950s or early '60s could envisage a surgical practice devoted entirely to cardiac surgery. During this period most surgeons in the Maritimes did a variety of operations which would now be done by specialists. It was not uncommon for general surgeons to have an office from which they did a general family practice.

While surgery on the major blood vessels in the thoracic cavity were practiced in some American and Canadian centres in the late forties and early fifties this did not occur in the Maritimes until 1947 when John W. Merritt (1901-1965) (Fig. 5:1)

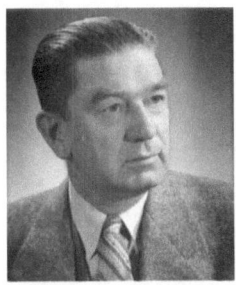

Fig. 5:1 Dr. John W. Merritt

is said to have done the first closure of a patent ductus arteriosus at the Victoria General Hospital. Dr. Douglas Roy recounts that as an intern in 1947, he was attending an autopsy when Dr. Merritt came in to look at the anatomy around the duct area. It was shortly after this that Dr. Merritt ligated the first ductus arteriosus. Dr. Merritt has been described as a renaissance physician. He was a gold medalist in medicine at Dalhousie University (1928), training entirely in Halifax with occasional visits to other North American hospitals. He had a interest in chest surgery and was one of several who worked at the TB hospital in Halifax as well as doing general surgery in the broadest sense at the Children's Hospital and the Victoria General Hospital. He was the first to attempt repair of a tracheo-esopohageal fistula in an infant. In addition to his surgical activities, he also maintained a family practice from his home in central Halifax.

He was a patron of the arts, being a founding father of the Neptune Theatre, a patron of the National Ballet, the Grands Ballets Canadiens de Montréal, a governor of the Maritime Conservatory of Music and a member of the Board of Governors of St. Mary's University.

Another surgeon, Victor Mader (1901-1959), a graduate of McGill University, is said to have done a mitral commissurotomy in the mid-fifties but this apocryphal story cannot be substantiated.

The first surgeon to devote his practice solely to cardiovascular conditions was Dr. F. Gerald Dolan. (Figure 5:2)

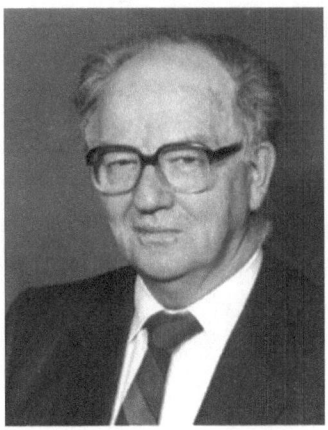

Fig. 5:2 Dr. F. G. Dolan

A quiet unassuming person with the fast technical skills that were important in the early days of cardiac surgery, Dr. Dolan was also known for his skills as a fly fisherman and one who would never divulge his best fishing holes. He graduated from Dalhousie Medical School and after his general surgical training went to Toronto. As recounted by Dr. Don Wilson, "We were doing some kind of vascular case on a Sunday afternoon when Gerry Dolan was visiting and asked me if he could watch. He didn't say anything until the case was over and then he said, 'That was interesting, is there any way I could get a job doing this kind of surgery?' 'Are you any good?' asked Dr. Wilson. 'Not bad,' said Gerry." With that conversation came an unexpected fellowship vacancy in Toronto, and with a McLaughlin Fellowship from Dalhousie, he spent two years with Dr. Wilson.

Incidentally, when Dr. Wilson started doing probably the first Canadian abdominal aneurysm repairs, there were no synthetic tubes available in Canada. Dr. Wilson said that he asked Dr. Dolan to go to Eaton's and buy a nylon shirt. From this, he and Dr. Dolan constructed a synthetic tube for the repair.

Dr. Dolan returned to Halifax in 1958. He began a practice of cardiac and vascular surgery within the general surgery department, being one of the first "general surgeons" to devote his practice to one anatomic area.

The next five years saw the expansion of cardiac surgery both at the Victoria General Hospital where mostly mitral commissurotomies were performed, and at the Children's Hospital where cases such as atrial septal defects, and pulmonary stenosis were done using surface hypothermia with inflow occlusion. At both hospitals the postoperative care was done in their recovery room areas, there being no special intensive care units. By 1962, Dr. Dolan reported his results of 105 cases of congenital heart surgery (*NS Med Bull* 41 (1962): 161).

It is important to note that the development of cardiac surgery in the Maritimes was dependent on events within the Department of Medicine. During the early fifties there were only a few internists who had a special interest in heart disease, men such as Lea Steeves and Sam Shane who began the first heart catheterization unit in 1958 using a combination of right-heart catheterization and fluoroscopy for diagnosis.

One of the first internists to do mainly cardiology was Douglas Roy.

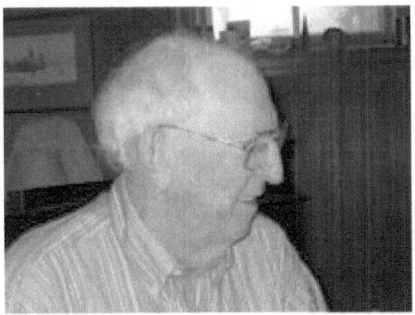

Fig. 5:3 Dr. Douglas Roy

He has a particular gift with cardiac auscultation in the diagnosis of heart problems and has recently produced a commercially available instructional CD on pediatric murmurs. He was instrumental in the development of cardiology at the Children's Hospital. In addition to his skills as a pediatric cardiologist he is an accomplished musician and an expert international sailor. As background, he graduated from Dalhousie Medical School but did his internal medicine training at the Royal Victoria Hospital, Montreal. This was at a time (1951) when the first cardiac catheterizations were being done by Dr. Arnold Johnson. The use of fluoroscopy was well established then but the introduction of serial X-rays while dye was injected into the heart was new. As Dr. Roy describes it, "We used to inject the dye and literally fire in the X-ray cassettes with a hockey stick." He returned to Halifax in 1952. He gradually switched from adult medicine to a full time pediatric cardiology practice. Diagnosis was done using fluoroscopy, then later catheterization at the adult hospital. The children were then transferred back to their hospital, often in a precarious hemodynamic condition.

The open-heart program began in 1962. The first heart-lung machine was purchased from Boston (Fig. 5:4)

B2

THAT WAS THE WEEK

Nov. 8-14, 1962:

Open-heart surgery step closer

By Lorna Inness

Open-heart surgery moved closer to use in Halifax hospitals with the ordering of a heart-lung machine from Boston. G.R. Matheson, president of the Nova Scotia Division of the Canadian Red Cross Society, said the machine was to be used to train surgical teams from the Victoria General and the Children's Hospital. He noted that during 1961, 894 heart operations had been performed in hospitals in 10 cities in Canada. Matheson added that the use of such operating techniques in Halifax would launch "a new and dramatic chapter" in Red Cross blood services.

Fig. 5:4 From the *Halifax Daily News*

and the first perfusionist was Mr. Alan Smith, from England.

Two important individuals returned to Halifax around this time. The first was Alex Gillis. (Figure 5:5)

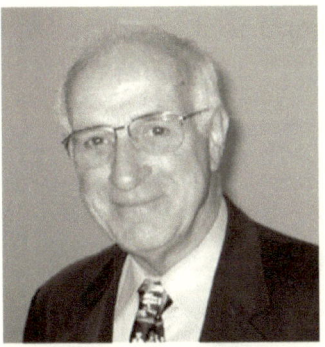

Fig 5:5 Dr. Alex Gillis

A graduate of Dalhousie University, he did all his surgical training at the Mayo Clinic starting on March 1, 1955, and by coincidence the very day that Dr. John Kirklin did the first open-heart at the Mayo Clinic. Dr. Gillis rotated through the cardiac service, it being like other centres, part of the department of general surgery. He became personal friends with Dr. Dwight McGoon who was a junior staff person there at the time. As he was finishing his time at the Mayo, he was looking at the few places available to train as a pediatric surgeon. Having received a nice letter of encouragement but no appointment from Dr. Willis Potts, he was a bit disheartened. While helping Dr. McGoon awhile later, there was a tall, quiet surgeon looking in from the gallery. When the case was finished, the visitor asked if a Dr. Gillis was around. It turned out that the guest was Willis Potts and there was an unexpected vacancy in the program: would Dr. Gillis like the job? Using a McLaughlin Fellowship to complete the two-year program, he returned to Halifax to become the first pediatric surgeon in the East. This also was not without some anxiety as there was some opposition to a young surgeon coming on staff to "steal away" the children's surgery from the general surgeons in the community.

The second surgeon to arrive was Dr. C. Edwin Kinley (Fig. 5:6),

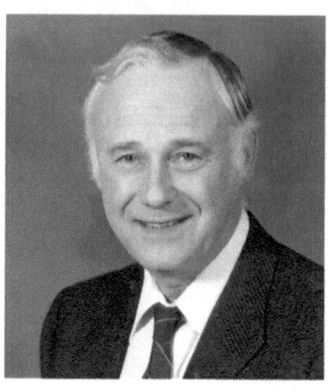

Fig. 5:6 Dr. Edwin Kinley

a Dalhousie graduate who pursued training in thoracic surgery with a particular interest in cardiac and vascular surgery. He had spent time in Birmingham, England, and at the Cleveland Clinic pursuing these interests. Both Drs. Gillis and Kinley then had personal experience with the heart-lung machine, which Dr. Dolan did not. Dr. Kinley was responsible for persuading the first perfusionist, Alan Smith from the Birmingham Children's Hospital, to move to Halifax to be part of the open-heart program. The three surgeons were involved with weekly trials on animals for about three months. The first operation using bypass was done at the Children's Hospital by Dr. Dolan and Dr. Gillis in 1963. It was a direct suture closure of a ventricular septal defect. For the next nine years cases were done intermittently at both hospitals. Dr. Gillis was initially limited to closed cases and did over fifty pulmonary bandings without mortality. As the other two surgeons became busier at the adult hospital doing vascular and thoracic cases, Dr. Gillis then did all the pediatric cases. During this period Dr. Robert Anderson (Fig. 5:7)

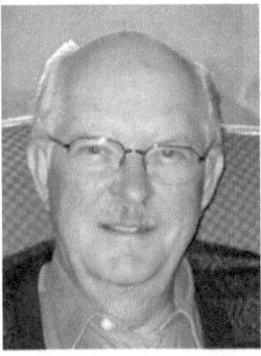

Fig. 5:7 Dr. Bob Anderson

recounts that surgical mortality at most heart centres was high and that only the sickest patients were referred to the surgeons. Probably because of this, the number of cases done in Halifax was small.

During this nine year period from 1963 to 1972 considerable progress was being made in cardiology, and this directly influenced the development of cardiac surgery in the Maritimes. Dr. Roy became full time at the Children's Hospital and Dr. Robert Anderson became the first full time cardiologist within the Department of Medicine in 1962. Dr. Anderson, who has now retired as head of the department, felt that the most exciting decade for him was the 1960s. He mused that it saw the first heart transplants, the first moon landing, and a time when long-haired students occupied the president's office at Columbia University. This decade also saw changes in Maritime cardiology.

Dr. Anderson was from a Prince Edward Island farming family. He graduated from Dalhousie Medical School 1954 and did general practice in North Sydney, Nova Scotia, for three years. He then spent two years doing internal medicine, a year with the cardiologist Paul Wood at the National Heart Hospital in London followed by a further year with Dr. Ramsay Gunton, a cardiologist at the Toronto General Hospital. Upon his return to Halifax, Dr. Anderson did some of the early left-sided cardiac studies using the Bjork technique of direct left atrial puncture and the direct apical ventricular puncture to measure left ventricular pressures.

Transeptal left heart catheterization was a shared learning experience for both Anderson and his Fellow, Dr. Brian Chandler. (Fig. 5:8)

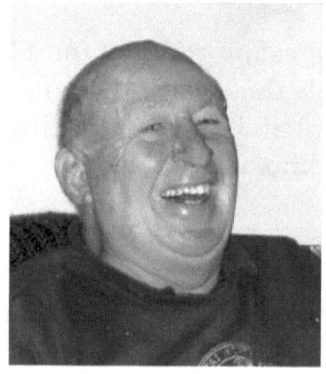

Fig. 5:8 Dr. Brian "Spud" Chandler

Dr. Brian "Spud" Chandler, from Prince Edward Island, graduated from Dalhousie Medical School in 1961 and went on to train in internal medicine at the University of Toronto. His interest was cardiac muscle biochemistry, studying in the United States, first in Pittsburgh with biochemist Robert Olsen and then at the NIH under Edmund Sonnenblick. His return to Halifax in 1967 added a second full time cardiologist. In his many leadership positions with the cardiology division he established the first coronary care unit in the Maritimes, modernized the cardiac catheterization facilities, and introduced coronary angiography and coronary angioplasty to the

Maritimes. He developed a cardiology residency program that produced six chiefs of cardiology in Canada. In addition to running the Division of Cardiology, he also had a string of standard-bred horses, which raced on the tracks around the Maritimes and in the USA.

There was a reluctance by surgeons in the Maritimes, as in other part of the country, to allow another specialty to evolve from the parent specialty of general surgery. It was a time when apart from urology and neurosurgery, all other surgical disciplines were under the general surgery umbrella in Halifax. Budgets, beds, resident assignments, and operating room deployment were strictly controlled. Allowing a cardiovascular specialty to develop within this milieu was a major challenge. Three individuals were influential in seeing this happen. Dr. Chandler was one of these: having developed the cath lab and the coronary care unit, he insisted on bringing cardiac surgery forward as part of overall cardiovascular care in the Maritimes.

Dr. Emerson Moffitt (Fig. 5:9) was the next important individual to be involved in cardiac surgical care.

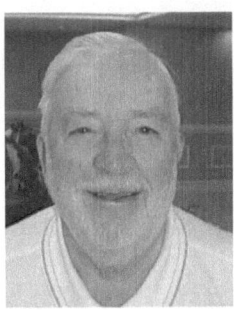

Fig. 5:9 Dr. Emerson Moffitt

Dr. Moffitt is a 1951 medical graduate of Dalhousie. He grew up in McAdam, New Brunswick, his father being a stationmaster for the CPR. He graduated from the University of New Brunswick and received his medical degree from Dalhousie University. As with many graduates at that time he spent four years in general practice in North Sydney, Nova Scotia. This included giving general anaesthesia using open drop chloroform and ether for the surgeons in that community. It was this experience that directed him to this specialty. He began his training in anaesthesia at the Mayo Clinic in 1954, eventually becoming head of the department at the 1,200-bed St. Mary's Hospital. During this period he started work with Dr. Jeremy Swan where they studied the physiological responses to open-heart surgery, which was just in its infancy. Dr. Moffitt persuaded Drs. John Kirklin and Dwight McGoon to leave a small catheter in the coronary sinus during surgery so they could study for the first time human cardiac metabolism during and after surgery. From 1957 to 1972, he published seventy-five papers on cardiac anaesthesia. Obviously he was a "catch" for Dalhousie when he decided to return there, becoming head of the anaesthesia department for five hospitals in Halifax and Saint John, NB.

In addition to influencing the practice of anaesthesia throughout the Maritimes, Dr. Moffitt's particular impact on cardiac surgery was enormous. He continued to do research on cardiac metabolism. Following a sabbatical with Dr. Swan of San Diego in 1979, he introduced the technique of preoperative coronary sinus catheterization with the Swan Ganz catheter. This resulted in another 128 publications. He inquisitiveness was contagious, as others joined in with him on these studies. Intraoperative clinical research in the operating room became comfortable on both sides of the "ether" screen. "Moff" had the ability to make puns on any statement. In defense, surgeons would do anything to cooperate with him. To the patient's advantage he taught the surgeons the philosophy that cardiac surgery was a joint responsibility and that the running of the "pump," for example, could be best done by sharing this activity with anaesthesia and the perfusionist. This then set the operative tone for cardiac surgical care in Halifax.

Cardiac surgery in other parts of Canada was by now sufficiently advanced that the Halifax medical community felt that it was time to have a surgeon devoted entirely to cardiac procedures. Dr. Alex Gillis recruited Dr. David Murphy to move from McGill and the Montreal Children's Hospital to do the cardiac surgery at the IWK Hospital in Halifax. Dr. Murphy (Fig. 5:10) received his Doctor of Veterinary Medicine from University of Toronto in 1956 and his medical degree from McGill in 1960.

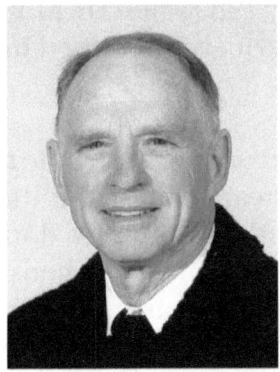

Fig. 5:10 Dr. David Murphy

He trained first in general surgery at McGill, then in pediatric surgery at the Boston Children's Hospital. Pediatric cardiac surgery training was in Boston and at Great Ormond Street, London, England. Shortly after Dr. Murphy moved to Halifax Drs. Moffitt and Chandler felt that the Victoria General Hospital should also have a surgeon who did just cardiac surgery. These two physicians threatened the then chief of surgery that they would refer their patients to Toronto unless he agreed to this. Because of his limited exposure to adult cardiac surgery, Dr. Murphy was persuaded by the two doctors to undertake a sabbatical upgrade in this specialty. After spending six months in Chicago at Rush Presbyterian Hospital he returned to Halifax in 1974.

There was reluctance by the Department of Surgery to make room for the new specialty. Patients were scattered throughout the surgical wards and it was foreign to have requests for the cardiac surgical patients to be admitted on a specific date with a specific day for surgery. There was also some reluctance to welcome a pediatric surgeon into the adult general surgical mix. Gradually, the patient open-heart load increased, from sixty cases in 1973, to over six hundred by 1989 when Dr. Murphy stepped down as chief. A number of events helped in the development of the service.

Dr. Kinley was able to secure a separate three-bed intensive care unit for the heart patients. Initially, postoperative care at the Children's Hospital was done by the surgeons. It was necessary to have an anaesthetist on the team with an interest in intensive care, but the anaesthetists on staff were reluctant to get seriously involved. To fill this gap, Dr. Chris Soder, trained both as a pediatrician and an anaesthetist, was hired. The cardiac surgeons were initially wary about this individual coming into the ICU to take over their jobs, but it was readily apparent that his skills were appreciated, particularly after the late night calls from the ICU stopped. He soon had the full cooperation of the entire surgical staff. Subsequently, Drs. Brian Macmanus and Sheri Litz, two other individuals with similar training, joined the unit.

In surgery, meanwhile, when Dr. Murphy left the IWK Hospital for Children in 1993, his position was filled by Dr. David Ross, a former resident who had spent two additional years doing pediatric cardiac surgery in Toronto and London, England. He subsequently became head of the cardiac surgical residency program and was instrumental in getting the program reestablished. He moved to Edmonton in 2001.

Surgical interns and residents were steered away from the Victoria General Hospital cardiovascular service. To solve this problem, in 1978, a new program of training former ICU nurses to assume intern duties, was developed, the first in Canada. While this move was never truly accepted by the nursing department, they continue to serve as role models and resource people for the other nurses on the cardiac floors. Job satisfaction has been high with only one new nurse in the past twenty-five years.

In 1975, the Maritime Heart Center was founded with the collaboration of cardiology, radiology, and anaesthesia. Its thrust was to enhance cardiac care facilities. The Canadian Heart Foundation supported research, the university supported education, but prior to this there was no single site to address the needs of cardiac patients. The first year's annual budget was sixty-five dollars but now it is a solid five-digit figure.

In 1989 homograft tissue for valve replacement was expensive, scarce, and was located in the United States. It was a complex system where the homografts were harvested locally, shipped to a company, CryoLife, in Georgia, USA, and kept there until they were needed. The pool of valves was shared by all participating United States and Canadian centres. Thus, they often did not have the right sizes available and it was difficult to get them delivered in an emergency. They would be shipped back to the surgeon at a cost of US$4,500 with a deduction of $500 off the cost for having donated the tissue in the first place. Meanwhile, the skin bank at the Victoria General Hospital was in its infancy. Lewis Page, who ran the bank alone, suggested that he could store our homograft tissues at much less cost, provided that the Maritime Heart Center would send him to the Virginia Beach Tissue Bank in the United States to learn their storage technique. From these beginnings in 1989, the first Canadian cardiac tissue bank was started. It now has a compliment of fifteen personnel, and has become the largest unit and supplier of preserved tissue in Canada.

The cardiac transplantation program was started by Dr. John Sullivan when he performed the first in the Maritimes in 1980. A perfusion technology program (Fig. 5:11) was started in 1963 and by 2003 there were eight full time perfusionists on staff.

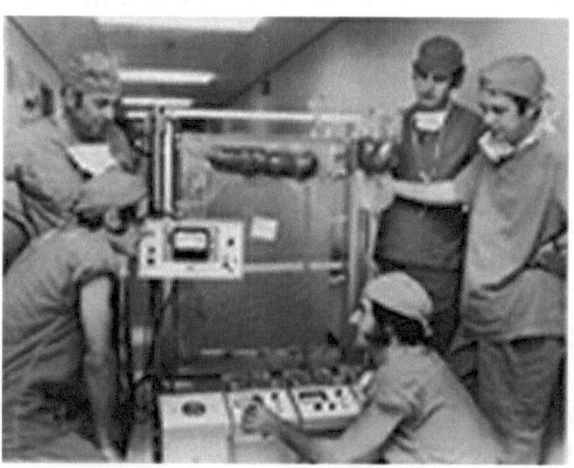

Fig. 5:11 The perfusion team 1973. Clockwise from bottom left: Ralph Ricketts, Rick Leadon, chief, Jim Macdonald, Gerard Myers and Clary Power.

Disc oxygenators gave way to Travenol bubble oxygenators in 1973 and then switched to Bentley type thereafter. Membrane oxygenators were introduced at the Children's Hospital in 1974 and their use was expanded to ECMO patients. The technology was crude. In order to get adequate forward flow through the membranes of the Landé-Edwards cube-shaped units, the bed had to be elevated by ten-inch blocks of wood under the four legs and the oxygenators placed on the floor. Figure 5:12 shows a patient on ECMO in 1974 and cleaners tidying up the walls after a mishap. (Figure 5:13)

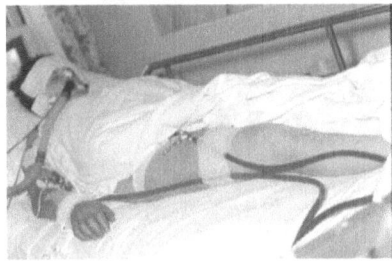

Fig. 5:12 Patient on ECMO using femoral vein to axillary artery.

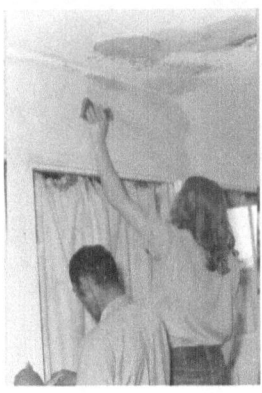

Fig. 5:13 The technology was crude. Cleaners after a membrane mishap.

A cardiothoracic residency program was established but was handicapped by limited funding of residency spots through the department of surgery. Five surgeons received their fellowships through the program and three now are members of the Maritime Heart Center. A research experience was mandated for the residents. In addition to spending a year or more in research at another centre, designated time each week was freed up to allow the residents to pursue research projects. Two PhD cardiac investigators (Drs. Drew Armour and Alan Marble) were affiliated with cardiac surgery and facilitated the resident training. Drs. Armour and Murphy began intraoperative studies on the cardiac autonomic nervous system, while Dr. Marble collaborated with Dr. Kinley in studying graft anastomotic rheology and stress factors causing false aneurysms.

Dr. Jim Parrott (Fig. 5:14) joined the center in 1976, having trained in cardiac surgery with Dr. Donald Hill in San Francisco.

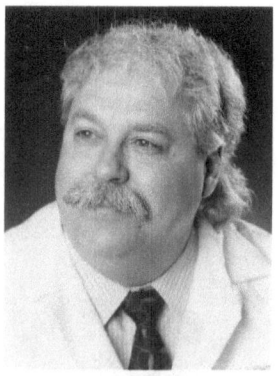

Fig. 5:14 Dr. James Parrott

It was decided that any new surgeon coming on the cardiovascular staff would first be asked to do some surgery in Halifax so their skills could be assessed. The date was set for Dr. Parrott's visit and the OR was alerted. As Dr. Parrott arrived in the operating room, it was noted that one hand was wrapped in a bandage. Despite this, he was hired. Alas, it was never found out whether he had really squashed his finger in the kitchen door as he had said. Through his interest in intensive care management the postoperative care of cardiac patients was improved and standardized. He had a way of making the surgeons in the lounge live his activities vicariously. It was not unusual for Jim to come to the lounge on Monday and say that he had just returned from New Orleans having seen the Mohammed Ali fight or that he had just got back from the Le Mans car race in Monte Carlo. Dr. Parrott left Halifax to head up the cardiac program at the university hospital in Winnipeg in 1981. Wistfully the surgeons' lounge was a quieter place for it.

Dr. Jeremy Wood, who had done his cardiothoracic training in Halifax joined the center after spending a year with Dr. Don Hill in San Francisco involved with their mechanical cardiac assist devices. Dr. Roderick Landymore (Fig. 5:15) was appointed head of the cardiac surgical division when Dr. Murphy resigned after fourteen years in this position.

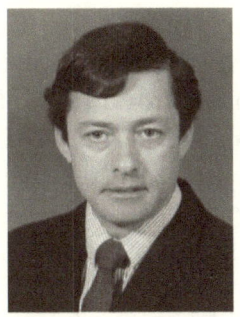

Fig. 5:15 Dr. Roderick Landymore

Dr. Landymore was a Dalhousie graduate who did his general surgical experience in Halifax and then qualified in cardiothoracic surgery with Dr. Frank Spencer in New York City. Research was his main interest and the clinical program increased with the patient needs from cardiology. The cardiothoracic surgical residency program was abandoned and the division's activities could be described as custodial. Dr. Landymore accepted a post in Saudi Arabia in 1994 and was replaced by Dr. John Sullivan. (Fig. 5:16)

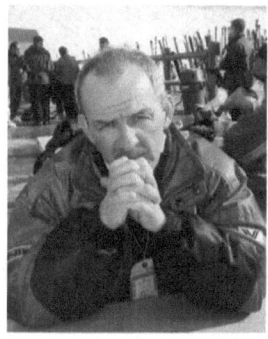

Fig.5:16 Dr. John Sullivan

Dr. Sullivan, a graduate of St. Mary's University and Dalhousie Medical School in 1974, did two years of general practice in Mabou, Cape Breton, where he was also required to give anaesthesia for surgical cases. He returned to Halifax in 1976 to complete his cardiothoracic training, which also included time at the Massachusetts General Hospital as a Canadian Heart Fellow. Upon his return, he set up the first noninvasive diagnostic vascular unit east of Montreal. Dr. Sullivan's skill as a vascular surgeon attracted a large referral practice and, with Dr. Kinley who also did vascular surgery, improved the calibre of this separately evolving specialty.

Dr. Sullivan was also able to reestablish the cardiac residency program, and with an emphasis on research training, two of his residents have received master's degrees and three their PhDs. There are six full-time and part-time research assistants. There are now six residents in the program, all from other Canadian universities.

In clinical care, new programs of laser transmyocardial revascularization, off pump cardiac revascularization, and total arterial graft coronary revascularization were introduced. The use of surgical nurse-practitioners was started. These RNs harvest radial arteries and, under endoscopic surgery, the saphenous veins for grafting. The case load of cardiac cases expanded to over 1,500 per year. In addition to Dr. John Sullivan the current staff of cardiac surgeons numbers eight. The group (2004) now includes the following surgeons: Drs. Jeremy Wood (1980), Idriss Ali (1991), Gregory Hirsch (1995), Imtiaz Ali (1998), Keir Stewart (1998), Camille Hancock-Freisen (2003), Stacy Oblenis (2003), and Jean François Legaré (2003).

The New Brunswick Heart Centre

The drive to develop a separate cardiac surgical centre in Saint John came from several former Dalhousie trained cardiologists. Drs. David Marr, Bob MacDonald and David Bewick felt that the waiting times for cardiac surgery were unacceptable for their New Brunswick patients. Additionally they had developed a state-of-the-art cardiac catheterization laboratory and then were dependent on Halifax to review the cases and enter them in the surgical list. Once they had a commitment from the New Brunswick government they asked Dr. Jim Parrott, then of Winnipeg, to head up the surgical section.

Dr. Parrott (Fig. 14) grew up in a small farming community west of Winnipeg. His family knew hardship. His bush pilot father died in a plane crash when Jim was three years old. His mother lived on welfare. To support himself through university, he played hockey as a goalie for the Wheat Kings, a New York Rangers farm team. A graduate of the University of Manitoba, he was able to obtain his MSc in cardiovascular physiology while pursuing his general surgery training. After spending four years in cardiothoracic training in San Francisco, he joined the Halifax group from 1976 to 1981. He then moved to Winnipeg Health Sciences Centre where he became head of the university section of cardiac surgery. Dr. Rand Forgie from New Brunswick who had trained at Dalhousie and the University of Alberta in Edmonton joined Dr. Parrott in 1991. In 1993, Dr. Craig Brown, who had trained with Dr. Parrott in Winnipeg, and then in San Francisco with Dr. Hill, moved to join the other two surgeons. Dr. Marc Pelletier recently returned from a Stanford University staff position to head the cardiac surgery team at the New Brunswick Health Centre.

Acknowledgement:

The following people were interviewed for this chapter and their recollections are appreciated. Douglas Roy, Robert Anderson, Emerson Moffitt, Alex Gillis, Brian Chandler, Janice Merritt, James Purvis, Bernard Steele, Alan Smith, Rick Leadon, Vida Clarke, Alan Marble, Lewis Page, Jim Parrott, and John Sullivan.

CHAPTER 6

CARDIAC SURGERY IN QUEBEC

Introduction

Jean E. Morin

Cardiac surgery in Quebec developed within the framework of the hospitals associated with the province's four medical schools: Laval, Sherbrooke, Montreal and McGill. The small number of surgeons originally involved gave them many opportunities to interact and support each other. They knew one another well and recollect those early days with much satisfaction, despite the many difficulties resulting from the embryonic state of knowledge and technology at the time.

We have chosen to present this history by focusing on the individuals who initiated cardiac surgery in their respective hospitals and those who have contributed to its development up to the present.

In 1962, a broad group of prominent cardiovascular and thoracic surgeons throughout the province founded the Quebec Association of Cardiovascular and Thoracic Surgeons. The association has since contributed significantly to the transfer of knowledge among its members. Its annual meetings helped to develop a sense of commitment and participation in the activities of the association. A section of this chapter is thus devoted to the history of this group.

To document the history of cardiac surgery in Quebec, I asked many of the discipline's founders and those who followed them to record their recollections. These reminiscences constitute the essence of this chapter.

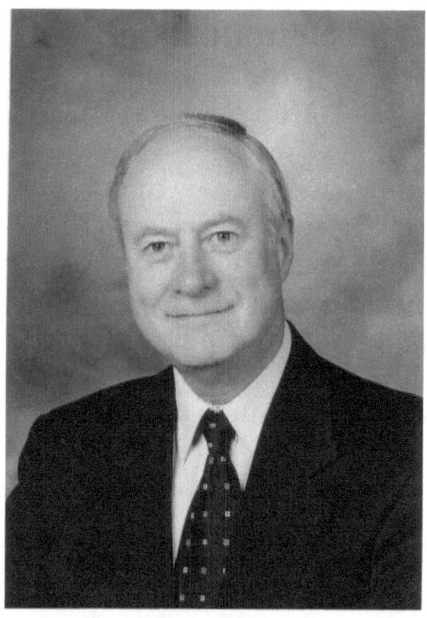

Fig 6:1 Jean Morin

QUEBEC ASSOCIATION OF CARDIOVASCULAR AND THORACIC SURGEONS

Jean E. Morin, MD

In 1962, cardiovascular and thoracic surgeons in Quebec realized that it would be beneficial to form a professional syndicate. Twenty-two surgeons representing the interests of the discipline throughout the province came together to form an association with the following objectives:

1. To group in an association all surgeons specialized in thoracic, vascular and cardiac surgery and recognized as such by the College of Physicians and Surgeons of the Province of Quebec.
2. To promote the scientific, economic, social and moral interests of surgeons specializing in thoracic, vascular and cardiac surgery.
3. To maintain, at the highest possible scientific level, the teaching and practice of thoracic, vascular and cardiac surgery.

The original directorship consisted of Eric MacNaughton, Gilles Lepage, Jacques Bruneau, Joffre-André Gravel, and Jean-Marie Lemieux, with Arthur Vineberg as the first president for a two-year term.

The group's request was well received by the government of Quebec and it was granted official status on September 6, 1962, as recorded in the *Quebec Official Gazette* of September 15, signed by Raymond Douville, undersecretary for the province.

Upon its formation, the association established rules for membership eligibility, annual fees, resignation criteria, disciplinary action, and the format for meetings. Since its establishment, the association has steadily pursued its original objectives, and all aspects of its mission have developed exponentially.

The members' economic interests have been successfully managed over the years. Many of the association's presidents (see appendix 1) devoted much time and energy in defending the status of cardiac surgeons before the assembly of delegates of the Federation of Medical Specialists of Quebec. The association's point of view was eventually recognized and cardiac surgeons now have a well-established place within the federation.

Scientific development was modest in the early days. In the mid-1970s, however, the value of continuing medical education became more widely acknowledged, and the association introduced more structured teaching sessions in 1975. At the spring meeting held that year at the Montreal Badminton and Squash Club, a surgical quiz was presented to the members to stimulate interest in professional development. Claude Grondin acted as the expert on cardiac issues and Jim Wilson on thoracic issues.

The annual meeting evolved at a rapid pace in subsequent years. It now consists of a full two-day gathering, at which cases are presented and topics of interest reviewed by faculty and residents. Leading cardiac surgeons from the United States and Europe regularly attend as guest lecturers, among them such prominent figures as John L. Ochsner, Lars G. Svensson, Jean-Paul Couetil, Didier Louelmet and François-Maurice Fontan.

In 2003, the Quebec Association combined its meeting with those of the Society of Cardiac Surgeons and the

Societat Catalana de Cirurgia (Catalan Society of Cardiac Surgery), giving it the international exposure that it wishes to promote.

The social aspect included in the association's original objectives has not been forgotten. While surgeons devote time to scientific sessions, family members enjoy the amenities of the resort chosen for the occasion. Members and industry representatives participate in all activities and share a sense of collegiality that is much appreciated.

In 1991, an award recognizing prominent Quebec surgeons was initiated by president Léon Dontigny. To date, fourteen surgeons have received the title of "Honoured Surgeon" by the Association (see appendix 2).

In short, the association has undoubtedly met the objectives set out in its 1962 charter. This document laid out the ground rules for its steady progress and unwavering focus on improved patient care.

Appendix 1: Presidents, Quebec Association of Cardiovascular and Thoracic Surgeons

Dr. Arthur Vineberg	1962-1963
Dr. Joffre-André Gravel	1964-1965
Dr. A. R. C. Dobell	1966-1967
Dr. Roger Paulin	1968
Dr. Pierre Grondin	1969-1970
Dr. Claude Mercier	1971-1972
Dr. Peter Blundell	1973-1974
Dr. Jean E. Morin	1975-1976
Dr. Luc Bruneau	1977-1978
Dr. Robert Cossette	1978-1980
Dr. Régent L. Beaudet	1980-1983
Dr. Claude Mercier	1984-1985
Dr. Gilles Lepage	1986-1987
Dr. Régent L. Beaudet	1988-1990
Dr. Léon Dontigny	1991-1993
Dr. Daniel Doyle	1994-2001
Dr. Richard Bauset	2002
Dr. Yves Langlois	2003-present

Appendix 2: Honoured Members, Quebec Association of Cardiovascular and Thoracic Surgeons

1991	Dr. Gilles Lepage
1992	Dr. Anthony Dobell
1993	Dr. Paul Stanley
1994	Dr. Arthur Pagé
1995	Dr. Ray Chiu
1996	Dr. Réjean Beaudet
1997	Dr. Pierre Grondin
1998	Dr. Paul Cartier
1999	Dr. Claude Grondin
2000	Dr. Jean E. Morin
2001	Dr. Claude Chartrand
2002	Dr. Normand Poirier
	Dr. Conrad Pelletier
2003	Dr. Michel Lemieux

CARDIAC SURGERY AT MCGILL

A. R. C. Dobell

The following chapter describes the development of heart surgery in the hospitals associated with McGill University. There was of course no grand design; progress depended on individual initiatives and advances in science and technology. Such advances often occurred after surgical meetings, particularly those of the American Association for Thoracic Surgery (AATS). Founded in 1917 during the First World War, the annual meetings of the AATS have included increasing reference to heart surgery since the Second World War. Cardiac surgery in Montreal was pioneered by surgeons with appointments at both McGill and hospitals affiliated with the University of Montreal, and there has always been some degree of liaison among the city's various medical facilities. For example we at McGill were enormously helped by the transplant pioneers at the Montreal Heart Institute.

The Pathfinders

Mercier Fauteux

Mercier Fauteux was the first surgeon associated with McGill University to investigate the possibility of operating on the heart. Born in 1898, Fauteux graduated from Laval University in Montreal and continued with two years' further training in France. He then practiced in several Montreal hospitals before becoming interested in coronary thrombosis. With the support of Edward Archibald, chief surgeon at the Royal Victoria Hospital (RVH), he began work in 1935 with Boris Babkin in experimental physiology and continued his investigations at the Peter Bent Brigham Hospital in

Boston between 1942 and 1946. Soon after returning to Montreal, Fauteux was appointed to found a department of cardiac surgery at the University of Montreal. He died suddenly in 1950 at the age of fifty-three.

Fauteux's experimental work was extensive. Though directed at coronary insufficiency, it gave him experience in cardiac resuscitation and defibrillation which led him to recommend that every operating room should be equipped with a defibrillator, long before safe defibrillators had been designed. Other conclusions, based on his 1947 report of over two hundred experimental heart operations:

• Cardiac irritability can be reduced with cocaine topically or intravenously.
• Hypoxia increases irritability.
• An electric shock can reverse ventricular fibrillation.
• The electrocardiogram will have a definite place in the operating room, and electrodes should be applied before the patient is anaesthetized.

These observations, made over half a century ago, would not be contested today and represent Fauteux's surgical legacy.

Three of his papers are notable in regard to coronary disease. The first was published in 1940[1] when accepted wisdom urged that ligation of the accompanying vein be carried out whenever an artery required ligation, presumably on the assumption that sluggish blood flow through the tissues would permit more complete oxygen extraction. Fauteux confirmed from seventy-five experiments with ligation of the anterior descending artery that concomitant ligation of the great cardiac vein was not harmful and might be beneficial.[2]

In a case report he described ligation of the great cardiac vein in a man of fifty-four with a "rigid and sclerotic" anterior descending artery, operated upon in April 1939. Following ligation of the great cardiac vein, the patient's crippling angina vanished. In an addendum he described five more patients operated upon after this first case.

Later while in Boston, Fauteux explored the benefit of pericoronary neurectomy[3] by resecting tissue over the left coronary artery and around the aorta and pulmonary artery in an attempt to block vasomotor reactions. Ligation of the great cardiac vein, however, remained the cornerstone of his operations for coronary disease.

In 1947,[4] he described attempts at intracardiac surgery with the venae cavae or the main pulmonary artery temporarily snared. These experiments at Harvard indicated that animals could tolerate circulatory arrest for five minutes but no longer.

Mercier Fauteux should be remembered as one of the pioneers of cardiac surgery, a man who, with a promising clinical future as he approached the age of forty, instead took up experimental surgery with a passion and directed his energy towards coronary artery disease. His legacy was to demonstrate that the heart could be manipulated surgically and to indicate precautions that would make cardiac surgery safer.[5]

Arthur Vineberg

Arthur Vineberg's worldwide fame derives from his strikingly original concept that an artery implanted into the myocardium might send off branches connecting with vessels in the heart musculature, thus providing additional blood supply. In a biographical essay he recorded that the idea first came to him during a lecture in pathology by Professor Horst Oertel who had pointed out that coronary atherosclerosis affected primarily the surface coronary arteries.

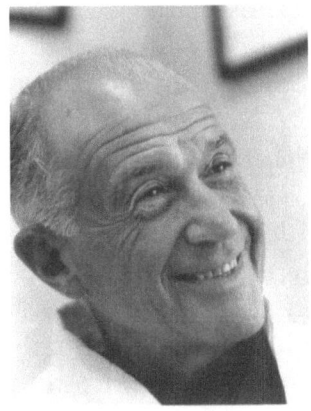

Fig 6:2 Arthur M. Vineberg

Later, when as a young surgeon living at home, his father suffered a myocardial infarction followed by angina and heart failure, Vineberg's passion to seek a surgical method of relieving these complications was rekindled. During his years as a demonstrator in anatomy he had noticed the close proximity of the internal mammary (currently termed the internal thoracic) arteries to the heart and so the remarkable concept evolved in his mind.

Five years younger than Fauteux, Vineberg graduated from McGill medical school in 1928 with a MSc in biochemistry as well as a medical degree. After a surgical internship at Bellevue in New York he was awarded a Rockefeller Fellowship in Experimental Surgery at McGill and, in 1930, registered in the graduate school of physiology while also serving as a surgical resident with

Edward Archibald at the RVH. Vineberg received his PhD for experiments on gastric physiology in 1933.

Under Archibald's tutelage, Vineberg became recognized clinically as a general and thoracic surgeon, and he treated pulmonary tuberculosis at several Montreal hospitals in the days when surgery for that disease consisted of thoracoplasty to permanently collapse the apex of the lung. He served in the Royal Canadian Army Medical Corps during WWII until his discharge in 1945.

Vineberg then returned to experimental surgery with a hypothesis clear in his mind and made his first report on the subject in 1946 in the *Canadian Medical Association Journal*.[6] In six animals the terminally ligated internal mammary artery (IMA) was drawn into a tunnel in the myocardium. Four months later, when radiopaque Schlesinger's solution was injected into the IMA and the excised heart X-rayed, one animal showed a connection between the implant and the coronary circulation. The injectate emerged retrograde from the orifice of the left coronary artery and it was necessary to ligate it to retain the fluid within the coronary system. The excitement engendered by this radiograph can be readily imagined and it was reproduced in several of Dr. Vineberg's papers.

Efforts were now expended to improve the consistency of the procedure. Myocardial ischemia was produced by ligating a branch of the anterior descending coronary artery and then the left IMA with a bleeding intercostal branch was drawn into a myocardial tunnel 2 cm long. In survivors the anterior descending artery was ligated at its origin up to six months after the initial procedure. Nine out of ten control animals without implants died immediately. Thirteen of the twenty-six animals with prior implants survived, although connections between the IMA and the coronary arteries were demonstrable in only half of them.

This report, published in *Surgery, Gynecology and Obstetrics* in 1950,[7] showed that Vineberg's procedure could protect against infarction and death following ligation of a coronary artery in an experimental animal. No previous operation could make this claim and the clinical possibilities were tantalizing. Vineberg continued his experimental work and developed a technique for slowly reducing the calibre of coronary arteries, using ameroid constrictors to provide a better experimental model.[8]

Clinical experience developed slowly, but between 1950 and 1958 Vineberg published twenty reports on the implant procedure. The operations were done for angina before coronary angiography was developed so no objective pre- or postsurgical test was available. Benefit was judged by symptomatic relief. It was only in 1963 that Mason Sones[9] demonstrated that contrast material injected into an IMA following Vineberg's operation flowed into the coronary system. This demonstration in a living postoperative patient led to a brief heyday for the implant procedure as it was evaluated by a number of surgeons.

Among these were Donald Effler at the Cleveland Clinic and Wilfred Bigelow in Toronto,[10] but shortly thereafter the Cleveland surgeons demonstrated the effectiveness of coronary bypass grafts and this operation immediately gained favour. It made surgical sense, instantly restored coronary blood flow and relieved angina, whereas the Vineberg operation did not increase coronary flow until the implanted artery arborized and connected to myocardial vessels. In addition, the IMA could not reach the posterior surface of the heart; the maximum number of implants was two, and finally the implant did not always successfully connect with the coronary system.

Some implants were shown to be patent in Cleveland, Toronto and Montreal, but some undoubtedly never functioned at all, as the animal work had demonstrated. Towards the end of his career, Vineberg added modifications he thought might expedite and expand the benefit of his operation. But innovations, such as the Ivalon sponge application and the omental wrap, were of doubtful benefit and quite possibly deleterious. It was difficult for Vineberg to stand aside as direct coronary surgery became the accepted operation for coronary artery disease. He was fiercely loyal to his country, his city, his university and his operation.

Pediatric Heart Surgery

Not long after Robert Gross reported[11] the first successful ligation of a patent ductus arteriosus in August 1938, Dudley Ross carried out the procedure on a child at the Montreal Children's Hospital (MCH). A few years later the resection of coarctations of the aorta and palliative shunts for cyanotic children were added to the armamentarium of surgeons caring for children and these too were carried out by Ross at the MCH.

In 1946, Arnold Johnson performed the first heart catheterization in Canada, and the cardiology department was established under his direction the following year. David Ross Murphy replaced Ross as surgeon in chief in 1954, and along with Gordon Karn he expanded heart surgery at the MCH. Patients were referred from the Maritime Provinces as well as upstate Vermont and New

York for standard operations that did not require a life-support system.

The problem was that most congenital heart defects require intracardiac repair. Simple atrial septal defects and pulmonary valve stenosis could be treated in the five-minute period of circulatory arrest provided by hypothermia; a number of these operations were performed at the MCH, permitting the surgeons to develop technical skills and establish close cooperation with the anaesthetists and nurses chosen for the surgical team. These procedures were done in 1957 after the hospital moved from its original mountain site to a location opposite the old Montreal Forum. It was at this point that its name was changed from the Children's Memorial Hospital to the Montreal Children's Hospital.

In 1956 Tony Dobell returned from Philadelphia after completing a residency in general and thoracic surgery, including a year (1953-54) in the experimental surgery laboratory working with what was at the time the only proven heart-lung machine in the world. He was appointed teaching fellow in surgery at the RVH and soon was invited to participate with David Murphy and Gordon Karn in developing open-heart surgery at the MCH. A DeWall-Lillehei disposable oxygenator system with noisy sigmamotor pumps had been assembled, and experimental work was done at night in one of the operating rooms of the old Children's Memorial Hospital. Animals were anaesthetized in the Donner Building which housed the experimental surgery facility on the McGill campus and then transported in the trunk of Dr. Murphy's car along with the heparinized donor blood needed to prime the heart-lung machine. The operations were used to familiarize nurses, anaesthetists and the perfusionist with the intricacies of intracardiac surgery and the management of cardiopulmonary bypass.

The move to the new MCH was carried out on December 1956. The site had previously been occupied by a division of the Montreal General Hospital (MGH). The old building was renovated and two new ones built alongside it to provide a modern general pediatric hospital. There was an excellent cardiology department, staffed by Arnold Johnson, Maurice McGregor, Wanda Jegier and James Gibbons; regular weekly conferences were held with the surgical team to review patient data, including heart catheterization results. Scott Dunbar, head of radiology, also added greatly to the group's expertise. The angiograms were displayed on cut films as cine-angiography was not then available.

The first pump operations were done in 1957. Only extremely ill children were approved for these procedures and the results were dismal. The surgeons were not happy with the bypass system and all were discouraged by the results; the operations were discontinued. A simpler Mark screen oxygenator was obtained, visits were made to the Mayo Clinic and Minneapolis, and patients were carefully screened for the next series of operations. Open-heart surgery thus became established at the MCH in 1958. These were not the first successful procedures performed under bypass in Montreal, as Édouard Gagnon had closed an atrial septal defect at the Montreal Heart Institute in July 1957. But since the early candidates for intracardiac surgery were primarily children with heart defects, open-heart surgery continued at the MCH on a regular basis. Many of the early patients had ventricular septal defects with heart failure or pulmonary hypertension. Some had congenital aortic stenosis. Fairly soon atrial defects were being repaired using cardiopulmonary bypass rather than hypothermia and primum defects were repaired as they were encountered. We puzzled over the first atrioventricular canal defects.

Our experience at the MCH was similar to that at other centres caring for children with congenital heart disease. With growing knowledge and improved technology more complex anomalies became reparable. Palliative shunts gave way to repairs for tetralogy of Fallot; when Bill Mustard showed how to reroute the venous circulation for transposition of the great arteries we adopted this procedure, or sometimes Senning's variant; prosthetic valves and conduits were used as needed. Scientific and technical knowledge increased in all areas: in myocardial protection; in postoperative management with the development of the intensive care unit and the training of intensivists; in anaesthesia; and in intraoperative and postoperative monitoring. Pump oxygenators improved: we went from a screen oxygenator to a disc, then to disposable bubblers, and finally to disposable membrane oxygenators. The contributions of industry were enormous. As a result of these advances, steady improvement in results was the rule. Progressively smaller children had their hearts repaired until babies were operated upon in infancy.

At the MCH we always had excellent perfusionists who worked closely with the surgeons. In the first operations the apparatus was run by John Gutelius, then a surgical resident, later head of surgery at Queen's. The first career perfusionist was Wolfgang Schroeder, a young German immigrant employed as an orderly, who left after several years to enter medical school. He was replaced by Claude Rancourt who later became a dentist with special training in facial surgery. The position was then taken by Maurice Martin, who after many happy years moved to London,

Ontario, as a career perfusionist, and then David Edgell who again after a lengthy stay moved to the Hospital for Sick Children in Toronto. All of them were diligent, highly responsible and innovative, and worked closely with the surgeons as perfusion flow and temperature were manipulated during operations.

The initial procedures were done by Murphy, Karn and Dobell together. The first two were experienced general pediatric surgeons who helped Tony Dobell as he gradually became a specialist in cardiac surgery. The three worked easily as a team, but in time the pediatric surgeons became increasingly occupied with noncardiac activities; David Murphy had administrative responsibility for the entire surgical department from 1954 until his retirement in 1974.

The team was expanded with the arrival of David Alton Murphy, originally trained as a veterinarian, then as a pediatric surgeon and subsequently a cardiac surgeon, who later had a distinguished career in Halifax. He was an exciting comrade during his few years in Montreal before he left for Chicago to complete his many-faceted qualifications with a residency in adult cardiovascular surgery.

Dobell continued with the surgical team at the Children's while simultaneously caring for adults at the RVH. More complex congenital anomalies were repaired and younger and smaller infants underwent surgery. An intensive care unit was created to manage the postoperative cardiac cases as well as other critically ill children.

In 1987, Christo Tchervenkov, who had completed his cardiovascular surgery training at McGill, was accepted as chief resident at the Boston Children's Hospital under Aldo Castaneda. This experience gave Tchervenkov a unique opportunity to adopt Castaneda's techniques and philosophy as he proved his hypothesis that infants with complex cardiac malformations were best operated upon in one stage at an early age, often soon after birth.

Upon his return a year later, Tchervenkov was immediately made an equal member of the cardiac surgical staff. Arterial switches were carried out with great success for transposition of the great arteries and ever-smaller infants with a variety of malformations underwent successful repair. The referral base widened as Tchervenkov's reputation expanded. He became chief of cardiac surgery in 1992 when Tony Dobell retired. Tchervenkov was joined in 1999 by Dominique Shum-Tim, a graduate of the McGill cardiothoracic program who had spent two fellowship years at the Boston Children's Hospital. Both Tchervenkov and Shum-Tim hold joint appointments at the MGH as well.

Since 2001, Tchervenkov and Marie Béland, chief of cardiology at the MCH, have spearheaded an international effort to standardize the nomenclature of congenital heart disease across the world.

In 2002, Renzo Cecere of the RVH staff was given a cross-appointment at the MCH to allow his expertise in transplantation and cardiac assistance to be applied in children. In 2002, the MCH team successfully implanted a Berlin artificial heart in a two-year-old child; the device functioned for 109 days before successful cardiac transplantation.

The Adult Hospitals

Once intracardiac surgery had been successfully introduced at the Children's Hospital in 1958, a screen oxygenator was purchased by the Royal Vic and a number of operations were performed by Drs. Vineberg and Dobell together. A few atrial septal defects were closed and initial experience was obtained in operating on the mitral valve. These were done with a beating heart and a competent aortic valve, and mitral valve annuloplasty yielded some success in severely dilated valves by tightening the anterolateral and posteromedial commissures to enable the valve leaflets to approximate each other.

These were our first experiences with acquired heart disease. Mitral stenosis was still treated by closed commissurotomy either with finger fracture or with a mechanical dilator. The first patients selected for open-heart surgery had enormous hearts and a very limited life expectancy, and although success was obtained there were also many disappointments as was generally true in this era. The primary focus of heart surgeons at the time was certainly on the treatment of congenital heart disease. Yet interest in acquired valvular heart disease was growing among both surgeons and cardiologists who were getting into the invasive investigation of heart disease.

In 1958, a joint cardiorespiratory service was established between the MCH and the RVH with Arnold Johnson as the head of the cardiac division. This move was of considerable benefit to both institutions not only clinically and in fostering research but also in attracting outstanding residents and fellows. Cardiology became in effect a full-time university department. Arnold Johnson later moved his office to the RVH and enrolled a strong team of cardiac physicians led by Maurice McGregor who was director of research and later physician in chief of the RVH and dean of the McGill Faculty of Medicine.

A similar reorganization of the department of surgery at McGill awaited the arrival of new surgeons in chief at both the MGH and the RVH. The first of these was H. Rocke Robertson, an outstanding surgical leader who moved from Vancouver to become chief at the MGH in 1959. He insisted that a surgical research facility be constructed before he would accept the position, and an entire wing was added over the operating rooms to become the University Surgical Clinic.

Henry James "Harry" Scott had for some years done the closed heart surgery at the MGH. This consisted in the main of mitral commissurotomy with an occasional patent ductus, coarctation or pericardiectomy, but obviously open-heart surgery was here to stay and the MGH needed to enter the field. Tony Dobell was invited to join with Scott in this endeavour and a disc oxygenator was purchased. Roger Samson, a laboratory technician who had served with the Red Cross in Korea, was appointed perfusionist, a position he was to hold for thirty-six years. A series of procedures was begun in the laboratory facility to evaluate the new pump oxygenator and to familiarize the entire team with the management of open-heart surgery. Experimental work continued in the laboratory even after clinical procedures began.

Between 1960 and 1964, Scott and Dobell worked together in a happy environment. Stewart E. A. Reid was director of cardiology at the MGH and staff cardiologists included Patrick "Pat" Cronin and Henry Mizgala. Most early patients referred to the surgical team suffered from valvular heart disease. Stenotic aortic valves were debrided and annuloplasty was done for mitral insufficiency. Most mitral commissurotomies were relieved by a closed technique, but as open-heart surgery was performed when an atrial clot was suspected, we also obtained experience in exposing and evaluating both left-sided valves.

The first prosthetic valves used were the Bahnson aortic cusps, in which the three leaflets were individually replaced by three fabric cusps. Although a competent valve could be constructed in this way, the fabric soon became invaded by fibrous tissue and the resulting stiffness caused obstruction. This was our first lesson in the body's reaction to implanted moving components in prosthetic valves. Several patients who had received Bahnson cusps were reoperated upon and the prosthetic cusps replaced with Starr valves sutured into the aortic root.

By chance some patients with idiopathic hypertrophic subaortic stenosis were operated upon, and as we were dissatisfied with septal muscle resection through the aortic valve, an approach was made through the mitral valve by way of a left thoracotomy. Looking back this seems like making a simple procedure unnecessarily complicated. Not surprisingly, no one was persuaded and the trans aortic route remained the popular approach. But perhaps this deviation reflected the mood of the times when operations were sometimes devised spontaneously to solve unforeseen problems.

As of 1964, Tony Dobell was on the staff of the three hospitals but operated primarily at the MGH and the MCH. That year he was invited to expand cardiovascular surgery at the RVH and began playing a greater role there, though he remained nominally involved at the MGH. Harry Scott was then joined by Peter Blundell, a recent graduate of Bill Bigelow's program in Toronto who had spent a year at the Mayo Clinic with Dwight McGoon doing research on valve replacements.

A new team was thus established at the MGH. In 1968, Ray C. J. Chiu entered the University Surgical Clinic there as a PhD candidate. He was brought to Montreal by Fraser Gurd, who had replaced Rocke Robertson on the latter's appointment as principal of McGill. Chiu had trained in general and thoracic surgery with Clarence Dennis at Downstate in Brooklyn and his research at the MGH was initially in the area of intestinal viability in low perfusion states. The low perfusion state was controlled experimentally by cardiopulmonary bypass and Chiu's mentor under Dr. Gurd was Harry Scott. Thus in time the cardiovascular and thoracic surgical service gained a valuable new area of expertise. Ray Chiu joined the clinical service in 1972, after completing his PhD and acquiring all the necessary qualifications. His imaginative contributions to research in cardiac surgery are documented elsewhere, but it should be emphasized that he was a full-fledged member of the surgical team at the MGH and McGill when the university's training program was initiated. Chiu divided his time between clinical work and research until his retirement from the former in 2000, but continues at the time of writing (2004) to work full-time in research.

While Ray Chiu was working towards his PhD David Mulder returned from his residency in cardiovascular and thoracic surgery under Hans Ehrenhaft at the University of Iowa. Mulder came to McGill for his residency in general surgery after a brilliant performance as a medical student at the University of Saskatchewan, and in 1970, joined the staff of the MGH in a harmonious relationship with Scott, Blundell and Chiu. While participating fully in cardiac and thoracic surgery he remained active in general surgery, particularly in the field of trauma, and was recognized from the first as a leading surgeon at McGill. He rapidly rose to become a full professor, surgeon in chief of the MGH and chairman of the university department of surgery, yet these duties did not seriously disturb the happy relationship that existed in CVT.

New appointments to the MGH staff were made as the volume of cardiac surgery expanded. Lee Errett was appointed after completing his training in 1985, but left for the United States in 1987, and later moved to St. Michael's Hospital in Toronto. Christo Tchervenkov received a joint appointment at the MGH when he joined the staff of the MCH in 1987. Hani Shennib completed the CVT program in1987, and after a year's fellowship at the Toronto General Hospital in the field of lung transplantation returned to MGH. Jean-Francois Morin was appointed in 1989 and left in 2002 to join the staff of the Jewish General Hospital. Morin was a mainstay of the clinical staff and enjoyed a joint appointment at the RVH.

Dao Nguyen completed the cardiothoracic residency at McGill in 1994. A brilliant resident, he was sent to the MD Anderson Cancer Center in Houston for two years as a clinical and research fellow before returning to the MGH. Regrettably, he was recruited by the National Institutes of Health in Bethesda, Maryland, where he is doing excellent research in thoracic oncology. Dominique Shum-Tim received a cross-appointment at the MGH when he joined the MCH in 1999, and continues an active research program at the University Surgical Clinic studying brain protection during deep hypothermic circulatory arrest.

Meanwhile at the RVH, Lloyd MacLean arrived in 1962 as surgeon in chief and set about modernizing the department. He had been selected by a committee chaired by Walter Mackenzie, dean of the medical school in Edmonton. A graduate of the University of Alberta, Maclean trained in surgery at the University of Minnesota under Owen Wangensteen and like others in that program was highly intelligent, inquisitive, and energetic. At the Royal Vic he immediately expanded the experimental surgery laboratories, established a sought-after training program and began a series of full-time appointments.

Though fully prepared in cardiac and thoracic surgery, MacLean decided to concentrate on the general surgery program at the RVH, and in 1964 he invited Tony Dobell to join the full-time staff there. Dobell had of course remained on the RVH staff and operated there as well as both the MGH and the MCH. At this time, of course, direct coronary artery surgery did not exist; prosthetic valves were under early evaluation (and several had proved disappointing); valvular surgery remained high risk because patients were referred in the final stage of their illness; and diagnostic tests such as echocardiography had yet to be developed. In fact the volume of heart surgery was modest, and all vascular procedures were done by the CVT services at both hospitals.

Noncardiac thoracic surgery was performed at the RVH by Darryl D. "Dag" Munro, chief surgeon at the allied Montreal Chest Hospital. CVT services remained classified as general surgical services at the two major adult hospitals and all junior residents in surgery rotated through them. There was no demand for further autonomy because CVT was so strongly supported by the two chief surgeons, Lloyd MacLean and Fraser Gurd. Tony Dobell's position at the three hospitals added further to the cohesion between the units and while Gurd was chairman of the McGill department of surgery he proposed the establishment of a university-based training program in CVT surgery. The evolution of this program is discussed below.

In 1968, Dobell was joined at the Royal Vic by Jean Morin, a graduate of Laval medical school who had trained in general and cardiovascular/thoracic surgery at Yale under William Glenn and Gustaf Lindskog. At the beginning of his career Morin cared for patients in all three subdisciplines of CVT, but later, after Dag Munro returned full-time to the Montreal Chest Hospital, he concentrated more on cardiac and thoracic surgery. In addition to clinical practice, Morin always had a great interest in health care organization and evaluation. An excellent administrator, he became chief of CVT at the RVH in 1978. He was a wise counselor to the institution. In 1980, Morin attended the University of Montreal during the summer to learn more about computer programming. Then with the support of private industry he designed a software program to record the parameters of patients undergoing heart surgery together with risk factors, operative findings, complications and outcomes. The RVH instituted this program in 1981, and it remains in operation today. After retiring from clinical practice in 2001, Morin founded the Réseau Québécois de Cardiologie Tertiaire (Quebec Tertiary Cardiac Network), an organization similar to the Cardiac Care Network of Ontario, which monitors cardiac service delivery and advises the provincial health minister on measures to be implemented to guarantee that all patients have access to quality care without undue delay.

In 1972, Normand Poirier joined the RVH staff after completing the McGill cardiovascular and thoracic surgery training program. A graduate of the University of Montreal, Poirier was a strong, indefatigable surgeon who gave superb care to his patients, some of whom were extremely challenging because of their advanced disease. He contributed greatly to the development of coronary surgery at McGill and to the transplantation program in which he was joined by Albert Guerraty, a valuable member of the RVH staff from 1984 to 1989. Guerraty had previously had extensive experience in heart transplantation at the Medical College of Virginia. Poirier later joined the staff of Notre-Dame Hospital in Montreal where he eventually became chief of cardiac surgery, while Guerraty joined Andrew Wechsler in Richmond and then in Philadelphia.

Later staff appointees to the RVH were all graduates of the McGill program and included Jean Allard, James Symes, Tom Salerno, and André Grignon, all of whom contributed greatly as coronary artery surgery achieved its potential. Allard received a research fellowship at the Cancer Research Institute (CRI) in San Francisco; he returned to the RVH in1978 but went back to California two years later. Symes was an excellent surgeon who later moved to St. Elizabeth's Hospital in Boston; during his stay at the RVH he conducted extensive research on angiogenesis for peripheral vascular insufficiency. Tom Salerno's extraordinary drive and energy stimulated all around him, particularly the residents in the experimental surgery laboratory. His output was phenomenal, and it was no surprise that he went on to head cardiac surgery services in Toronto, Buffalo, and at present in Miami. Grignon, who joined the RVH in 1979, later moved to Iowa where he died tragically.

The last graduates of the McGill CVT program to join the RVH were David Latter, Benoit de Varennes and Pat Ergina. Like several other graduates Latter held a postgraduate fellowship at Stanford with Norman

Shumway and his outstanding associates and took over the cardiac transplant program when he returned in 1991. Latter was joined in July of 1991 by Benoit de Varennes, who joined the faculty immediately after completing the residency in CVT at McGill. These two became the primary surgeons in the transplantation program and enjoyed great success. Through their involvement surgery for heart failure started to prosper. Dr. de Varennes soon developed an expertise in mitral valve surgery and has established a database for mitral valve repairs. He is currently chief of cardiac surgery at the RVH. Patrick Ergina was recruited from the CVT program in 1993 and became an active member of the group. His strong interest in surgical education led to his appointment as core program director for the department of surgery.

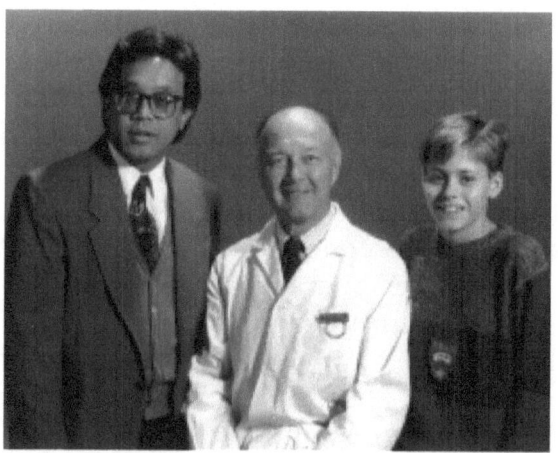

Fig. 6:3 From left to right: Patrick Ergina, Tony Dobell and postoperative patient

Two recent graduates of the cardiothoracic program established at McGill in 1992 have since joined the RVH staff. Kevin Lachapelle spent a fellowship year with Sir Magdi Yacoub in London concentrating on complex valve surgery; Renzo Cecere did his postgraduate training with Leonard Bailey at Loma Linda where he focused on cardiac transplantation and mechanical assistance for failing hearts. Both profited enormously from this extra experience and are excellent mature surgeons. Cecere has taken over the transplantation program and with the cardiologists has established a heart failure clinic. Both he and de Varennes have a strong interest in long-term mechanical circulatory support.

Jean Morin acted as mentor to these young individuals until his retirement from active practice in 2001. He then took on administrative responsibilities as surgeon in chief of the Royal Victoria Hospital and president of the Reseau Québecois de Cardiologie Tertiare.

It seems desirable to provide a brief description of the McGill program in cardiovascular and thoracic surgery and its evolution over the years.

The McGill Training Program

McGill's proposal to the Royal College of Physicians and Surgeons in the mid-1960s was fully supported by all participants and approval was rapidly obtained; the program was shortly approved as well by the American Board of Thoracic Surgery. From the first the program was centred at the university and not the hospitals. It consisted of six-month rotations as chief resident in each of the four affiliated hospitals MCH, MGH, RVH and the Montreal Chest Hospital); all cardiac, vascular and thoracic surgery performed in these hospitals was done on the CVT service. The prerequisite was complete training in general surgery, and clearly McGill trainees had the inside track since they became known to the CVT faculty during their rotations through the service during their general surgical training. Interested and capable residents usually did their lab year (part of the general surgery program) under one of the CVT faculty as well, and as this was almost always was a productive and exciting experience for both faculty and resident, the progression into CVT after general surgery was assured.

The first trainee was E. J. P. Charrette who received an appointment at Queen's University in Kingston after completing his training in 1967 and later became chief of CVT there. In the ensuing twenty-eight years, forty-one surgeons went through this program. Nineteen of them moved or returned to the United States, some in private practice and some in academic positions. One returned to his native Venezuela. The remainder have spent their professional lives in centres across Canada. Of the total, at least eleven have become full professors.

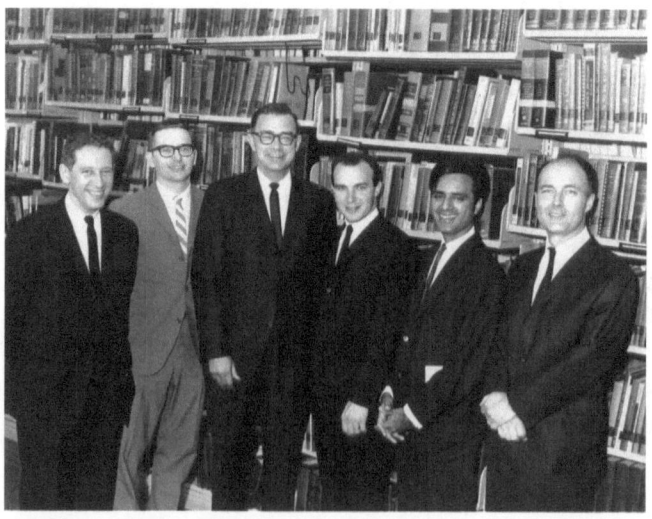

Fig 6:4 McGill CVT Trainees; L to R: Claude Mercier, Ed Busse, David R. Murphy, Edward Charette, M. S. Chughtai, and Anthony Dobell

Specialists in vascular surgery had joined the faculty and in 1992 this discipline was split off from CVT which continued as a cardiothoracic training program. From 1992 to 1998, ten surgeons completed the cardiothoracic program; four of them are currently on the McGill faculty, three have joined other Canadian medical schools, two are in the United States, and one returned to Saudi Arabia. Noncardiac thoracic surgery became a separate service in 2000, and David Mulder was appointed as chief of the thoracic program. A six-year training program in cardiac surgery had been inaugurated in 1992, while the cardiothoracic program still existed. This included two years of core surgery pertinent to cardiac surgery, one year of research and four years of heart surgery. To date seven surgeons have graduated from the new program: four are attached to other medical schools in Canada, and three are in the United States. Since the entry level follows immediately after medical school, applicants are forced to apply to specialist programs during their undergraduate medical education. This seems completely unrealistic in terms of their lack of experience; one hopes adjustments may be made during the core years.

Organization

Cardiac surgery at McGill was for many years a component of the division of CVT surgery. This requires a little explanation. The service was from the first a university-based program in clinical care as well as education, but surgery was originally organized into hospital-based units, and each of the two major adult hospitals had in fact its own training program. Thus when the university-based service was set up, I called it a division. Division of what? Division of the McGill department of surgery would seem the appropriate answer, though this was never defined and there were no other formal divisions. At any rate the organization worked smoothly, in large part because it was so strongly supported by the two chief surgeons, Fraser Gurd and Lloyd MacLean, who rotated every five years as chairs of the department of surgery.

I was fortunate to be in a position to be chief or chair of this division from its inception until 1992. In fact the title was not put to much use, but the system worked due to the quality and commitment of the faculty members and the continuing expansion and improvement of cardiac surgery which made the era so exciting. The leadership was taken over in 1992 by Ray C. J. Chiu who had been promoted to a full professorship in 1981 in recognition of his important contributions to research in cardiac surgery. Upon his retirement, it passed to David Mulder. A former surgeon in chief of the MGH and chair of the university department of surgery, Mulder was then approaching his thirtieth year of surgical leadership at McGill.

An important asset to the division was the establishment in 1968 of the Stikeman Visiting Professorship. Set up in memory of a young man who died of a malignancy more than a year after undergoing a radical pleuropneumonectomy by D. D. Munro, this bequest made it possible to bring a surgical leader to McGill annually. The visit was made in the late spring each year when the finishing resident(s) could be recognized but with the passage of time it became an annual reunion when former residents returned from their current institutions across the United States and Canada. These return visits have been greatly appreciated by the McGill faculty, and the visiting professors invariably stimulate intense interest and reflection among residents and faculty alike. In addition the program has enabled visiting professors to learn about McGill, which has often proven helpful for graduates seeking fellowships elsewhere.

Notes:

1. M. Fauteux, "Experimental study of surgical treatment of coronary disease," *Surg Gynecol Obstet* (1940), 71: 151-55.

2. M. Fauteux and J. Palmer, "Treatment of angina of atheromatous origin by ligation of the great cardiac vein," *Can Med Assoc J* (1941), 45: 295-98.

3. M. Fauteux and O. Swenson, "Pericoronary neurectomy in abolishing anginal pain in coronary disease: Experimental evaluation," *AMA Arch Surg* (1946), 53: 169-81.

4. M. Fauteux, "Chirurgie intracardiaque: arrêt temporaire de la circulation par occlusion des veines caves ou de l'artère pulmonaire comme temps préliminaire : Étude expérimentale," *Union Med Can* (1947), 76: 1036-48.

5. M. Fauteux, "Cardiac resuscitation," *J Thor Surg* (1947), 16: 623-39.

6. A. M. Vineberg, "The development of an anastomosis between the coronary vessels and a transplanted internal mammary artery," *Can Med Assoc J* (1946), 55: 117-19.

7. A. M. Vineberg and P. H. Niloff, "The value of surgical treatment of coronary artery occlusion by implantation of the internal mammary artery in the ventricular myocardium: An experimental study," *Surg Gynecol Obstet* (1950), 91: 551-61.

8. J. Litvak and A. M. Vineberg, "Experimental gradual arterial occlusions with in vitro and in vivo observations," *Surgery* (1959), 46: 953-63.

9. D. B. Effler et al., "Increased myocardial perfusion of the internal mammary artery implantation: Vineberg's operation," *Ann Surg* (1963), 158: 526-34.

10. W. G. Bigelow, H. Basian, and G. A. Trusler, "Internal mammary artery implantation for coronary heart disease: A clinical follow-up study one to eight years after operation," *J Thorac Cardiovasc Surg* (1963), 45: 67-79.

11. R. E. Gross and J. P. Hubbard, "Surgical ligation of a patent ductus arteriosus: report of first successful case," *JAMA* (1939) 112: 729-31.

Appendix 1: Faculty Members of McGill Programs in Cardiovascular and Thoracic Surgery (1965-1992), Cardiothoracic Surgery (1992-2000), and Cardiac Surgery (1992-2003)

Anthony R. C. Dobell	1965-1992
Darryl D. Munro	1965-1983
James A. Wilson *	1965-1997
David R. Murphy	1965-1974
Gordon M. Karn	1965-1981
Harry J. Scott	1965-1989
Lloyd D. MacLean	1965-1989
Arthur Vineberg*	1965-1968
Peter Blundell	1965-1998
Jean E. Morin	1968-2000
David A. Murphy	1968-1973
David S. Mulder	1970-2003
Ray C. J. Chiu	1972-2000
Normand Poirier	1972-1978, 1989-1989
James F. Symes	1975-1992
Jean Allard	1978-1980
André Grignon*	1979-1984
J. Earl Wynands	1980-1988
Albert Guerraty	1984-1989
Tomas A. Salerno	1982-1983
Lee Errett	1985-1987
Christo I. Tchervenkov	1988-2003
Pierre L. Pagé	1988-2003
Hani Shennib	1988-2003
Jean-Francois Morin	1989-2003
Benoit DeVarennes	1991-2003
David Latter	1991-1996
Patrick Ergina	1993-2003
Dao Nguyen	1996-1999
Kevin Lachapelle	1997-2003
Dominique Shum-Tin	1999-2003
Renzo Cecere	2000-2003

* Deceased

Appendix 2: Graduates of McGill Programs

1967 Edward J. P. Charette *	Kingston, Ontario **
1967 Claude Mercier *	Montréal
1968 M. S. Chughtai	McGill
1968 Edward F. G. Busse	Regina, Saskatchewan **
1970 J. Asirvathem	
1971 M. A. James Sheverini	
1971 Guilermo Malavé	Caracas, Venezuela
1972 Normand L. Poirier	Montréal **
1973 Guy Lemire	Long Beach, California
1973 Eric D. Foster	Albany, New York **
1975 James F. Symes	Boston, Massachusetts **
1975 Ronald M. Becker	Chico, California
1976 Jean R. Allard	Inglewood, California
1977 Tomas A. Salerno	Miami, Florida **
1978 James W. Dutton	Victoria, British Columbia **
1978 A. Steven Cain	Ogden, Utah
1979 André Grignon *	Des Moines, Iowa
1980 Dennis Modry	Edmonton, Alberta **
1980 Lynda Mickleborough	Toronto, Ontario **
1980 Elias Abdulnour	Montréal
1982 Richard W. Long	Erie, Pennsylvania
1983 Davis C. Drinkwater	Nashville, Tennessee **
1983 Fraser M. Keith	Tampa, Florida
1983 Arun K. Jain	
1985 Alex J. Bayes	Calgary, Alberta
1985 Lee E. Errett	Toronto, Ontario
1986 Christo I. Tchervenkov	McGill **
1987 Richard J. Novick	London, Ontario **
1987 Giles S. Hedderich	Lincoln, Nebraska
1987 Hani Shennib	McGill **
1988 Michael L. Dewar	New Haven, Connecticut
1989 David A. Latter	Toronto, Ontario
1989 Jonah N. K. Odim	Los Angeles, California
1990 Thomas A. Burdon	Stanford, California

1990	Garrett L. Walsh	Houston, Texas **
1991	Benoit DeVarennes	McGill
1991	Gary Kochamba	Los Angeles, California
1992	Jerome B. Riebman	San Jose, California
1992	William T. Kidd	Calgary, Alberta
1993	Patrick Ergina	McGill
1994	Daniel Marelli	Kansas City, Kansas
1994	Dao Nguyen	Bethesda, Maryland
1995	Kevin Lachapelle	McGill
1995	Dominique Shum-Tim	McGill
1996	G. Baslaim	Saudi Arabia
1996	Felix Ma	McGill
1997	Renzo Cecere	McGill
1997	Gary Salasidis	Toronto, Ontario
1998	Stephanie Helmer	Delray Beach, Florida
1998	Mackenzie Quantz	London, Ontario
1999	John Tsang	Regina, Saskatchewan
1999	Steven Tahta	Missoula, Montana
2000	Mark Pelletier	Toronto, Ontario
2001	Victor Chu	Greenville, North Carolina
2001	Natalie Roy	California
2002	Steven Korkola	Regina, Saskatchewan
2003	Edward Chedrawy	Stanford, California

* Deceased
** Professor or department head

CARDIAC SURGERY AT HOSPITALS AFFILIATED WITH THE UNIVERSITY OF MONTREAL

Notre-Dame Hospital
(Hôpital Notre-Dame)

Dr. Normand Poirier and Dr. Léo La Flèche

The history of cardiac surgery at Notre-Dame is closely associated with the development of the other hospitals within the University of Montreal network. In the beginning, surgeons would operate at several sites pursuing their careers in various hospitals at the same time.

Dr. Edouard Gagnon (1900-1976) graduated from the University of Montreal in 1942. He began his surgical training at Notre-Dame Hospital and Ste. Justine Hospital, then served in the Canadian navy for two years before resuming his training at the University of Toronto from 1945-1948, being enrolled in the highly respected Gallie Course. Returning to Montreal, he joined the surgical staff of Notre-Dame Hospital and the University of Montreal Medical Faculty, orienting his career in general and thoracic surgery. After a visit to Charles Bailey in Philadelphia, Dr. Gagnon performed the first mitral commissurotomy in Quebec at Notre-Dame Hospital along with cardiologist Paul David in February 1950, about the same time as Wilfred Bigelow's first such operation in Toronto.

In 1954 Dr. Gagnon became the first chief of the newly created section of cardiothoracic surgery at Notre-Dame. He was a co-founder in 1954 of the Montreal Heart Institute; where on July 3, 1957, he performed, with the assistance of Dr. Léo La Flèche, the first open-heart operation in Quebec using extracorporeal circulation. (The operation took place at Maisonneuve Hospital where the institute was then located with a separate administration.) The patient was an adolescent boy with an atrial septal defect and the result was excellent.

Cardiac surgery was in its infancy and subsequent cases of open-heart surgery were less successful. It was thus decided to put the program on hold for a period of time and Dr. Gagnon decided to focus on thoracic surgery at Notre-Dame Hospital. He remained however the senior consultant in surgery at the Heart Institute from 1954 to 1959. At Notre-Dame he made important contributions in the treatment of traumatic rupture of the tracheobronchial tree. In addition to his surgical contributions, he was an excellent ambassador for Quebec. He was at ease in both French and English and greatly enjoyed the inter-relationship with the anglophone community as well as with the Canadian and American Associations. He was a strong participant in the affairs of national and international associations and was considered by many as the voice of French Quebec in cardiac surgery.

Gagnon gradually built the team of cardiac surgeons at Notre-Dame by bringing with him Dr. Léo La Flèche, and then Drs. François Telmosse and Alfred Joassin. Léo La Flèche was a 1950 graduate of McGill University and obtained his entire surgical training at Tulane University-Charity Hospital in New Orleans (1950-1955) under Dr. Alton Ochsner. When he returned to Montreal in 1955, he spent an additional year as chief resident at the Montreal Heart Institute and then joined their staff from 1956-1959. At the same time, he held an appointment at Notre-Dame, and this is where he would pursue his career after 1959, becoming chief of thoracic surgery between 1972 and 1978. Beginning in 1970, he was also appointed to the surgical staff of the Montreal Chest Hospital and was later granted operating privileges at the Montreal General Hospital. Most of his contributions were in the field of thoracic surgery. As the organization of cardiac and thoracic surgery at Notre-Dame was difficult during that period, he also practiced much of his surgery at the Montreal Chest Hospital after 1974. In addition to thoracic and vascular surgery, his interests included medico-legal issues. Between 1970 and the present, he has been very active in the field of medico-legal expertise, having evaluated over five thousand cases.

In 1978, cardiac surgery at Notre-Dame was performed by Drs. Telmosse and Joassin with the help of surgeons from the Montreal Heart Institute, primarily Drs. Yves Castonguay and Gilles Lepage. Regent Beaudet was recruited by Dr. Pierre Daloze, the new chief of the department of surgery at Notre-Dame Hospital, to rebuild the service. He was a graduate of the University of Montreal who had obtained the majority of his training under Frank Spencer at Bellevue Hospital-New York University. At first, upon his return to Montreal in 1972, he had started to work at Hôtel-Dieu but this period was brief. Upon his arrival at Notre-Dame, he completely took over the service. It became obvious that there was no longer any need for the help of the Montreal Heart Institute surgeons and he performed all the cardiac surgeries. Soon thereafter, however, the workload increased and he recruited Dr. Normand Poirier who was practicing at the Royal Victoria Hospital. Following these changes, Dr. Joassin concentrated his activities mainly in thoracic and vascular surgery. Dr. Telmosse also concentrated in the other two specialties and provided assistance in cardiac surgery.

As director of the program at Notre-Dame, Beaudet shared his workload with Poirier. Beaudet was concentrating increasingly on cardiac surgery but Poirier at this time remained a broad cardiovascular and thoracic surgeon, sharing his time between all three aspects of the discipline.

Poirier graduated from the University of Montreal in 1965. He completed his surgical training at McGill in CVT and then pursued a six-month fellowship in Boston in 1973. In Boston, he worked with Drs. M. Buckley and E. Mundt pursuing experiments on cardiogenic shock and left ventricular-assist techniques in the Myocardial Infarction Research Unit of the Massachusetts General Hospital. Returning to the Royal Victoria Hospital in Montreal he introduced the first intraaortic balloon pump in Quebec. He joined Beaudet at Notre-Dame in 1978.

In 1981, Dr. Albert Guerraty joined the service at Notre-Dame. Born in Chile, Guerraty received his medical degree from the University of Chile. He then completed his surgical residency at the University of Montreal. Beaudet organized a two-year fellowship for him in the Department of Surgery-Medical College of Virginia. He wanted him to come back to Notre-Dame and initiate a cardiac transplantation program. Guerraty worked for two years with Richard Lower in Richmond, Virginia, and when he returned to Notre-Dame, he was more than ready to start the program.

The following years saw two more additions to the service. The first one was Dr. Daniel Doyle who had trained at the University of Montreal and was sent for a fellowship with Dr. John Ochsner in New Orleans. He was soon followed by Dr. Denise Normandin who was also a product of the University of Montreal. After training in Montreal, she undertook fellowships in Toronto and San Diego, increasing her knowledge and skills in cardiac surgery as well as in intensive care management. When she returned to Notre-Dame, she completed a very strong team that worked well together.

Under Beaudet's direction, Notre-Dame was chosen to be the centre for clinical evaluation of the Medtronic-Hall mechanical valve. In order to achieve good follow-up, they put in place a service called the "Click Track Clinic." The sound of the disk was registered and compared with the registration of the preceding visit. If there was a change in the sharpness of the sound, the formation of a clot could be suspected and the patient was investigated more thoroughly. Eventually, this procedure was deemed insufficiently reliable and it was discontinued. (The documentation was done meticulously by the wives of Poirier and Doyle.) Poirier persisted in using this Medtronic-Hall valve prosthesis despite transfers between Notre-Dame and the Royal Victoria Hospital on two occasions. He would eventually present, in 1999, his twenty-year experience with this valve in Vienna. The following year, his work was published in the *COR Europaeum*. At the time, his personal series was the largest in the world with the longest follow-up, including data on more than 95 percent of his 650 implanted valves.

The transplantation program performed admirably. Unfortunately, this service underwent a turbulent period in the 1980s and many surgeons departed. Doyle went to Quebec City, Normandin left Notre-Dame. In 1984 Poirier and Guerraty moved to the Royal Victoria Hospital to pursue their work on heart and heart/lung transplantation. Nelson Nadeau, a skilled vascular surgeon, replaced Beaudet as the chief of service, which was then divided into three different components.

Dr. Denis Gravel, the newly appointed chief of the department of surgery, called upon Poirier at the Royal Victoria Hospital, offering him the opportunity to become the new chief of cardiac surgery and to rebuild the service. Poirier accepted and returned to Notre-Dame. His years at the Royal Victoria Hospital had been very rewarding. With Christo Tchervenkov, they had presented in 1984 at the American College of Surgeons a new type of coronary artery bypass, using the gastro-epiploic artery. There was angiographic follow-up on the patency of the bypass. At the same time, John Pym in Kingston had found similar use for the gastro-epiploic just a few weeks before Poirier.

Soon thereafter, Beaudet decided to take a sabbatical leave. His interest turned towards politics; he was elected to the National Assembly of Quebec in 1994 and would never return to the practice of cardiac surgery.

Returning to Notre-Dame in 1989 was not easy for Poirier despite the benefit of his experience in cardiac transplantation with Guerraty. There were many reforms going on across the province, budget cuts were taking place, and discussions were starting for the formation of a new University Hospital Centre for the University of Montreal. Hôtel-Dieu, St. Luc and Notre-Dame were to become one university centre. Discussions are still ongoing and it is undecided how cardiac surgery will eventually be structured in this context.

Nevertheless, clinical care had to continue and patients treated. Dr. Louis Normandin, a University of Montreal graduate, went for a fellowship in Paris. He returned to Notre-Dame in 1993 and became progressively more involved in cardiac transplantation and in lung and heart-lung transplants. Michel Martin, another graduate of the

University of Montreal, took his fellowship in Buffalo with Tomas A. Salerno and then traveled to South America and Italy. Upon his return to Notre-Dame in 1997, he started the beating heart coronary artery bypass program. Working with the cardiologists, they would combine coronary artery bypass to the LAD and dilatation to the other vessels. During this time, the lung transplant program was closed at McGill and had to be reorganized in another institution. After an initial attempt to develop lung transplantation at Laval Hospital in Quebec City, it was realized that it would be more suitable to have this program in Montreal, as the majority of patients were from that area. It was thus decided to centralize the lung program at Notre-Dame where it was already operating as the only program in Quebec. Dr. P. Ferraro started his training at the University of Montreal, then went to Laval in Quebec with Dr. Deslauriers and after a year at the Mayo Clinic he completed his training with Dr. Bartley Griffith at the University of Pittsburgh. He then returned to Montreal to take over the lung transplant program at Notre-Dame Hospital and continued its development in close partnership with Dr. L Normandin of the cardiac service with excellent results. A very close inter-hospital relationship now exists between the newly structured thoracic surgery service under André Duranceau and the cardiac surgery service. Normandin played an important role in this program from a cardiac point of view.

In March 2001, the tragic, sudden death of Martin at age forty-two greatly affected his close partners. Soon after, Poirier, also disabled by illness, had to discontinue his clinical activities. Again, the service was rebuilt by the addition of Jos Helou and Bao-Do. The Notre-Dame unit has gone through a lot of changes since its beginning but looks towards the future to play an important role in the structure of the University of Montreal Hospital Centre.

Hôtel-Dieu Hospital
(Hôpital Hôtel-Dieu)

Paul Cartier

Mercier Fauteux is described elsewhere as one of the genuine pioneers of cardiac surgery in the late 1930s and 1940s. In April 1939, he performed a ligation of the great coronary vein at Hôtel-Dieu for the relief of angina. He subsequently performed a few more such procedures with the addition of a pericoronary neurectomy.

Jacques Bruneau (1913-1985) had an immense influence on the development of thoracic surgery in Quebec. He was the director of the department of surgery at the University of Montreal between 1950 and 1956 and chief of surgery at Hôtel-Dieu from 1957 to 1970. A graduate of the University of Montreal, Bruneau began his training at Hôtel-Dieu under Armand Paré. He continued with a three-year fellowship in general and thoracic surgery at Barnes Hospital, Washington University in St. Louis from 1940-1943 under Evarts Graham and Peter Heinbecker. Graham was at the time one of the dominant figures in American surgery, renowned for his contributions to thoracic surgery including the first successful pneumonectomy for lung cancer. Jacques Bruneau was one of the first French-Canadian surgeons to train in the United States; previously most had gone to Europe and especially to France to acquire surgical skills.

When Bruneau came back to Hôtel-Dieu in 1943, it was obvious that his training had been different from that of his predecessors. He emphasized diagnostic precision with a thorough investigation and considered all the options before deciding on operative intervention. At operation dissection was meticulous and tissue trauma was minimized. He enjoyed teaching and, like Graham, did not tolerate mediocrity. Bruneau's self-imposed discipline produced excellent patient care and was an example to all associated with him. These characteristics were soon noted by his colleagues, who realized that he was transforming the surgical department in his institution. His operative technique greatly influenced the training of residents as he offered trainees the same discipline he had experienced in the United States.

Bruneau was the first surgeon at Hôtel-Dieu to close a patent ductus. A visionary of health care delivery and teaching hospital organization, he proposed in 1950 a five-hundred-bed teaching hospital on vacant land adjoining the University of Montreal, but the plan was never implemented.

Paul Cartier completed his training in Montreal and followed this with a fellowship in Cleveland under Claude Beck who devised several operations aimed at indirectly improving blood flow to the myocardium. The Beck #1 operation consisted of applying an abrasive talc to the epicardium in the hope of creating inflow through inflammatory adhesions. The Beck #2 procedure was one of the most difficult Cartier was to witness. It consisted of a direct anastomosis between the descending aorta and the coronary sinus with the goal of producing retrograde perfusion of the coronary vasculature. Special clamps were designed to allow approximation of the aorta to the coronary sinus without interposing a bypass graft.

Cartier visited Charles Bailey in Philadelphia in the early 1950s to observe closed mitral valve surgery and did the first mitral commissurotomy at Hôtel-Dieu in 1953. Cartier later introduced the Vineberg internal mammary implant to Hôtel-Dieu. Jean Migneault, a prominent cardiologist at the hospital, studied a postoperative patient angiographically and showed an anastomosis between the implanted mammary artery and the left coronary artery. In 1958, Cartier performed a coronary endarterectomy, one of the first direct coronary operations ever done.

In 1958 Paul Stanley returned from his training at the University of Minnesota and started open-heart surgery at Ste. Justine's children's hospital the following year; subsequently, in 1963, he initiated direct valve surgery at Hôtel-Dieu. Réjean Baudet, another graduate of the University of Montreal, who had continued his postgraduate training with Frank Spencer at New York University, returned in 1973 and developed coronary bypass surgery at Hôtel-Dieu. When he moved to Notre-Dame Hospital, cardiac surgery at Hôtel-Dieu was taken over by Ignacio Prieto and Fadi Basile who performed the first coronary revascularization on a beating heart there in 1981.

Surgery at Hôtel-Dieu has always been a very strong department which attracted highly innovative surgeons. Their influence in Quebec is felt to this day.

Sacré-Coeur Hospital
(Hôpital du Sacré-Coeur de Montréal)

Robert Cossette and Arthur Pagé

Sacré-Coeur Hospital in the northern part of Montreal was founded by the Sisters of Providence in 1926. The hospital gained worldwide recognition as Dr. Norman Bethune worked there for three years after leaving the Royal Victoria Hospital, where he had become the first chief of thoracic surgery in 1933.

The birth of cardiovascular surgery at Sacré-Coeur in 1971 resulted from the work of two progressive individuals: Dr. André Proulx, chief of medicine, and Dr. Arthur Pagé, chief of surgery.

Pagé, a graduate of the University of Montreal, pursued his surgical training at Notre-Dame. During that time, he was exposed to the evolution of cardiac surgery by having the opportunity to work with Dr. Edouard Gagnon. In 1960, to complete his training, he went to Houston and spent an entire year with Michael DeBakey, Denton Cooley, and Stanley Crawford. Upon his return to Montreal, Pagé was at the forefront of the specialty. Before his arrival at Sacré-Coeur, the institution was a general hospital with a specific interest in pulmonary and orthopedic diseases. Arthur Pagé initiated arteriographic techniques and did the first aortic graft at Sacré-Coeur in July 1961.

A cardiovascular and thoracic surgery section was created in 1966 with Pagé as chief. In 1967 he was joined by Dr. Claude Mercier (1931-1987), a diploma course graduate of McGill, who had spent two years at Georgetown University with Charles Hufnagel. Mercier and another McGill graduate, Edward Charrette, obtained the first certificates as specialists in cardiovascular and thoracic surgery from the Collège des Médecins de Québec (Quebec College of Physicians) in 1967, the memorable year of Expo 67 in Montreal. Mercier performed the first permanent pacemaker implantations at the hospital. The quality of the surgical service under Pagé's direction was excellent, especially in the fields of vascular and thoracic surgery. The residents in the University of Montreal's CVT training program were already having rotations at Sacré-Coeur.

Cardiology patients were sent to Maisonneuve Hospital to undergo heart catheterization. Its Hemodynamic

Laboratory was at the time directed by Dr. Jacques Proulx, brother of André Proulx at Sacré-Coeur. When the Montreal Heart Institute relocated from Maisonneuve to Bélanger Street in 1965, it left a large vacuum at the mother hospital. Cardiac surgery continued at Maisonneuve under Dr. Roland Lévy, but to a much lesser degree. As the number of cases was rapidly diminishing, it was noted that approximately half of the referrals were coming from Sacré-Coeur. In addition, the population north of Montreal was increasing and it seemed opportune to develop a full cardiac surgery service at Sacré-Coeur. Lévy worked at both hospitals until 1975 when he returned exclusively to Maisonneuve (known since 1972 as Maisonneuve-Rosemont following its merger with Saint-Joseph de Rosemont Hospital).

In 1971, the infrastructure for cardiac surgery at Sacré-Coeur was put in place with the development of a catheterization lab and a cardiac operating room. This was made possible through generous contributions from private foundations. The first heart catheterization was performed in May 1971. During the same month, Roland Lévy successfully performed two mitral commissurotomies, in addition to the facility's first open-heart surgery with extracorporeal circulation, a successful homograft mitral valve replacement. On June 1, 1971, Lévy performed the hospital's first aortocoronary bypass. This great achievement was made possible with cooperation from Maisonneuve Hospital: Jean-Pierre Bertrand, a technician in hemodynamics, and perfusionist Yvon Roy worked at both institutions for a short period of time before coming permanently to Sacré-Coeur.

Robert Cossette was born in Tillbury, Ontario, and graduated from the University of Montreal. He pursued his surgical training at the University of Montreal and obtained a McLaughlin traveling fellowship that allowed him to train in Boston for a year. Upon his return to Montreal in 1970, Cossette worked at Maisonneuve-Rosemont until 1976, when he became chief of cardiovascular and thoracic surgery at Sacré-Coeur.

Dr. Léon Dontigny arrived in 1971. Following his undergraduate and specialist training at the University of Montreal, he completed his apprenticeship with a two-year stay at the Cleveland Clinic. In addition to cardiothoracic surgery, he was responsible for the Advanced Trauma Life Support Program in the province of Quebec and often lectures on the subject of trauma.

Dr. L. Conrad Pelletier, who has had a widely varied career, joined Sacré-Coeur in 1972. After his graduation and initial surgical training at the University of Montreal, he spent two years in the department of physiology at the Mayo Clinic in Rochester, Minnesota. His clinical career took place at Sacré-Coeur and the Montreal Heart Institute, where he became chief of surgery in 1979. He was also chairman of the department of surgery at the University of Montreal from 1986 to 1994. Pelletier eventually obtained an MBA from the École des Hautes Études Commerciales (HEC Montréal), affiliated with the University of Montreal. His interest in administration led him to key administrative positions at Sacré-Coeur, the Montreal Heart Institute, Ste. Justine Hospital, and finally, with the Quebec Ministry of Health. Recipient of a large number of awards, he is still active in health care planning.

Alain Verdant has also been a prominent figure at Sacré-Coeur since 1974. Born in France, he trained at the University of Montreal and the University of Toronto. His interest in the pathology of the great vessels resulted in widely recognized achievements in the treatment of thoracic aortic disease. Verdant gave the Bigelow Lecture at the 1995 Canadian Cardiovascular Society Meeting on the surgical treatment of descending thoracic aneurysms.

Pierre Pagé joined this group in 1982. He had developed a special interest in anti-arrhythmia surgery during his fellowship at University of Alabama. Upon his return to Sacré-Coeur, he developed an excellent working relationship with Dr. Réginald Nadeau, a respected cardiologist also interested in electrophysiology. Together, they developed a surgical approach to anti-arrhythmia surgery for which Pagé received international recognition.

Finally, Richard Baillot was on the hospital's staff from 1984 to 1995. His meticulous work and dedication to coronary artery surgery allowed him to obtain excellent results. He had gained this expertise from a two-year fellowship at the Cleveland Clinic.

Cardiac surgery in Quebec has greatly benefited from the influence of Sacré-Coeur. Robert Cossette was for many years director of the University of Montreal's Cardiovascular and Thoracic Surgery Residency Program. In this capacity, he influenced many trainees and contributed to their career development. As a new century begins, the hospital is looking towards expanding its expertise into robotic surgery.

St. Luc Hospital
(Hôpital St-Luc)

Guy Roberge

Cardiac surgery at St. Luc, which forms part of the University of Montreal Hospital Centre along with Notre-Dame and Hôtel-Dieu hospitals, followed the initial development of a Hemodynamic Service by Drs. Guy

Roberge and Oswaldo Ricco in 1974. By 1987, the service was performing a thousand cases of heart catheterization annually and it had become difficult to obtain enough surgical referrals. It was estimated at the time that four hundred patients per year would require surgery.

The case to develop a cardiac surgery program at St. Luc was presented to the regional authority and the provincial government. As early as 1989, it was recognized that the Quebec health care system's surgical capacity was insufficient and that expansion had to be considered. As a result, many new centres were opened for cardiac surgery throughout the province, among them St. Luc Hospital, which received approval from the Ministry of Health in 1992.

Cardiac surgical services had in fact been introduced gradually as early as 1990, when Drs. Yves Leclerc and Yves Castonguay from the Montreal Heart Institute performed a few procedures. In 1992, a formal surgical service was established at St. Luc. Dr. Keir Marshall Stewart came from Vancouver and took on the initial cases; he was joined soon afterwards by Drs. Pierre Ghosn and Yves Castonguay. Since that time, the service has continued to grow with seven hemodynamicians and two cardiac surgeons performing approximately 2,500 heart catheterizations, 850 angioplasties and 270 open-heart procedures annually.

Ste. Justine Hospital
(Hôpital Ste-Justine)

Claude Chartrand

Ste. Justine Hospital is a large institution combining a tertiary pediatric hospital with a full department of obstetrics and gynecology. Its first heart operation was performed in 1953 by Paul Cartier, whose primary affiliation was with Hôtel-Dieu.

In 1958, Paul Stanley joined the hospital on a full time basis. A quiet, hard-working bachelor, he devoted his entire time and attention to caring for children suffering from cardiovascular disease. After graduating in medicine from the University of Montreal in 1951, Stanley began his surgical training in the hospitals associated with the university, followed by a fellowship at the University of Minnesota, then in its heyday as a leader in intracardiac surgery. Supported by a McLaughlin Fellowship, he traveled for almost a year through the United States and Europe to observe the techniques and philosophies of leading surgeons. His first open-heart procedure took place in 1959 and he was designated chief of the cardiovascular surgery service in 1963. Stanley achieved excellent results throughout his career and is an unsung pioneer in the development of pediatric heart surgery in Canada.

Claude Chartrand was a strong addition to the service when he joined Stanley in 1971. After his graduation and specialist training in the University of Montreal network, he spent two years as a research fellow at Stanford University gaining first-hand knowledge from the leaders of heart transplantation. Another recipient of a McLaughlin Fellowship, he traveled extensively for a year visiting the University of California, University of Utah, Cambridge University and La Sorbonne. On returning to Ste. Justine, Chartrand established an experimental laboratory and was a Medical Research Council of Canada scholar from 1971 to 1976. He produced a large number of valuable papers documenting advances made in his laboratory with a major focus on cardiac transplantation.

Stanley and Chartrand, working as a team, established cardiac surgery at Ste. Justine and in 1984 performed the first pediatric heart transplant in Canada. The tradition they began is continued today at Ste. Justine by cardiac surgeons Suzanne Vobecky and Nancy Poirier.

CARDIAC SURGERY AT THE MONTREAL HEART INSTITUTE

Claude M. Grondin

The following is a brief account of a group of individuals who gathered in Montreal in 1954 under the roof of a small newly created heart centre which would inspire physicians and health-care planners in North America and abroad. While the development of cardiac surgery in the mid-1950s rested on the shoulders of a handful of pioneers worldwide, the Montreal Heart Institute (MHI) was created almost solely by a single individual, its founder, Paul David (1919-1999).[1]

In 1949, Albani Paquette, health minister in the Duplessis cabinet, agreed to build a five-hundred-bed hospital in northeastern Montreal, to be owned and run by the Order of Grey Nuns. Maisonneuve Hospital was incorporated the following year and construction began in May 1950. The hospital opened in early 1954.

Meanwhile, Paul David, a young cardiologist on the staff of Montreal's Notre-Dame Hospital, was approached in 1951 by Mother Thérèse Courville, superior general of the Order, to lead the cardiology service of the new facility. David had spent his college years in Paris before the war and obtained his medical degree from the University of Montreal in 1944. He had been at Notre-Dame since 1947, following two years of residency in some of the best training programs in the field: in Boston, with Paul Dudley White at the Massachusetts General Hospital, and in Paris, with Jean Lenègre at Lariboisière Hospital. Upon his return to Montreal, David had made a name for himself in collaboration with thoracic surgeon Édouard Gagnon, who performed a surgical correction for a coarctation of the aorta in 1948, and more significantly, the first mitral commissurotomy in Canada in February 1950.[2]

In 1952, in response to the Grey Nuns' offer, David suggested that he be allowed to operate a cardiology unit administratively independent from the main hospital, on the model of the Montreal Neurological Institute (MNI). Founded in 1934 by American-born neurosurgeon Wilder Graves Penfield (1891-1976), the MNI had by then acquired a worldwide reputation for excellence. David and the nuns would also have known of the world's first heart centre, the National Institute of Cardiology (Instituto Nacional de Cardiología) in Mexico, founded by Ignacio Chávez in 1944. The nuns promptly agreed to David's plans and added a tenth floor to the building already under construction. The unit would consist of forty-two beds, a cardiac catheterization laboratory, an operating room, a clinical laboratory and an outpatient facility. One smaller floor above the tenth floor was to house the surgical experimental lab and a conference room. No hospital in Canada held this many cardiology beds. One man's dream was about to come true.

The Montreal Heart Institute opened for business on January 11, 1954, as the world's second cardiac *institute*, though in fact it had another elder sibling in Minneapolis. The Variety Club (an American nonprofit organization) had raised $1.6 million with the help of Hollywood's film industry led by Ronald Reagan, and built a four-storey unit next to the University of Minnesota Hospital, on the banks of the Mississippi River. The Minneapolis Variety Club Heart Hospital, with eighty beds, was officially opened in March 1951 by Oscar-winning actress Loretta Young. A long corridor linked the facility to the main hospital, where the operating rooms were located and where the world's first cardiopulmonary bypass operation was to take place precisely one month after the opening of the heart centre.[3] Whether David or the nuns had visited this close cousin or the one in Mexico is not known, but it was felt at the time that the forty-two beds planned for the MHI would suffice.

From the outset, David surrounded himself with people he had known at Notre-Dame Hospital: in surgery, Édouard Gagnon (soon to be joined by Arthur Vineberg from the Royal Victoria Hospital); in cardiology, by Osman Gialloreto, Yvan Lessard, and Yves Desrochers, all from Notre-Dame; and by Ghislaine Gilbert in pediatric cardiology. Gilbert had just completed her residency at Johns Hopkins with Helen Taussig (who had helped Alfred Blalock develop his operation on blue babies and, at times, did not object to taking credit for it). Other members of David's staff included Léon Lebel, cardiologist at Hotel-Dieu; John Gauthier, in photography; André Grenier, in charge of the surgical lab; Henriette Tenaille, a social worker just in from France; and Sister Lucille Ouellette who was to head nursing. Finding himself short one hundred thousand dollars just before the facility was due to open, David paid a visit to federal health minister Paul Martin, Sr. The institute opened on schedule! Long after the establishment of Medicare, in the 1960s and seventies, David would continue to erase the hospital's perennial deficits through personal visits to the health minister's office.

Cardiac Surgery at the Montreal Heart Institute in 1954

The multiple techniques used in early open-heart procedures—Lewis's hypothermia, Gross's atrial well, Lillehei's cross-circulation, and Gibbon's cardiopulmonary bypass (CPB)—their complexity, and the subsequent abandonment of most of them, may partially explain the delay in adopting open-heart surgery (OHS) at the Montreal Heart Institute. The heart-lung machine was first used there on July 3, 1957, some time after Mustard's initial attempt in Toronto. John Callaghan was the first Canadian to use CPB for open-heart surgery. After training in Toronto with Wilfred Bigelow, Callaghan had moved to the University of Alberta and had done his first case in 1956 using the DeWall apparatus.[4] To better understand the delayed adoption of OHS in Montreal, one has to take into account not only the high failure rates of the various techniques but also the strong rivalries among the individuals who pioneered them.

At the end of October 1955, Tom O'Neil, Charles P. Bailey's assistant in Philadelphia, came to Montreal at David's suggestion (as well as, presumably, Édouard Gagnon's invitation) to demonstrate the atrial well technique. David had met O'Neil in Paris at the first World Congress of Cardiology in 1950. He had served as a translator between O'Neil and the French surgical team which performed France's first mitral commissurotomy.[5] In 1955, neither O'Neil nor Bailey had much faith in CPB, as both were staunch advocates of Gross's atrial well for the closure of ASD. O'Neil did four ASD closures while at the institute and impressed everyone with his skill. (He did not perform any closed heart operations as Gagnon was an expert in that field.) Did O'Neil's visit dampen enthusiasm for true open-heart surgery and delay the use of CPB? Was this part of the plan for the invitation? Probably not, although in those days quite a number of physicians and surgeons were opposed to CPB, some for religious reasons. Did not one play God with cardiac arrest? Gagnon was certainly not part of this marginal group, yet he was never a fervent proponent of CPB either, although along with several others he pioneered the technique in Canada.

Surgical Recruiting and the First CPB at the Institute

As mentioned previously, Paul David had enticed Édouard Gagnon into coming to the institute. Gagnon had kept his appointment at Notre-Dame Hospital, where he did thoracic surgery, as had Vineberg at the Royal Vic. There were thus no full-time surgeons at the MHI in 1954. At that time a cardiology service, even one with forty-two beds, could hardly keep two cardiac surgeons busy. (In Minneapolis, perhaps it would, but not in Montreal.) Gagnon and Vineberg assisted one another for the institute's first mitral commissurotomy in February 1954 and Vineberg did his first internal mammary artery implantation there one month later. The following March, Gagnon interposed a segment of human aorta to correct a long coarctation, a première in Québec. He and Léon Katz had just established the first homograft bank in the province.

The institute's surgeons were not impressed with Lewis's inflow occlusion or Swan's masterly use of hypothermia, and even less so with Lillehei's cross-circulation technique or Gibbon's machine. The latter appeared complex and cumbersome. On the other hand Katz, who would eventually set up the heart-lung machine in the lab and later in the operating room, was impressed with DeWall's device and his publications on the subject. David and Gagnon agreed to have him examine it in Minneapolis. Upon his return, Katz was convinced he could construct a machine similar to DeWall's and ultimately use the apparatus in humans. Several other early investigators had gone this route before and built units akin to the Minneapolis device.

A brilliant engineer, Léon Katz had previously assisted David in the construction of the institute's OR and its surgical and cardiac catheterization laboratories. In setting up the cath lab, Katz had obtained the assistance of Osman Gialloreto, a young Italian cardiologist whom David knew from Notre-Dame. Gialloreto, a graduate of Padua, had begun a residency at Notre-Dame in 1951. He had trained in cardiology in Switzerland with Mahaim and between 1948 and 1950 at Boucicault Hospital in Paris with Lenègre. Cardiologist André Cournand, who would be awarded a Nobel Prize in 1956 for his contribution to the development of cardiac catheterization,[6] was a frequent visitor to Boucicault and had been instrumental in setting up Lenègre's cath lab. Unable to obtain an appointment in war-torn Europe following his two years with Lenègre, Gialloreto emigrated to Canada and although fully trained, applied for a residency in cardiology at Notre-Dame. A short time later, he teamed with Paul Brodeur and Jean-Louis Léger of the radiology department in setting up an angiography room with the Picker Company's new X-ray apparatus.[7] This system allowed the rapid taking of six pictures following peripheral injection of contrast material. Impressed with the young man's knowledge and background, David convinced Gialloreto to establish the institute's cath lab in 1954. Following a four-month stay in Sweden, Gialloreto arranged to install the first Schönander biplane angiography system in North America. A team from the National Heart Institute in Bethesda, Maryland, visited the MHI to observe its cath lab before buying their own Schönander biplane. At the institute, Gialloretto also took care of teaching and recruiting residents and staff. Ultimately, David appointed him as joint director of the institute.[8]

In the summer of 1957, after multiple trial runs in the lab with Katz's modified version of the DeWall-Lillehei machine, everything appeared ready for the first clinical procedure. In the interim, David had recruited a third surgeon to help Gagnon and Vineberg. The candidate, Jean-Louis Lamy, had spent some time in Minneapolis observing OHS on Lillehei's service. By 1957, OHS had become a daily routine in Minneapolis. Lillehei and Varco had their own service—Green and Orange surgery—and were surrounded by future leaders in the field. In addition to Dick DeWall, these included Norman Shumway, Walt's brother Richard Lillehei, Herb Warden, Morley Cohen, Vince Gott (who would a few years later take over Blalock's chair at Hopkins) and Christiaan Barnard, just in from Capetown. Aldo Castaneda would soon join from Guatemala. Yet Lamy and Gagnon had some difficulty in establishing rapport from the very beginning. The previous year, Leo Laflèche had also joined the group as a resident, probably upon Gagnon's recommendation. These two got along well. Laflèche, a McGill graduate, had trained for five years at Charity Hospital in New Orleans, where Michael DeBakey had taken his training, before returning to Montreal in 1956 as Gagnon's chief resident at both Notre-Dame and the institute.[9]

On July 3, 1957, eight-year-old Pierre Whissel underwent direct closure of a large secundum ASD with CPB, using a modified version of the DeWall apparatus. Laflèche worked with Katz on the heart-lung machine while resident Sam Liang scrubbed and assisted Gagnon. (Lamy had not yet been appointed.) The patient did well and was discharged two weeks later. This proved to be Québec's first successful attempt at OHS with cardiopulmonary bypass.

Anthony Dobell, trained in Philadelphia with Gibbon, was the second surgeon in Québec to use a heart-lung machine. On November 17, 1957, Dobell closed an ASD, also of the secundum variety. The same year also witnessed the beginning of open-heart surgery with CPB in Toronto, Winnipeg and Vancouver.[10] In March 1959, Joffre Gravel in Québec City operated on his first patient (presenting with pulmonary stenosis) using CPB, with Dobell in attendance.

In 1958, David recruited a second candidate, Gilles Lepage, whose surgical training had made a strong impression on him. Lepage had spent three years in general surgery at Vanderbilt University in Tennessee and was about to return from England after two years of training in cardiothoracic surgery, including a year with Russell Brock in London. The new recruit would begin in early 1959. According to David, Lepage was even-tempered and easy-going. Unlike Gagnon and Lamy, he got along with everyone from day one. Eventually, these particular qualities would help him become one of the founding members of the Quebec Association of Cardiovascular and Thoracic Surgeons. Gilles Lepage and the similarly affable Wilfred Bigelow also cooperated on several ventures and became close friends.

At the end of 1958, Gagnon, whose philosophy more often than not appeared to be at odds with that of David (who kept a close eye on the daily workings of all services including surgery) decided to return to Notre-Dame full-time. He was followed *the very same day* by both Laflèche and Vineberg who returned, respectively, to Notre-Dame and the Royal Vic. David promptly appointed Lamy head of cardiac surgery. Gagnon soon brought Katz to Notre-Dame to begin an OHS program there. Katz also assisted cardiologist André David (no relation to Paul) set up its cardiac cath lab. The institute thus needed to recruit a new technician to run the heart-lung machine. Jacques Lussier, who had established the cath lab at the Ste. Justine pediatric hospital, joined the MHI surgical team in early 1959 and began a long career as the head of perfusion, establishing in the process the first training school for perfusionists in the province. Laflèche, for his part, limited his work at Notre-Dame to thoracic surgery and closed heart operations. Vineberg, who never performed open-heart surgery at the MHI and only a handful of cases at the Royal Vic, pursued his work on mammary artery implantation at McGill and attained fame for these procedures in the early 1960s.

Édouard Gagnon would ultimately return to the institute in 1975 to undergo coronary artery bypass grafting. He developed deep venous thrombosis and succumbed to a pulmonary embolus a few months later. This Canadian pioneer of open as well as closed heart surgery was only sixty!

Following Gagnon's departure from the MHI, Lamy began to put his personal mark on the service. In the lab, where he had been allowed to spend ample time during his former boss's tenure, he had begun working with the Kay-Cross oxygenator. (Many other investigators had also adopted the Kay-Cross, including Gross in Boston who was not about to kneel at Minneapolis's altar, as his request for a residency in Wangensteen's program had once been denied.) Lamy boldly decided to do away with the "bubbler," and published the institute's first fifty OHS cases using Cross's machine and discounting those performed by his predecessor with the DeWall oxygenator.[11, 12]

Lepage had not really worked with Gagnon's team since he arrived shortly before its departure. He accepted

Lamy as his new chief and went about creating his own niche: the postoperative care of OHS patients (he had been in charge of the surgical intensive care unit on Brock's service in London), and the implantation of cardiac pacemakers for atrioventricular (AV) heart block. In those days, complete AV block was not uncommon following surgical closure of a VSD. There was in addition the more common "medical" AV block that occurred in older patients. Paul Zoll in Boston had begun to address the problem of this form of block a few months earlier.

Implantation of Pacemakers

Lepage implanted the first pacemaker at the MHI (Electrodyne, transthoracic) on July 21, 1961, a few weeks after the first Canadian implantation by Bigelow's group in Toronto. Between 1961 and 1973, this patient underwent nine operations for lead breaks or battery failures before technology improved in these two areas. Claude Meere, who joined the MHI team in 1969, established a pacemaker clinic made necessary by the high volume of pacemaker implantations: greater than two hundred annually, beginning in 1974. In 1979, the Sixth World Congress on Pacing—coinciding with the first issue of *Pace*, a medical journal devoted entirely to cardiac pacing[13]—was hosted by Meere in Montreal. Meere, along with Seymour "Sy" Furman, Victor Parsonnet and others, was elected to its editorial board. Fittingly, the Toronto group led by Bernard S. Goldman also joined the editorial board. In time, transthoracic pacemakers were replaced by the transvenous ones which ultimately became the domain of invasive cardiology (in the early 1990s). Toward the end of the nineties, the converter-defibrillator followed suit and was implanted in the cardiac cath lab.

Cardiac Surgery and the MHI: Both at a Crossroad

During 1958, with Gagnon, Laflêche and Vineberg controlling OR time, Lamy had had little opportunity to do open-heart operations, perhaps as few as six or eight cases! But in 1959, on his first year as head of the department, Lamy performed over sixty OHS cases with Lepage. Lepage, on the other hand, acted as the primary surgeon on barely a half dozen of them. The two surgeons did an equal share of closed heart operations, but Lamy, like Gagnon, kept the upper hand in all cases necessitating CPB. In that sense, Lamy treated his associate the same way Gagnon had treated him. During the 1950s, such a policy was accepted or tolerated. But with the revolutionary 1960s at the gate, this high-handed behaviour was bound to create havoc.

Predictably, at the end of 1961, Lamy could no longer go on running the department in this autocratic fashion and hinted in a letter to David (a fatal faux-pas on his part, as it turned out) that he might quit if David did not do "something" about the situation or—between the lines—about Lepage, his assistant. David promptly accepted the written offer of resignation from his head of surgery. Lamy had to step down![1] In part because of his limited clinical experience at the time, Lepage did not want to burden himself with what appeared to be a hot seat whose tenants were being ejected every other year. David therefore had to look outside the institute for a new chief of operations. This appointment would come from an unexpected source.

By early 1959, other changes were brewing at the MHI. Discussions began about the facility being too small and the need to look elsewhere for larger quarters, either on the parking lot of Maisonneuve Hospital or perhaps, on the University of Montreal campus where construction of a university hospital was to begin (supposedly soon). David was hesitant about the latter option, as the University wanted control over the institute's affairs. David met with premier Duplessis, who had been at odds with the University's rector for some time and thus preferred to have the institute build elsewhere. Duplessis offered David one million dollars to purchase land on the northeast side of Montreal, somewhat close to Maisonneuve but not on its grounds. But David's sister happened at the time to be the director of the small Marie-Enfant Hospital, a couple of blocks from Maisonneuve on Bélanger Street on a tract of land even larger than that of Maisonneuve Hospital.

David ultimately opted for the Bélanger Street site as the University insisted on controlling all matters, a nonnegotiable issue in the eyes of the institute's director. Construction began in 1964 on a 110-bed hospital, somewhat smaller than the two-hundred-bed unit planned for the university campus, but David planned to proceed in a stepwise fashion and enlarge the facility later on. In the interim, however, he knew that he first needed to find a new head of surgery, as Lamy had just "agreed" to move on.

Gaston Choquette, a young cardiologist, ended up acting as a go-between. Choquette happened to work at both MHI and Jean-Talon Hospital, where a request for vascular surgery privileges had been received from a French-Canadian surgeon training in Houston with Michael DeBakey and Denton Cooley, both world authorities in vascular and cardiac surgery. Informed of this by Choquette, David paid a visit to Cooley who operated at both Methodist Hospital with DeBakey and St. Luke's Episcopal Hospital, where Pierre Grondin, the "candidate," was the chief resident. David was both overwhelmed and devastated by this experience. To begin with, he was not even introduced to the head of cardiology, but instead was presented with a surgical service run entirely by surgeons, doing five or six open-heart operations a day (the equivalent of the institute's monthly caseload), all with no glitches or haste. David was thrown for a loop: at the institute in Montreal, everything "had" to be run by cardiology, for one thing, yet on the other, its surgical outcomes were only middling in his eyes, certainly not on a par with those he was privileged to witness in Texas. The message of "too many cooks" would eventually sink in.

Cooley knew about David's visit and let his chief resident operate on a lot of heart patients during the two weeks the director spent in Houston. The surgical cases were complex but the results were simple: the patients did well. David knew he had found his man. Grondin would arrive in January 1963. The new chief had been a general practitioner for three years before training in general surgery in Los Angeles and had then run a busy general surgery practice for another three years before going to Houston. He had experience, poise, and was coming from the world's busiest heart surgery program. David had no doubt the candidate would succeed in helping the institute open new vistas. It happened.

The Surgical Service Takes Off: The New MHI Is Built

In 1961, Lamy performed the institute's two hundredth open-heart operation. This, after four years of experience with CPB, amounted to one case a week, a modest output! Grondin and Lepage would do two hundred cases *a year* beginning in 1965. The one thousandth procedure was performed in 1967, and by 1984, the magic number of one thousand patients annually was reached. The MHI would long remain Canada's busiest OHS centre, until the Toronto General took over this distinction in the mid-1980s. Currently, between 1,800 and two thousand patients undergo OHS annually at the institute, yet to meet current needs and eliminate backlogs, this output should be increased to over 2,500. This would require fifteen to twenty additional surgical beds. An expansion project, launched in 2000, has been approved. Construction should begin in 2004-2005.

With the advent of coronary artery surgery, the volume of OHS grew rapidly. This increase coincided with the construction of a new five-storey wing on the east side of the main building that added fifty beds to the existing 110. The number of operating rooms doubled to four, with new intensive surgical and coronary care units and one additional cardiac cath room. The new facility opened in the fall of 1976. At about the same time, the institute received five million dollars from Jean-Louis Lévêque, a well-known Montreal financier whose initial million-dollar donation a decade earlier had launched the research service. Lévêque's donations ultimately totaled ten million and led to the construction of the six-storey research centre that bears his name.

In the mid-1960s, cardiac surgery at the institute as elsewhere was equally divided between acquired adult (valvular) and pediatric (congenital) procedures. In the early 1970s, the pediatric cases moved to the Ste. Justine Children's Hospital. As a result, the number of juvenile patients at the MHI dwindled and the pediatric service closed down in the midseventies. Still, some adult congenital cases remained—ASD, VSD, old tetralogy of Fallot patients palliated with Blalock shunt procedures. In the mid-to late 1980s, Yves Leclerc, who had trained in Birmingham, Alabama, and Toronto, began taking charge of the adult congenital caseload. More recently, the MHI has become the operating centre for Ste. Justine's over-aged patients to the point that nearly a hundred adult congenital cases are referred for surgery to the institute each year. Nancy Poirier, who trained at the Hospital for Sick Children in Toronto and at the Cleveland Clinic, has taken over this task. She also devotes slightly over half of her time to pediatric cardiac cases at Ste. Justine Hospital.

Valvular Heart Surgery

The first Bahnson's partial aortic cusp replacement at the MHI took place in September 1962, and the first total cusp replacement three months later. The first aortic valve replacement (AVR) with a Starr-Edwards prosthesis occurred in June 1963. (Six years later, it needed to be replaced due to ball variance.) The first mitral replacement was carried out seven months after the first AVR, following several unsuccessful attempts. (One of these occurred in Gagnon's patient, Canada's first mitral commissurotomy, whose symptoms had recurred after thirteen years.) Patients with long-standing mitral valve disease often represented a greater operative risk than those with aortic valve disease, due to the presence of pulmonary hypertension. Intraoperative myocardial protection may also have played a role: Aortic replacement required direct canulation and perfusion of the coronary arteries, whereas during mitral replacement intermittent unclamping of the aorta was used to insure coronary perfusion. The intermittent unclamping of the aorta often filled the coronary vessels with air bubbles resulting in myocardial ischemia. The first tricuspid valve replacement with a ball valve prosthesis was performed in December 1963. Double replacement, with a Starr-

Edwards prosthesis for the mitral valve and a Magovern prosthesis for the aortic valve, took place the following May. The first triple valve replacement, a technical feat in that era, occurred in June 1968—although this "exploit" was overshadowed by the institute's first heart transplantation one month earlier, as discussed below.

In the early 1970s, biological prostheses were used with greater frequency at the institute, which led some years later to frequent reoperations for wear and tear on the leaflets. This occurred at about the same time that reoperations became necessary in patients with saphenous bypass grafts to the coronary arteries. Thus, in the mid-to late '70s, reoperations of all sorts became a speciality in themselves and accounted for nearly 20 percent of the surgical workload. This percentage has dropped by more than half in the last decade due to greater use of the internal mammary as a conduit in CABG and, in valvular heart disease, to more frequent use of valvuloplasty and of mechanical prostheses.

The first resection for acute dissecting aneurysm of the aorta at the MHI was performed in November 1963. Although diagnosed—and approached—as an acute type B dissection (descending aorta), presenting with thoracic and abdominal pain accompanied by disappearance of unilateral leg pulse and limb ischemia, in retrospect it is clear from the operative findings that the patient had a type A dissection of the ascending aorta. The procedure was done through a left thoracotomy and partial (left atrium to femoral artery) bypass. As recommended by DeBakey, the proximal anastomosis was to the outer layer of the dissection (thus allowing reentry) and the distal one to the inner layer. All signs and symptoms disappeared after surgery, including the limb pulse which returned to normal. When last seen in 1999, the patient was doing well, thirty-six years after the operation. The first Bentall at the MHI was performed in 1973, although a few patients had previously had replacements of the ascending aorta for type A dissection without replacement of the aortic valve, the first in 1968. Not infrequently, such dissections led to a false lumen or recurrence as a leak at the anastomotic sites would fill the ascending aorta, left in place and wrapped around the graft to insure hemostasis. In the past few years, preservation of the valve has more frequently been achieved in cases of aneurysm of the ascending aorta and valvular insufficiency, whether or not accompanied by acute or chronic dissection. Bentall's procedure has remained a sound choice for chronic dissection in the case of Marfan's syndrome.

Cardiac Transplantation at the MHI: Canada's First

At the MHI, preparations for a heart transplantation program had been underway since Christiaan Barnard's initial success on December 3, 1967. After performing the first successful heart transplant in the United States on May 2, 1968, Denton Cooley did several more in the span of a few days. Before the end of the year, he would write five papers on his expanding series, and in January 1969, he reported seventeen transplants[14] including one with a ram's heart. Enthusiasm in Montreal mounted with Cooley's successes. Pierre Grondin visited his former mentor in Houston. Upon his return, he began to instruct and prepare the team of physicians, nurses and technicians. He soon went back to Houston with members of the team. In the interim, while presiding over the Inter-American Congress of Cardiology, Paul David met with Christiaan Barnard, who convinced him of the feasibility of heart transplantation. Everyone and everything appeared ready, including tissue typing and anti-lymphocyte serum. Surrounding hospitals were put on alert as potential donor sources. The first two donors came from nearby Jean-Talon Hospital.

The first transplantation took place on May 31, 1968. The donor's heart was unable to take over circulation satisfactorily and the patient died two days later. A second attempt three weeks later was successful: Gaétan Paris survived nearly six months and enjoyed life to the fullest with all the publicity and press clippings before succumbing to sudden death on November 30. The heart institute likewise shared the limelight. It boasted the world's second largest series (next to Cooley's) by the end of the year.[15] Heart transplantation put the MHI on the map, so to speak. The news astonished the Canadian medical community but it should not have, as it was natural for the country's most active open-heart surgery centre to lead the way.

The institute's reputation would remain but not the transplantation program. By the end of the year, several patients had died due to rejection. In early December, just after Paris, the longest survivor, passed away, David suggested that the transplant team suspend its clinical program until further notice. The hiatus would last fifteen years. Despite the moratorium, the Second World Heart Transplantation Meeting was held in Montreal in May 1969, under the auspices of the city and its colourful mayor, Jean Drapeau. The three-day meeting, organized and led by Grondin, was a success despite the doubtful future of heart transplantation. Scientific sessions were held in the institute's auditorium and social gatherings took place at the Biosphere on the Expo 67 grounds. Yousuf Karsh, the famous Ottawa photographer, was there to immortalize Barnard's profile. Elliott Rapaport, *Circulation*'s chief editor, was also in attendance but turned down a request to publish the meeting's proceedings in his journal. The proceedings appeared instead in the *Laval Medical Journal*. There would be no Third World Congress on Heart Transplantation (planned for Paris under Dubost's direction).

Heart transplantation resumed in 1983 with the Stanford group's report on cyclosporin as an effective agent in the prevention or treatment of graft rejection. (The drug had been found useful in kidney transplants in earlier studies.) Conrad Pelletier and Yves Castonguay, the latter a participant in MHI's earlier endeavour, began the transplant program anew in April 1983, after a briefing with the Stanford team in Palo Alto. Five patients underwent transplantation that year. Numbers reached twenty by 1987 and have remained in that range since. Although only about fifty heart transplants are performed per year in the whole province (forty-five in 2002), results have improved considerably with survival at one year greater than 80 percent and at five years greater than 70 percent. By 1983, Grondin and Lepage, the local pioneers, had departed. Grondin had gone to the United States and Lepage was partially retired. Michel Carrier spent two years in training with Jack Copeland at the University of Arizona and took over the program around 1988, a post he still holds today.

The Artificial Heart

In January 1983, Yves Hébert became the first North American physician allowed to visit Barney Clark, the patient whose heart William DeVries at the University of Utah had replaced with a Jarvik-7 artificial heart device the previous month.[16] Hébert and Michel Carrier implanted the first artificial heart at the institute in September 1987. Wilbert Keon in Ottawa had implanted Canada's first mechanical heart the previous year.)

Hébert and Carrier had spent several days along with their team in Utah, and then awaited the purchase of the expensive device by a donor as the provincial government was unwilling to foot the bill at the time. Since February 2000, the Thoratec mechanical heart (or an occasional Novacor model) has replaced the Jarvik series. A little over twenty-five patients had received a total mechanical heart as a bridge to transplantation as of May 2003, with a success rate of 70 percent. In most cases of failure, the patients have succumbed to multiple organ failure before transplantation could take place.

Between 1999 and June 2003, a total of sixty mechanical hearts have been implanted throughout the province of Québec, including fifty-three as a prelude to transplant. Of the latter, thirty-three patients received a new heart through transplantation and twenty-seven of them are still alive.

Coronary Artery Bypass Grafting

Scores of mammary artery implantations were conducted at the MHI between 1963 and 1969. Their number grew further after postoperative angiography demonstrated their efficacy.[17] Direct revascularization began in September 1969 with a saphenous vein bypass to the right coronary artery by Pierre Grondin, a few weeks after Paul Field in Sudbury, Ontario performed the first saphenous vein bypass in Canada.[18] A few weeks earlier, on May 29, a right coronary stenosis had been treated at the institute with a saphenous vein patch and, three years earlier, a vein bypass from the aorta to the left anterior descending artery had been fashioned to correct a congenital anomalous origin of the left coronary artery from the pulmonary artery. In the latter case, an angiographic study established the patency of the graft seven years later.[19] This 1966 operation preceded those of both René Favaloro and Dudley Johnson but not the one reported by Edward Garrett and co-workers.

In the fall of 1969, bypass grafting was also applied to the left anterior descending and the circumflex arteries. Sequential anastomoses[20] and circular vein grafts[21] to four or five branches were subsequently used. Later, beginning in 1972, the internal mammary artery was used as a bypass conduit.[22] Some years later and on a much smaller scale, the radial, the gastro-epiploic and the epigastric arteries were also utilized[23, 24] While the institute trailed the large U.S. centres chronologically in the development of CABG, it rapidly closed the gap through early postoperative angiographic evaluation of grafts and by publishing the results in major medical journals. In fact, it was myocardial revascularization and these postoperative studies, more than any other undertaking including heart transplantation that raised the MHI's profile in the scientific community. Multiple papers appeared in the literature and numerous presentations were given at various major medical meetings all through the 1970s and eighties on this single topic. This scientific endeavour established the facility as one of the major heart centres in North America.

The very first presentation on the subject came in fact from the institute's department of surgery at the American Heart Association's annual meeting of November 1970 in Atlantic City,[25] barely one year after the start of its direct myocardial revascularization program. The study underlined the relationship between graft flow rate at operation and postoperative graft patency. The abstract appeared in *Circulation* in October 1970. Two months later, Jacques Saltiel in radiology wrote on the improvement of postoperative left ventricular function after bypass grafting.[26] Numerous subsequent publications from the cardiology, radiology, and surgery services earned Martial Bourassa, Jacques Lespérance and Claude Grondin—and their respective department heads—the Lenègre prize in Paris, honouring the year's best work in cardiology from French-speaking countries worldwide. The prize also honoured the memory of France's most renowned cardiologist, Jean Lenègre, whose untimely death from aortic stenosis had occurred a few months earlier.

Once MHI's reputation was well established in America and overseas, an era of international exchanges began, which has continued to this day. France and Spain, among other countries, started to send young physicians for residency training in Montreal. Established cardiologists and cardiac surgeons as well as nurses and technicians crossed the Atlantic to learn from and exchange with Institute staff. This interaction likewise provided manpower to the MHI and ensured a steady flow of residents to the hospital. In the past, reliance on the University of Montreal for residents had often been affected by the mood of the University's committee on education, or that of the Dean—both of whom, as a matter of policy, did not look favourably on institutions such as MHI that were based out on the periphery (i.e., away from a full-service general hospital). Competing towers of Babel in their eyes.

The Spanish Adventure

The exchange between Spain and the MHI proved most beneficial to all parties. The accord, a product of friendly links between Pierre Grondin and Ramiro Rivera, head of surgery at Madrid's largest hospital, La Ciudad Sanitaria Provincial, began officially in 1972 between both provincial governments. Grondin had previously helped Rivera perform Spain's first Vineberg procedure, ultimately leading to that country's direct revascularization program. The accord was especially dear to the Canadian ambassador to Spain as it represented, in essence, Canada's first real exchange with Franco's Spain, spurned since the war by most countries including our own. Exchanges were eventually established at several levels so that coronary angioplasties in Spain also began under the guidance of the MHI. Over the years, more than fifty Spanish physicians have spent a year or more of residency training at the institute. In Spain, the accord extended to cities other than Madrid and to other medical specialties. In Canada, it likewise included other hospitals in Montreal and Quebec City and other medical fields such as general surgery and nephrology. In 1973, Rivera established Spain's first Society of Cardiac Surgeons and appointed Grondin its first president. It is safe to say that modern surgical and medical treatment of coronary artery disease in Spain began with this accord. It benefited the institute's physicians as well and provided them an avenue for teaching and research as well as access to a rich European culture. This humanitarian exchange may have been precisely what Paul David had in mind during the planning and construction of the Institute. Agreements with other countries were also established, including Santo Domingo, Belgium and Argentina; countries that, like Spain, continue to send young physicians for residency training at the Institute.

Coronary Artery Grafting (continued)

In 1984, a ten-year angiographic follow-up study comparing internal mammary artery and saphenous vein bypass grafts showed the distinct superiority of the former procedure.[27] This investigation, conducted at the institute, proved to be the first in the literature to establish this point clearly and would alter the techniques of coronary surgery in surgical centres around the world. It prompted a long editorial article by the writer in the specialty's most important periodical, the *Journal of Thoracic and Cardiovascular Surgery.*[28] A second editorial two years later by the same author in this journal served as the opening picture and background of *ABC World News Tonight* with Peter Jennings in July 1986 as a preview for a segment clip on coronary artery surgery in the United State.[29]

From the beginning, coronary artery grafting was carried out with CPB. Early on, some surgeons, Jay Ankeney[30] in Cleveland for one, recommended bypassing the right and sometimes, the left anterior descending arteries without CPB. The idea was rapidly abandoned, however, only to be rekindled years later, in the mid-1980s, mainly outside the United States.[31, 32] The idea took time to spread,[33, 34] while mini-invasive techniques (smaller incision, limited access) began to appear. In New York, Valvanur A. Subramanian, a former Lillehei trainee, began combining the mini-invasive approach and off-cardiopulmonary bypass (off-pump) grafting. Both novelties were severely criticized by the surgical establishment.[35, 36] Yet Raymond Cartier, who one day went to New York to observe Subramanian perform a triple bypass without CPB (though through a standard incision) was impressed. Upon his return, Cartier devised retaining instruments to stabilize the beating heart, something Subramanian was not making use of at the time, and began doing multiple grafts off-bypass. He soon extended the technique[37] to all his patients, whereas in most centres it was still reserved for older patients, who were more subject to temporary or permanent subtle cerebral dysfunction due to CPB. Cartier's instruments are now available in 70 percent of Canadian heart centres and are also used in Europe. (In the United States, disposable—and expensive—stabilizing instruments have taken over the market.) Since 1995, the technique has spread to most centres. Nowadays, off-bypass grafting is probably used in 25 to 30 percent of older patients in America. A recent randomized study may dampen the enthusiasm for this technique, however, as it showed a significant drop in postoperative patency in off-pump versus on-pump bypass grafting. Robotic cardiac surgery, which began during the same decade, has yet to be accepted and widely used. Skeptics are not convinced of the value of this procedure, which for the moment, remains a technique of the future.

Arrhythmia Surgery

Surgical treatment of cardiac arrhythmias (other than heart block) began in North Carolina in 1968 with the interruption of abnormal pathways in the Wolf, Parkinson and White Syndrome (WPW). In the case of atrial fibrillation (AF), the most common form of arrhythmia, modern treatment—through cardioversion—began earlier. The MHI surgical service may have pioneered this initiative not only in Québec but also in Canada.

Whereas *defibrillation* implies the application of an electrical shock using a direct or alternating current to the heart to terminate VT or VF, *cardioversion* attempts through a similar mechanism (but at a lower current intensity) to end an abnormal atrial rhythm such as AF or flutter. Cardioversion must be synchronized to the QRS to avoid a jolt in the vulnerable period of the electrical cycle. In VT or VF this is of no concern, as the heart has already "stopped."

True Surgical Treatment of Arrhythmias

Two individuals at the institute were to provide the impetus for the surgical treatment of arrhythmia: Denis Roy of the department of cardiology and Conrad Pelletier from the surgical service. Roy had applied for residency at Duke on Pelletier's recommendation, but the Carolina program was full at the time. John Gallagher there suggested that Roy apply to Maastricht where Hein Wellens was running the electrophysiology (EP) service. A phone call did the trick. After a year in Holland, Roy spent a year in Philadelphia with Mark Josephson, Leonard Horowitz and surgeon Alden Harken, Dwight's grandnephew. Roy returned to Montreal in 1982. Prior to coming to the MHI, Pelletier had rubbed shoulders with Reginald Nadeau, the local arrhythmia expert, during his seven years at Sacré-Coeur Hospital. He had been intrigued by the emerging surgical specialty, although no arrhythmia surgery was being performed at the time at Sacré-Coeur. So, on March 28, 1983, Pelletier and Roy joined forces and performed the first intraoperative mapping (and endocardial resection) in a fifty-year-old male with a large ventricular aneurysm and ventricular arrhythmia. Although postoperative study showed no evidence of recurrence, the patient died of cardiogenic shock two months later. Six months afterwards, they performed the first successful interruption of abnormal AV tracts in a young man with WPW. Interruption of these tracts in the EP lab was to take place six years later at the MHI, on May 1, 1989. The first surgical implantation of a cardioverter-defibrillator was done by Yves Leclerc on January 15, 1988. The first implantation of a defibrillator in the cath lab occurred a decade later on July 1, 1998.

In 1996, Pierre Pagé who like Leclerc had trained in Alabama (with Albert Waldo) and had introduced arrhythmia surgery at Sacré-Coeur Hospital joined the institute and began using Cox techniques for AF. The first Maze procedure was performed on June 8, 2001, and scores of others have been done since, all along with other operations for either valvular or coronary artery disease

The Formation of the MHI Surgical Service

From the beginning, the department of surgery was fashioned by Paul David, the institute's director and founder. During MHI's first decade, every appointment to the surgical staff was indeed his doing, including Édouard Gagnon, Arthur Vineberg, Léo La Flèche, Jean-Louis Lamy, Gilles Lepage, and Pierre Grondin. By the time Grondin arrived in 1963, the first four had departed. Yves Castonguay, who joined the group in 1965, was recruited by Lepage and Grondin. Subsequent heads of the service were appointed by a committee presided over by the University of Montreal, yet formed at David's discretion until he retired in 1985. In the early 1970s, the University board decided that all appointments to its affiliated hospitals were to be for four years and nominations would last only two terms. Thus, in 1975, Lepage replaced Grondin who had in fact spent three terms at the helm. As Lepage did not wish to serve a second term, the search committee then drafted Conrad Pelletier from Sacré-Coeur Hospital. All subsequent directors of the department have stayed on for two terms; thus, Yves Leclerc succeeded Pelletier in 1987, and was followed by Michel Carrier in 1995 and Michel Pellerin in 2003.

Through the years, several directors of the surgical service took it upon themselves to renew the troops with strong "draft choices." Following their cardiothoracic training in University of Montreal hospitals, these individuals were sent to major surgical centres in Europe as well as in the United States to obtain additional expertise in specific fields of activity in both research and clinical practice. In this regard, the work and vision of Pelletier and Carrier must be praised, for the results leave little doubt as to their foresight and wisdom. As a case in point, the growth in the number of OHS cases in recent years has paralleled that of papers published annually by the surgical staff in major medical journals. It is apparent also that nearly all members of the service have participated in this effort. In 2002, for instance, more than half of the dozen papers published by the service in refereed American journals came from different authors. The hiring in the meantime of general practitioners to provide coverage on the ward and in the OR, along with an increase in the number of surgical residents, has helped free surgeons for research and publishing. Moreover, in the interim, vascular surgery has diminished (by general consensus) and pacemaker implantations have all but disappeared from the daily surgical schedule. These changes have also provided the surgical staff with more time for research.

Several new members have joined the service in the last dozen years as others have left or retired. Each decade has coincided with the addition, more or less, of three new members. Thus, in the late 1960s and early seventies, Claude Meere, J. P. Martineau, and Claude Grondin joined the group who had arrived in the 1960s (Pierre Grondin, Yves Castonguay) or late fifties Gilles Lepage). In the late 1970s, William Jones, Conrad Pelletier, and Yves Hébert came on board, followed in the 1980s by Yves Leclerc, Michel Carrier, Denise Normandin, and Raymond Cartier. During the 1990s, Michel Pellerin, Pierre Pagé, and Louis Perrault came onboard, and since 2000, Denis Bouchard, Nancy Poirier, and Philippe Demers have been recruited.

Over the years, meanwhile, various individuals have left the service. Gagnon, Vineberg, La Flèche and Lamy departed between 1958 and 1961. Jones and Normandin were to stay only two years before moving on to other institutions. By then Pierre Grondin had already left: In 1978, he became head of cardiovascular surgery at St. Francis Hospital in Miami. Lepage retired in 1990 as did Martineau in 1995. Castonguay and Meere both moved before retiring, Castonguay to Montreal's St. Luc Hospital in 1994 and Meere to the University of Sherbrooke two years later. Claude Grondin left in 1986 to succeed Fred Cross as head of cardiovascular surgery at St. Luke's Hospital in Cleveland. Both had graduated from the University of Minnesota surgical program under Wangensteen, Varco, Lillehei and company (Cross and Lillehei had in fact been co-trainees).

The last dozen or so members of the institute's surgical service took their cardiovascular training in Montreal. All except Hébert (a brilliant recruit, fully trained technically and academically), underwent two or more years of additional training in major American or European centres as planned, each gaining exposure to a particular field of cardiac surgery: Cardiac transplantation was covered by sending Carrier to Arizona with Jack Copeland, congenital heart operations by Poirier spending a year apiece in Toronto and at the Cleveland Clinic, and mitral valve repair by Pellerin working for two years in Paris with Alain Carpentier. Pelletier and Cartier spent two and three years respectively at the Mayo Clinic including a year or more in research. Pagé and Leclerc went to John Kirklin's program in Alabama, the former to work with Waldo in arrhythmia and the latter for adult and congenital heart surgery. (Before returning, Leclerc spent an additional three years in the Toronto program). Perrault spent three years in France obtaining a PhD, working with Menasché in Paris and Vanhoutte in Strasbourg. Bouchard went to the Cleveland Clinic for two years to learn mitral valve repair with Toby Cosgrove and all aspects of adult cardiac surgery at the busiest heart surgery centre in the United States. More recently, Philippe Demers returned after two years at Stanford University with special emphasis on surgery of the aorta with Craig Miller and on transplantation. An additional candidate is currently being trained in robotic surgery in Holland. Thus, most aspects of cardiac surgery appear well covered by candidates whose formation took place in the best surgical centres in the field, a testimony to wise advance planning by the department directors.

All of these individuals have followed in the footsteps of the handful of pioneers who opened the way here and elsewhere. These pioneers have not been forgotten. They are frequently awarded recognition in historical reviews, even in those of lesser length. Other participants in this endeavour must also be remembered. Special tribute should indeed be paid to one group of individuals whose contribution was invaluable, namely the patients of the early pioneers.

Often, in the narrative of firsts or breakthroughs, medical history neglects the contributions of those who made these achievements possible. Some participants even paid with their lives so that others who were to follow would survive. These are the unsung heroes, the unknown soldiers whose memory must be honoured, for they are responsible as much as the pioneers themselves for the successful development of open-heart surgery May they not be forgotten. Surgeons and heart surgery would not have overcome nature's limits without them.

Notes:

1. A. Jacques, *Une âme, une équipe: Docteur Paul David, Institut de cardiologie de Montréal* (Montréal: Édition Laporte et Cie, 1985).
2. E. D. Gagnon, "Commissurotomy in mitral stenosis," *Can Med Ass J* (1950), 63: 537-40.
3. G. W. Miller, *King of Hearts: The True Story of the Maverick Who Pioneered Heart Surgery* (New York: Times Books, 2000).
4. J. C. Callaghan et al., "The acid-base aspect of extracorporeal circulation," in *Extracorporeal Circulation*, J. Garrott Allen, editor (Springfield, Illinois: Charles C Thomas, 1958), 179-92.
5. C. P. Bailey et al., "Commissurotomy for aortic stenosis," *J Int Coll Surg* (1953), 20: 393-402.
6. A. Cournand and H. A. Ranges, "Catherization of the right auricle in man," *Proc Soc Exper Biol Med* (1941), 46: 462-66.
7. P. Brodeur, O. Gialloreto, and P. David, "L'angiocardiographie," *L'Union Med du Canada* (1953), 82: 373-79.
8. H. N. Segall, *Pioneers of Cardiology in Canada* (Willowdale, Ontario: Hounslow Press, 1988).
9. Léo Laflèche, personal communication (June 2003).
10. J. E. Wynands, "History of cardiac anaesthesia: the contribution of Canadian anaesthetists to the evolution of cardiac surgery," *Can J Anesth* (1996), 43: 513-84.
11. J. L. Lamy and L. Katz, "Chirurgie cardiaque à ciel ouvert et circulation extracorporelle: Notions théoriques et considérations sur les applications expérimentales et cliniques," *L'Union Méd du Canada* (1958), 87: 1027-32.

12.   J. L. Lamy et al., "Chirurgie à cœur ouvert. 50 cas cliniques," *L'Union Méd du Canada* (1959), 88: 1360-76.

13.   "The VIth World Symposium on cardiac pacing, Montreal, Canada, October 2-5, 1979: Abstracts," *Pacing Clin Electrophysiol* (1979), 2: A1-29.

14.   D. A. Cooley et al., "Organ transplantation for advanced cardiopulmonary disease," *Ann Thorac Surg* (1969), 8: 30-46.

15.   P. Grondin, in discussion of Cooley, *supra*.

16.   W. C. DeVries et al., "Clinical use of the total artificial heart," *New Engl J Med* (1984), 310: 273-78.

17.   M. G. Bourassa et al., "Criteria for internal mammary artery implantation based on cine coronary arteriography," *Can Med Assoc J* (1970) 103: 720-23.

18.   P. Field et al., "Direct myocardial revascularization: saphenous bypass grafts to the distal coronary artery. Technical details and postoperative hemodynamics," *Ann Thorac Surg* (1970), 10: 112-20.

19.   B. R. Chaitman et al., "Anomalous left coronary artery from pulmonary artery: An eight year angiographic follow-up after saphenous vein bypass graft," *Circulation* (1975), 51: 552-55.

20.   C. M. Grondin and R. Limet, "Sequential anastomoses in coronary artery grafting: technical aspects and early and late results," *Ann Thorac Surg* (1977), 23: 1-8.

21.   C. M. Grondin et al., "Optimal patency rates obtained in coronary artery grafting with circular vein grafts," *J Thorac Cardiovasc Surg* (1978), 75: 161-67.

22.   C. M. Grondin et al., "Coronary artery grafting with the saphenous vein or internal mammary artery:

Comparison of late results in two consecutive series of patients," *Ann Thorac Surg* (1975), 20: 605-18.

23.   L. P. Perrault et al., "Clinical experience with the right gastroepiploic artery in coronary artery bypass grafting," *Ann Thorac Surg* (1993), 56: 1082-84.

24.   L. P. Perrault et al., "Early experience with the inferior epigastric artery in coronary artery bypass grafting: A word of caution," *J Thorac Cardiovasc Surg* (1993), 106: 928-30.

25.   C. M. Grondin et al., "Aortocoronary vernous bypass grafts: Initial blood flow through the graft and early postoperative patency," *Circulation* (Oct. 1970), suppl 3, 42: 106.

26.   J. Saltiel et al., "Reversibility of left ventricular dysfunction following aortocoronary bypass grafts," *Am J Roentgen Rad Ther Nucl Med* (1970), 110: 739-46.

27.   C. M. Grondin et al., "Comparison of late changes in internal mammary and saphenous vein grafts in two consecutive series of patients 10 years after operation," *Circulation* (1984), 70 (3, pt 2): 1208-12.

28.   C. M. Grondin, "Late results of coronary artery grafting: Is there a flag on the field?" (Editorial) *J Thorac Cardiovasc Surg* (1984), 87: 161-66.

29.   C. M. Grondin, "Graft disease in patients with coronary bypass grafting: Why does it start? Where do we stop?" (Editorial) *J Thorac Cardiovasc Surg* (1986), 92: 323-29.

30.   J. L. Ankeney, "To use or not to use the pump oxygenator in coronary bypass operations," *Ann Thorac Surg* (1975), 19: 108-9.

31.   F. J. Benetti, "Direct coronary surgery with saphenous vein bypass without either cardiopulmonary bypass or cardiac arrest," *J Cardiovasc Surg* (1985), 26: 217-22.

32.   E. Buffolo et al., "Direct myocardial revascularization without cardiopulmonary bypass," *Thorac Cardiovasc Surg* (1985), 33: 26-29.

33.   A. J. Pfister et al., "Coronary artery bypass without cardiopulmonary bypass," *Ann Thorac Surg* (1992), 54: 1085-92.

34.   V. A. Subramanian et al., "Minimally invasive coronary bypass surgery: a multicenter report of preliminary clinical experience," *Circulation* (1995), 92 (suppl): I-645.

35.   B. W. Lytle, "Minimally invasive cardiac surgery," *J Thorac Cardiovasc Surg* (1996), 111: 554-55.

36.   D. J. Ullyot, "Look, Ma, no hands!" *Ann Thorac Surg* (1996), 61: 10-11.

37.   R. C. Cartier et al., "Systematic off-pump coronary revascularization in multivessel disease: Experience of 300 cases," *J Thorac Cardiovasc Surg* (2000), 119: 221-29.

38.   N. E. Khan et al., "A randomized comparison of off-pump and on-pump multivessel coronary artery bypass surgery," *New Engl J Med* (2004), 350: 21-28.

39.   P. L. Pagé, personal communication (May 2003).

Appendix

Members of the MHI Surgical Service:

Édouard Gagnon	1954-1958
Arthur Vineberg	1954-1958
Léo Laflèche	1956-1958
Jean-Louis Lamy	1957-1961
Gilles Lepage	1958-1988
Pierre Grondin	1963-1978
Yves Castonguay	1965-1994
Claude Meere	1968-1996
Claude Grondin	1969-1986
Jean-Paul Martineau	1971-1995
William Jones	1977-1979
Conrad Pelletier	1979-2000
Yves Hébert	1980-
Yves Leclerc	1985-1999
Michel Carrier	1987-
Denise Normand	1987-1989
Raymond Cartier	1988-
Michel Pellerin	1995-
Pierre Pagé	1996-
Louis Perrault	1997-
Denis Bouchard	2000-
Nancy Poirier	2000-
Philippe Demers	2003-

Important Dates:

Opening of MHI (at Maisonneuve hospital)	January 11, 1954
Opening of new center on Bélanger	January 6, 1966
Building of new wing (110 to 160 beds)	September 1976

First mitral commissurotomy at MHI	February 15, 1954
First IMA implantation (Vineberg) at MHI	March 1954
First CPB (Closure of ASD)	July 3, 1957
First closure of VSD	April 6, 1959
First correction of tetralogy of Fallot	October 12, 1959
First correction of Transposition (Mustard)	May 4, 1968

First Pacemaker implantation	July 21, 1961
First correction of acute dissecting aneurysm	November 9,1963

First aortic valve replacement	June 18, 1963
First tricuspid valve replacement	December 19, 1963
First mitral valve replacement	February 7, 1964
First double valve replacement	May 14, 1964
First triple valve replacement	June 11, 1968

First selective coronary arteriography	April 1964
First cardiac transplantation	May 31, 1968
First total replacement with mechanical heart	September 29, 1987
First coronary artery bypass	September 24, 1969
First bypass with IMA	June 12, 1972

First surgical correction of WPW	October 31, 1983
First correction of WPW in EP lab	May 1, 1989
First pacemaker in EP lab	October1987
First converter-defibrillator in OR	January 15, 1988
First converter-defibrillator in EP lab	July 1, 1998

First coronary angioplasty	February 13, 1980
First treatment of aortic stenosis in cath lab	September 19, 1986
First treatment of mitral stenosis in cath lab	March 4, 1987
First closure of ASD in cath lab	April 7, 1999
First closure of post MI VSD in cath lab	August 29, 2002

SHERBROOKE UNIVERSITY HOSPITAL CENTRE

Javier Teijeira, Gabriel Laberge, and
Bertrand Scalabrini

The University of Sherbrooke's Faculty of Medicine
and university hospital were founded during the "Quiet
Revolution" in Quebec. During this period, great reforms
were undertaken in education and socio-economic
development. The Faculty of Medicine, opened in 1964,
adopted a highly innovative practice plan for medical
personnel, and attracted teachers and researchers from
throughout North America and Europe. From the
beginning, surgical specialists were asked to develop a
cardiovascular and thoracic surgery department that
would offer services to the region and contribute to the
university's teaching and research mission.

On March 24, 1970, Claude Labrosse performed the first
open-heart intervention in Sherbrooke. This consisted
of the repair of an atrial septal defect with anomalous
venous return. He was assisted by Dr. Bernard Goldman
from the University of Toronto. The first chief of CVT
surgery in Sherbrooke was Sheldon Bergman, who was
followed by Claude Labrosse, Javier Teijeira, Daniel
Bonneau, again Javier Teijeira and Xavier Muller. Under
their leadership, the clinical service has progressed
steadily since its inauguration and four open-heart
procedures are currently performed annually.

Vascular and thoracic surgeries were performed mainly
at the Hôtel-Dieu, St. Vincent de Paul and Sherbrooke
hospitals, all affiliates of the Sherbrooke University
Hospital. Gabriel Laberge, Bertrand Scalabrini and
Robert Paulette contributed to the development of the
specialties at these centres. In 1995, the four hospitals

amalgamated to form the present "Centre Hospitalier Universitaire de Sherbrooke (CHUS)" at the Notre-Dame and Fleurimont (university) sites, under the direction of Javier Teijeira.

In addition to providing clinical services, the Sherbrooke Faculty of Medicine has contributed to training and research activities since its inception. Members of the CVT department were especially interested in surgical repair of the mitral valve, minimally invasive coronary bypass with all arterial conduits and endovascular management of aortic aneurysm. Over the years, the Unit has contributed to the dissemination of knowledge through publishing and through the organization of national and regional meetings.

QUEBEC HEART INSTITUTE (LAVAL HOSPITAL)

Michel Lemieux

Founded in 1918, Laval Hospital was, from the start, to be entirely devoted to the care of pulmonary disease— mainly tuberculosis, which at the beginning of the twentieth century was responsible for the death of two hundred Quebecers per hundred thousand annually. As was customary in education and health care at the time, it was administered by a religious order, the Sisters of Charity of Quebec. The site chosen was in the west end of Quebec City, up on the hill; the site was believed to be salutary as open and windy areas were considered essential in the treatment of tuberculosis.

In the mid-1950s, just as large TB sanatoria were being built across Quebec, an effective treatment for the disease was discovered, rendering these new institutions obsolete before construction was completed. Indeed, the central pavilion of the Laval Hospital, which today houses cardiology and cardiac surgery was completed in 1955. Laval thus became a general hospital and the western pavilion of the old TB Hospital was given to a new private corporation which called itself the Quebec Heart Institute.

In 1956, cardiology was a relatively new medical specialty, and although a fair number of people were diagnosed with heart disease, investigation was limited to auscultation and oxymetry: Cardiac surgery was practiced in only a few centres and made world news with every advance.

As in many other centres treating TB, chest surgery in Quebec was practiced mainly by orthopedic or general surgeons. There were few, if any, specialists in chest surgery at the time. As the need for surgical treatment of tuberculosis came to an abrupt end, surgeons became interested in other organs of the chest cavity, notably the heart and the great vessels which had until then, remained inaccessible to all but a few pioneers, and considered by many a no man's land.

The first and only formally trained chest surgeon in Quebec City, Maurice Beaulieu, had completed his training in 1955. He had been fortunate enough to observe Charles Bailey performing mitral commissurotomies in Philadelphia and in the neighboring state of New Jersey where Beaulieu had pursued part of his training. That was the extent of his training in cardiac surgery when he joined the Quebec Heart Institute in 1956.

However, the pioneering work of Bailey and Harken in the United States and of others in England and Sweden gave birth to the new surgical specialty of cardiac surgery and awakened the interest of many a young surgeon seeking work in overcrowded general surgical services. Indeed, cardiac surgery in the mid and late 1950s was a challenge suited only for the bold. Joffre-André Gravel was such a surgeon. He had completed his general surgical training in Quebec and was seeking a new field in which to establish a practice. After spending six months in Stockholm observing the work of Clarence Crafoord, Gravel went to London where Russell Brock was doing marvels in closed heart surgery. Upon his return, he joined the staff of the new Quebec Heart Institute as the second member of the cardiac surgery team. Gravel was quick to put his newly acquired knowledge into practice as he and Beaulieu performed the first cardiovascular procedure at the institute, repairing a coarctation of the aorta. Although the Institute's first interventions were successful, operations were few and far between and were limited to closed-heart procedures such as coarctation repairs, mitral commissurotomies and an occasional Vineberg procedure.

Beaulieu, however, was a full-time physician, earning $14,500 a year and spending a lot of time in the research laboratory setting up an extracorporeal circuit similar to the one described by Gibbon in Philadelphia. Here he gained the experience that eventually made the system suitable for clinical use. Finally, in October of 1959, Beaulieu, Gravel, and Jacques Matte, their technician from the beginning, felt ready for an open procedure which was to be a pulmonary valve commissurotomy. This first open cardiac procedure in Quebec City was to be quite an event. First, in order to have enough blood to prime the extracorporeal circuit, a call was issued on the air and a special blood donor clinic set up at the hospital. (As it turned out, most donors came from the army base at nearby Valcartier.) The patient, a man in his late twenties, was given the last rites the night before surgery and on the day of the operation, special prayers were said in the operating room by the Mother Superior in the presence of the surgical staff. Finally, and most importantly, Anthony Dobell, who had recently joined the surgical department at the Montreal Children's Hospital, was present in the operating room to share his expertise for the institute's first open-heart operation. Dobell's family had strong historical ties with Quebec City, as his great-grandfather, James Sewell, was dean of Laval University from 1863 to 1883, and his family was very involved in the local lumber business. He had trained in Philadelphia under the guidance of John Gibbon, who had first conceived a heart-lung machine that would make open-heart surgery possible. The operation, a day-long affair, was successful and the patient left the hospital a month later.

Despite these initial successes with the closed technique and one initial open-heart operation, due to lack of experience and the growing pains of cardiac surgery it remained at low volume throughout the early sixties.

André McClish was an anaesthetist who upon completing his training in Quebec and following a few visits to Montreal to observe cardiac surgery, decided to acquire expertise where it was needed, i.e., extracorporeal circulation. He enrolled in the Cardiac Surgery Program in Minneapolis where he not only observed and participated in the pioneering work of Lillehei and others, but primarily developed his own expertise in the physiology of extracorporeal circulation under Richard DeWall's guidance. Upon his return to Quebec City in 1960, he set about the task of developing an extracorporeal system at the institute. With the help of local engineers, he conceived his own system using a new nondisposable bubble oxygenator which was first used in patients in 1963. Although there were many structural problems with the system, the concept of a bubble oxygenator in 1963 was innovative and the principle withstood the test of time. It was, however, abandoned a few years later for lack of improvement as disposable bubblers became widely available.

Cardiac surgery in the early 1960s was mostly oriented towards the correction of congenital heart defects. The pioneering work of Lillehei, Varco, Kirklin and others, and the development of extracorporeal circulation had shown that open-heart surgery could be performed with relative safety in children and young adults. Adult cardiac surgery, however, awaited the development of reliable valvular prostheses.

Jean-Paul Després had trained in general surgery in Quebec and was offered a full-time appointment (still at $14,500 a year) in the department of surgery at the Quebec Heart Institute, on condition of acquiring further training in cardiac surgery. Since there was as yet no formally structured training program in the discipline, knowledge and expertise were acquired through preceptors. One such mentor for Després was Anthony Dobell at the Montreal Children's Hospital. Després visited regularly on days when Dobell was performing congenital surgery. Another was Gilles Lepage at the Montreal Heart Institute. Després traveled every week to Montreal for a full year, to either the Children's Hospital or the Heart Institute. In the winter of 1960-61, he visited Edmonton, Alberta where John Callaghan had just settled, and spent six months acquiring additional knowledge and experience in the surgical treatment of congenital heart disease, mainly the correction of tetralogy of Fallot. Després returned to Quebec in the summer of 1961.

For many reasons, including the lack of clinical expertise and appropriate equipment, cardiac surgery was slow to develop in Quebec City in the 1960s. The clientele consisted mostly of children referred by the one pediatrician in the area with training in pediatric cardiology, and every year the caseload reached barely a dozen. Consequently, each case remained a major event, and the scenario described for the first open-heart case was repeated long afterwards. However, the experience acquired during these early years, along with the arrival of new staff in both pediatric and adult, and the advent of adult cardiac surgery with the development of viable valve prostheses, made the difference and allowed the service to progress from infancy to adolescence.

Coronary surgery began after the pioneering work of Dudley Johnson, René Favaloro and George Green in the late 1960s, and was to be the signal for major development in all spheres of cardiac surgery. Indeed, no surgical specialty and few medical specialties, with the exception of cardiology in the past five years, had known such rapid development.

In 1968 and 1969, caseloads for heart surgery in Quebec City were seventy-seven and ninety procedures respectively. Approximately one-third of these operations were performed for the correction of congenital malformation, and the rest in adults for valve replacement or for myocardial revascularization by way of the Vineberg procedure. The advent of direct coronary surgery with aortocoronary bypass was to change all of that.

Major changes occurred during the latter half of the 1960s and in the early 1970s. Gravel, who with Beaulieu had pioneered heart surgery in Quebec, left the institute in 1968 to devote all his time to general surgery. He was replaced by Claude Labrosse, who had just completed his training in Toronto under Bigelow. Labrosse was well-trained in both pediatric and adult cardiac surgery, and was the first formally trained cardiac surgeon to join the local team. Although he was a welcomed addition to the group, his stay in Quebec was to last only two years as he left in March 1970 to take charge of cardiac surgery at the Sherbrooke University Hospital Centre after his predecessor decided to return to the United States.

The first myocardial revascularization by direct aortocoronary bypass in Quebec City was performed in 1970: a single venous graft implanted on the LAD. Michel Lemieux, a graduate of Laval University, had trained in general surgery at the New York University Medical

Center. After a year in the surgical research laboratory at the Peter Bent Brigham Hospital in Boston, he completed his training in cardiovascular and thoracic surgery in New York under Frank Spencer and returned to Quebec in July 1970. His contribution was to be in coronary surgery which he introduced in September the same year.

Until 1970, the service was truly cardiovascular and thoracic as pulmonary and vascular surgeries were performed on a daily basis in two operating rooms designated exclusively for that purpose. The service had also organized a six-bed surgical intensive care unit in collaboration with the department of anaesthesia, designated exclusively for postoperative cardiac and vascular patients. With the expected increase in caseload due largely to coronary surgery, however, the service had to be restructured. Maurice Beaulieu, a chest surgeon by training, decided to devote all of his activities to thoracic surgery, and the group abandoned peripheral vascular procedures, thus becoming exclusively a cardiac surgery service.

Despite having adequate facilities for the time, cardiac surgery in Quebec City still had some problems to settle before reaching maturity. Indeed, in order to answer the challenge of coronary surgery with its great annual increase in volume, the service could no longer depend exclusively on one colleague from the department of anaesthesia and one perfusionist. The intensive care unit, until then a closed unit, also depended on the availability of one physician-anaesthetist. The struggle to develop a more functional administrative structure resulted in further delays and kept the caseload low until 1974. At that point, having resolved all of these problems, cardiac surgery in the city outgrew its provincial competitors and soon became one of the largest services of its kind in Canada.

The rapid development of cardiac surgery during this period, along with the aura and prestige surrounding it, attracted many surgical trainees to the specialty, and there were career opportunities for all. In 1973, Denis Désaulniers, who had trained in the University of Montreal's program and spent an extra year in Birmingham, Alabama, became the third member of the team. Two years later, Jacques Metras, trained in general surgery in Quebec, spent two years in New York City training in cardiac surgery under Frank Spencer. Upon his return, Metras played a major role in the development of adult cardiac surgery at Laval, mainly coronary procedures.

While development in Montreal took place at many sites (indeed at one time there were more cardiac surgery units in the city of Montreal alone than in the province of Ontario), in Quebec City, it evolved at a single facility, Laval Hospital, which revived its Quebec Heart Institute in 1976. As a result of the tremendous increase in heart procedures, a third operating room was allocated to cardiac surgery in 1980, and postoperative facilities were modernized and expanded to eight intensive care beds and ten for intermediate care.

Gilles Raymond joined the team in 1979. Raymond had trained in Montreal in general and cardiac surgery, followed by a year in Philadelphia with L. Henry Edmunds. Upon his return to the province, he settled in Sherbrooke, replacing Claude Labrosse as head of the service there until he relocated to Quebec City a few years later.

Laval Hospital was and remains one of only a few centres where both pediatric and adult cardiac surgery are practiced. Pediatric procedures were performed until

1973 by Jean-Paul Després and then by Denis Désaulniers until 1983, when Paul Cartier took over after completing his training. Cartier was originally from Montreal, where he had trained in general surgery. Cartier graduated in cardiac surgery from the New York University program in 1982 and spent an extra year with Aldo Castaneda and Richard VanPragh in Boston before opting to practice in Quebec City. Paul Cartier was to have a short but brilliant career at Laval. He soon acquired a reputation as an excellent and innovative surgeon in both pediatric and adult heart surgery. His pioneering work, in establishing a tissue bank in Quebec City and in the use of homografts, brought him international recognition and the respect of cardiac surgeons everywhere. Paul Cartier died suddenly on January 2, 2001, at the age of forty-eight. His contributions to the discipline were recognized when the Canadian Cardiovascular Society established the "Paul Cartier Cardiac Surgery Resident Research Award," presented each year at the annual meeting to the resident whose research project was deemed to be the best contribution to the development of cardiac surgery in Canada.

Jean Perron, a Cartier protégé, trained in Toronto, Boston and Paris. Upon his return to Laval, he was given the task of performing all pediatric cardiac surgery, to which he responded with remarkable zest and brilliance. His accomplishments, notably in the treatment of babies born with a single ventricle (the Norwood operation) have been outstanding and earned him a place of honour amongst the top-ranking pediatric heart surgeons.

In spite of being one of the largest cardiac surgery centres in the country, for a long time Laval Hospital did not hold a government permit to set up a heart transplant program, an anomaly considering that it already had a special clinic for patients with heart failure and that the infrastructure for heart transplantation was already in place. In fact, Quebec City had an active kidney transplant program at Hôtel-Dieu Hospital and thus acquired a wide experience in transplant immunology. After obtaining a positive decision through a lengthy and sometimes torturous political process, Laval's heart transplant program was set-up in 1993 under Daniel Doyle, who had arrived from Montreal's Notre-Dame Hospital, which had an active transplantation program under the leadership of Albert Guerraty. Doyle, a general surgery graduate from the University of Montreal, had pursued training in cardiac surgery at the Ochsner Clinic in New Orleans under the tutelage of John Ochsner and Noel Mills. Upon his return to Montreal, Doyle had acquired experience in heart transplantation as the program at Notre-Dame Hospital was organized. Doyle performed the first heart transplantation in Quebec City in May 1993.

Laval Hospital's monopoly in cardiac surgery came to an end in 1990. For reasons that to this day are still unclear, a second program had been organized at Quebec City's Hôtel-Dieu Hospital and a team of two cardiac surgeons led by Pierre Grondin was now competing not only for a portion of the clientele, but worse, for a portion of the budget allocated to heart surgery in the city. Pierre Grondin, back from Miami, organized the program at Hôtel-Dieu in 1990 and retired in 1995, but only after recruiting two excellent young cardiac surgeons, Richard Bauset and Richard Baillot. Both had come out of excellent programs and set up practice elsewhere, Bauset in Sherbrooke and Baillot at Sacré-Coeur Hospital in Montreal. Shortly after their arrival in Quebec City, negotiations began to form a single team operating at one site. These deliberations went on exclusively among the surgeons for nearly two years before an agreement was signed in August 1997 and the Minister of Health informed of the decision. A single team was to work at Laval Hospital as of January 1998. The logic of this agreement was beyond challenge, and in the fall of 1997 the facilities at Laval were expanded so that by January a fourth operating room was ready and the caseload set at forty per week. In addition, plans were immediately drawn up for a further major expansion. A fifth operating room was to be added and the intensive care unit expanded to twenty-five beds in order to accept an eventual caseload of fifty cases per week and two thousand cases per year by 2003.

The decision to form a single unit in Quebec City was beneficial to all parties, both politically and administratively. It also proved to be a positive move for all surgeons concerned, allowing for improvements in the quality of practice and ultimately in patient care.

Jean-Paul Després, a pioneer in cardiac surgery in Quebec, retired in 1995 after spending thirty-five years at the Quebec Heart Institute as one of its original members. We owe today's success to the courage and determination that he showed in the early years. His death from cancer in 2002, only five years after his retirement, was a sad event for all of us.

With the advent and rapid evolution of Interventional Cardiology, particularly in the treatment of coronary disease, the field of cardiac surgery was also expanding. Technical developments in the field of left ventricular assist devices (LVADs) and more recently in the mechanical heart, and the knowledge acquired particularly from the Rematch Project, have opened the possibility of new alternatives to heart transplantation. Improvements in graft materials and increased knowledge in the technique of extracorporeal circulation have made the replacement of the aortic arch and the thoracic aorta safer procedures. François Dagenais, a cardiac surgery trainee from the University of Montreal, spent two years at Stanford, where under the guidance of Craig Miller he was to acquire knowledge and experience in the surgery of the aorta as well as in the field of heart transplantation and in the use of various LVADs. His return to Quebec City in the year 2000 was an important addition to the team in that he filled a much-needed position in the heart transplant program. He was also to be the key figure in developing the new aortic surgery program and in implantation of mechanical heart devices. Our goal of achieving a holistic approach to the surgical treatment of cardiovascular disease, which is generally favoured in institutions such as ours, was now deemed to have been met.

Clinical research, through participation in multicenter projects or the clinical evaluation of new prostheses and grafts at the premarketing stage, was carried out by various individuals in the group with the participation of all, making for a rapid accumulation of useful data for eventual dissemination and publication. All findings on every procedure performed since 1990 have been stored in a data bank which can currently supply scientific and statistical data for nearly twenty thousand patients. In most cases, data was stored from the time of surgery to the last follow-up visit. The database project now employs a staff consisting of a full-time epidemiologist and a full-time nurse supervised by cardiac surgeon Richard Baillot.

Laval Hospital was the first institution in Quebec City with facilities for experimental surgery. As previously mentioned, experimental work leading to the initial use of extracorporeal circulation and to the development of a new disposable bubble oxygenator used throughout the 1960s and into the early 1970s, was performed in the animal laboratory. Throughout the years, various projects have been carried out involving myocardial perfusion and more recently myocardial tolerance to ischemia. Patrick Mathieu is the latest addition to the cardiac surgery team in Quebec. Mathieu, trained in cardiovascular surgery in Montreal, maintained a keen interest in surgical research and chose to broaden his knowledge in transplant immunology by spending an extra two years in Nantes under the tutelage of Soulillou and Anegon. Upon returning to Quebec, Mathieu has pursued research in fundamental aspects of surgery involving transplant immunology and the study of vascular endothelium in transplanted hearts and vascular allografts.

The cardiovascular service of the former Quebec Heart Institute, now known as *The Institute of Cardiology and Pneumology of Laval University at Laval Hospital,* has thus made great strides in the last thirty years. The initial crew has now gone into retirement and the second wave is well established. They leave behind a major league facility, now performing over two thousand heart procedures annually in five operating rooms with a support unit of twenty-five intensive care beds. The service is now able to cover every aspect of cardiovascular surgery and is well supported by a staff of specialized and dedicated personnel as well as by fellows and residents. The cardiac surgery service at Laval Hospital has become one of the busiest in Canada.

It would be most unfair to single out any one person as responsible for this great success. It is the result of a combined team effort. Each new surgeon has been asked to bring, through subspecialty training, a specific contribution to the service. The excellent support and collaboration of a dedicated and highly professional nursing staff has always been a major asset.

Finally, this brief review cannot be completed without acknowledging the special contribution of two members of the team who have passed away. Jean-Paul Després, a colleague whose determination and courage allowed the institute to survive its early and painful beginnings, and Paul Cartier, to whom we at the institute, our patients, and cardiac surgery in Quebec owe so much.

CHICOUTIMI HOSPITAL

André Brassard

The Cardiovascular-Thoracic Surgery Service in Chicoutimi was officially inaugurated in 1958 at the Hôtel-Dieu St. Vallier (later known as Chicoutimi Hospital) under the direction of Dr. Émile Bertho. The new service had both a clinical and a research laboratory arm with animal quarters that could accommodate up to 250 dogs and other animals. The organization of the clinical service was gradually established and open-heart surgery under cardiopulmonary bypass (CPB) was initiated in 1961. CPB was first achieved using a Lillehei-DeWall bubble oxygenator with multiple sequential digital compressions instead of the current roller pumps.

Initially, the service's activities focused mainly on valvular and congenital heart disease. Myocardial revascularization was performed only with the Vineberg technique. In subsequent years, its level of activity varied greatly due to difficulty in recruiting and retaining physicians. To maintain CVT surgical services in Chicoutimi, outside surgeons came to help on many occasions until 1973, when two new surgeons, Drs. André Brassard and Alberto Perez, arrived, thereby increasing the productivity of the service and placing it on a more stable footing.

The experimental laboratory closed in 1974 as a result of administrative and financial constraints. Thereafter, Dr. Émile Bertho left the hospital in 1974 and Dr. Perez in 1978. Closing the cardiac surgery service in Chicoutimi was considered during this period because of its small caseload, its distance from other major centres and insufficient budgetary allocations. But its activities were maintained with the help of surgeons from the Montreal Heart Institute.

Dr. Gabriel Laberge joined the staff in 1979 and was succeeded by Dr. John Francis Mathieu in 1981. Dr. Pierre Michaud, whose main interests were vascular, thoracic and esophageal surgery, arrived in 1983. Finally, Dr. Jean-Marc Farinas joined the group in 2000.

Today, the Chicoutimi Hospital Centre is a general hospital serving the needs of a population of approximately three hundred thousand scattered over a very large territory. It provides services in all the major medical and surgical specialties. Cardiology services include cardiac catheterization, coronary angiography, angioplasty and pacemaker insertion. In surgery, approximately 250 open-heart procedures are performed yearly.

Acknowledgements

We wish to recognize the generous contributions of:

- Ms. Jocelyne Prince, for transcribing the manuscript
- Dr. Jean Couture, Laval Hospital
- Mrs. Françoise Godbout, CVT Association
- Dr. Benoit de Varennes, McGill University Health Centre
- Dr. Christo Tchervenkov, McGill University Health Centre
- Dr. Harry Scott, McGill University Health Centre
- Mrs Hélène Servant, Laval Hospital
- Dr. Luc Bruneau, Hôtel-Dieu
- Dr. Ignacio Prieto, Hôtel-Dieu

References:

Delarue, Norman C. 1989. *Thoracic surgery in Canada: A story of people, places, and events; the evolution of a surgical specialty.* Toronto: B. C. Decker.

Segall, Harold N. 1988. *Pioneers of cardiology in Canada, 1820-1970: The genesis of Canadian cardiology.* Willowdale, Ont.: Hounslow Press.

CHAPTER 7

CARDIOVASCULAR RESEARCH:
THE VIEW FROM MCGILL UNIVERSITY

Ray C. J. Chiu

Prologue

In this chapter, I have chosen to emphasize how novel ideas conceived by people at McGill led to new discoveries and innovative surgical procedures in cardiac surgery. The thought process, which is central to scientific investigation, is not always apparent in readily available published scientific papers which report only the results of research. This emphasis on the creative process rather than on the data and results obtained may have skewed the choice of investigators and their projects described in this chapter, since it depends on the author's own familiarity with how each idea evolved. This also caused the inclusion of a heavy dose of personal reflections. Thus, it should be noted at the outset that this is not an all inclusive account of McGill research, and many McGill investigators not covered in detail here have also contributed significantly to cardiac surgery, both by their clinical observations and laboratory research.

From "Holmes Heart" to Innovations in Congenital Cardiac Surgery

The Abbott Collection

Maude Abbott,[1] as a young medical graduate from McGill, first met Sir William Osler[2] in 1898 at Johns Hopkins Hospital, almost a decade after Osler moved to Hopkins in Baltimore following an illustrious career as a physician and pathologist at the Montreal General Hospital, McGill University. Abbott had been appointed as an assistant curator of the Pathology Museum at McGill, and was sent by the Faculty of Medicine to Washington to see the Walter Reed Army Medical Museum and other institutions en route to help her plan for the museum at McGill.

According to a description by Tony Dobell years later,[3] the memorable meeting of these two medical luminaries from McGill took place when Abbott joined Sir William's ward rounds, with the customary crowd of students, interns and guests in tow. Osler noted that her finger had been accidentally crushed in a door and injured. He became concerned, saw that the finger was dressed, and invited her to one of his student night dinners. Osler discussed some classic writings in medicine, then at the end turned to Abbott and said,

> *I wonder if you realize what an opportunity you have. That McGill Museum is a great place. As soon as you go home, look up the British Medical Journal for 1893 and read the article by Mr. Jonathan Hutchison on "A Clinical Museum."* . . . *It is the greatest place I know for teaching students in. Pictures of life and death together. Wonderful. You read it and see what you can do.*

And so, as Abbott later wrote: "He gently dropped a seed that dominated all my future work."

In organizing the museum back at McGill, she came upon a fascinating cardiac malformation specimen prepared and described in 1824 by A. F. Holmes, the first Dean of McGill Medical School. Studying in detail this specimen, known today as the "Holmes heart," piqued her interest in congenital heart disease. Eventually she collected and examined one thousand cases and used the data gathered as the basis for her classic monographs in several texts between 1908 and 1940. She became an authority on congenital heart diseases during the first half of the twentieth century, as she meticulously correlated anatomical deformities with embryological mal-development, as well as subsequent physiological abnormalities, and clinical manifestations. Since such knowledge is fundamental to pediatric cardiac surgery which started to develop in the mid-1950s, the impact of Abbott's contributions to the birth of cardiac surgery was enormous.

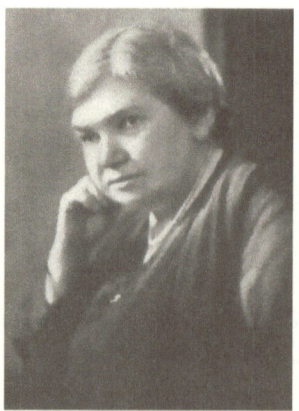

Fig 7:1 Dr. Maude Abbott. Osler Library Portrait Collection, McGill University

One interesting anecdote in the saga between these two medical giants: Osler invited Abbott to write the section on congenital heart disease in the first edition of his famous *Textbook in Medicine.* Abbott asked how she should treat this subject, and Sir William replied, "Statistically." That was in the year 1905.

Tiny and Complex

One admirer and major beneficiary at McGill of Abbott's pioneering work was Tony Dobell. He was a resident in John Gibbons's service at Jefferson Medical College in Philadelphia when Gibbons performed the historic first successful open-heart surgery in a young woman with atrial septal defect in 1953.[4] He soon returned to McGill University, founded the new division of cardiovascular and thoracic surgery, and was its director for nearly two decades. Dobell contributed significantly to the progress and maturation of cardiac surgery by publishing more than one hundred papers in leading journals, both on clinical and experimental topics, especially those related to pediatric cardiac surgery[5] and cardiopulmonary bypass.[6] For years, he virtually single-handedly developed one of the finest services in congenital cardiac surgery at the Montreal Children's Hospital, later served as president of the Society of Thoracic Surgeons, and was a founder of the Canadian Association of Cardiovascular and Thoracic Surgeons. Besides such leadership roles, Dobell's most unique gift was his ability to instill in his students a deep sense of humanity and honesty, while encouraging both technical excellence and academic devotion. He inspired many of his trainees to excel, some later to become leaders elsewhere in Canada and beyond, while others remained at McGill to pursue his vision. Upon his retirement in 1992, the pediatric cardiac surgery service at McGill, which had been synonymous with Tony Dobell for decades, was passed on to one of his students, Christo Tchervenkov. Under his skilful hands, and with his younger associate Dominique Shum-Tim, they continue to take on some of the most complex and high-risk congenital heart procedures in very young infants. The innovative spirit has been maintained in their work on the neonatal aortic arch reconstruction without circulatory arrest;[7] biventricular repair in neonates with hypoplastic left heart complex;[8] as well as in single stage repair of transposition complexes with systemic obstructions.[9] These novel approaches and excellent clinical outcomes are recognized internationally.

Snake Heart, Laser Punctures and Beyond

The Vineberg Legacy

Arthur Vineberg was an imaginative, bold and stubborn man. Without these attributes, he could not have accomplished what he did, and be recognized as a true pioneer in the surgical therapy for myocardial ischemia, the most common disease and cause of death in developed countries.

Vineberg was born in Montreal in 1903, educated and trained at McGill University. He practiced and carried out research at the Royal Victoria Hospital from 1935 to 1965, and was chief of the division of cardiac surgery from 1956 to 1965 at that hospital. He died in 1988 after publishing over 250 articles and three books. His internal mammary (IMA) implantation procedure to treat myocardial ischemia, widely known as the *Vineberg operation*, was first described in 1946.[10] It consisted of freeing the internal mammary artery distally, and tunneling it through the ischemic myocardium between two incisions, with the distal end ligated but the intercostal artery branch left open to allow bleeding into the myocardium.

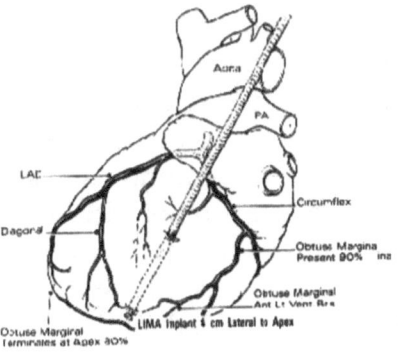

Figure 3. (b) Anterolateral implantation site.

Fig 7:2 Vineberg operation (from Vineberg AM: *Myocardial revascularization by arterial/ventricular implants.* Boston: John Wright / PSG Inc., 1982, p. 260)

Following extensive studies in a canine model, the first clinical IMA implantation was carried out in 1950.

For more than a decade, Vineberg published extensively to show his operation was effective, both experimentally and clinically. In his initial paper, using the injection of Schlesinger solution into an IMA implant four months post-op, he reported that the injectate could be seen in the coronaries and the aorta, indicating the development of an IMA to coronary artery anastomosis. In a canine chronic myocardial ischemic model, IMA implants were found to improve exercise tolerance. Since the beneficial effects observed appeared not to occur immediately but only six weeks to six months later, Vineberg subsequently added epicardiectomy and Ivalon sponge application as adjunctive procedures to promote revascularization. His patients, who came not only from various parts of Canada but also from foreign countries, often reported improvement in symptoms and well being, although no prospective randomized studies were ever attempted. Some patients experienced improvements lasting many decades after implantation. Although he published extensively on such results, for years the Vineberg operation was viewed skeptically and was not widely adopted. Common sense dictates if one leaves an implanted artery open within a skeletal muscle mass, it will bleed and form a hematoma, which soon clot and the arterial implant thrombose. But if this is not the case in Vineberg's myocardial implant, why?

The reason, Vineberg believed, was that the myocardium had a spongelike structure and contained numerous sinusoids, which provided a ready run-off for the blood from the implant. This view was based on an observation by Wearn et al.[11] nearly ten years earlier in 1933. These sinusoidal spaces were lined with endothelial cells and were in continuity with coronary arterial and venous systems, as well as with "luminal sinusoidals" communicating directly with ventricular cavities.

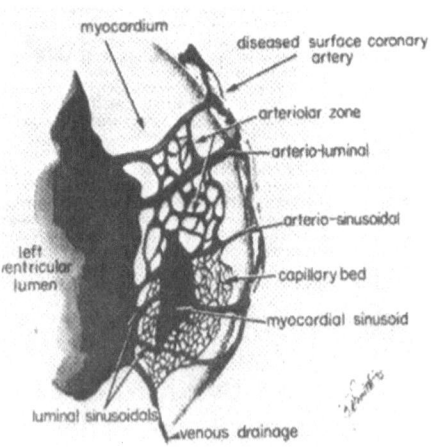

Fig 7:3 Myocardial sinusoids (from Vineberg AM: *Myocardial revascularization by arterial/ventricular implants.* Boston: John Wright / PSG Inc., 1982, p.16).

Thus, the Vineberg operation was dubbed by some as a "snake heart operation" since in the amphibian hearts, such as those of the snakes, myocardial circulation is indeed provided by channels which brings the blood back and forth from the ventricular cavity into the spongelike myocardial sinusoids, as a coronary vascular system had not evolved. Such a myocardial perfusion system is less efficient than that provided by coronary circulation; nevertheless it is sufficient for cold-blooded species like the snake with low metabolic rates. Using injection cast models, Vineberg demonstrated that the flow through the arterial implant could indeed distribute readily and promptly to a wide segment of myocardial mass, which appeared to support his thesis that these sinusoids could provide an efficient run-off for the inflow from the implants. In spite of such explanations, skepticism persisted until the development of Sones's technique for coronary angiography in the early 1960s. A patient who received a Vineberg implant many years earlier showed up at the Cleveland Clinic and to the surprise of many, the internal mammary artery implant did remain patent all those years. Furthermore angiography demonstrated vascular anastomosis between the implant and the left anterior descending coronary artery (LAD) distal to its occlusive lesion. Such evidence of revascularization was highly convincing,[12] and Vineberg was finally vindicated![13] As Vineberg's operation became credible, the underlying myocardial sinusoidal concept, which provided the anatomical rationale for this operation, was accepted and included in textbooks of cardiac surgery. By the late 1960s, a prospective randomized clinical trial of the Vineberg procedure was initiated in the Veterans Hospital System in the United States. However, it was not completed due to the advent of direct coronary artery bypass grafting (CABG) which quickly superceded the classic Vineberg procedure.

Challenging a Dogma

In 1968, upon finishing residency training in the United States under Clarence Dennis who attempted the first open-heart surgery with cardiopulmonary bypass in 1951, I arrived at McGill to pursue a PhD in experimental surgery, while going back to the textbooks to prepare for my cardiac surgery specialty Board and Royal College Fellowship examinations.

Unexpectedly, I noted a perplexing dilemma. In my textbooks on cardiac surgery, the spongelike myocardial sinusoidal system in the mammalian heart was clearly depicted as the rationale for the Vineberg operation, but in my textbooks of anatomy and histology, this was totally absent. I wondered how anatomists and histologists could miss such a prominent and important myocardial structure. Thus I went back to review scientific evidence available in support of the existence of myocardial sinusoids. It appeared there were two lines of findings for this theory. The first was the histological sections reported by Wearn et al. in 1933,[11] which showed endothelial lined irregular lumens connected to coronary vascular branches. I suspected that the limited technical sophistication available in the early 1930s could have distorted venules to appear like "sinusoids." Another series of data provided by Vineberg and associates between the 1940s to sixties were based on plastic casts as described above, for which the vinyl-acetate solution was injected, and upon the solidification of the polymer cast, the myocardial tissue was dissolved by immersing the specimen in a high concentration alkaline solution. Consequently, any endothelial cells, which were supposed to line the sinusoidal space filled by the cast, were destroyed, thus their presence could not be determined.

In what was to be known as the "chicken blood" experiment in our lab, we bought two chickens and obtained their blood by cardiac punctures. A Vineberg procedure was carried out in a canine model, and the chicken blood, whose avian red cells are nucleated, was injected into the myocardial implant under physiological pressure. The myocardial specimens were removed and fixed either in formalin or glutaraldehyde promptly, and processed for histological and electromicroscopic examinations. The canine red cells, which have no nuclei, were found within the coronary vascular spaces lined by endothelial cells as expected, but the nucleated avian red cells were virtually all outside of the vascular space and in between muscle fibers. It was clear that the so called sinusoidal spaces outlined previously by vinyl-acetate casts were in fact extracellular interstitial spaces between the muscle layers, which could explain why Vineberg's casts appeared to arrange in palisades.

Subsequent review of the more recent embryology and cardiology literature revealed that in fact in the early embryonic stage, mammals like amphibians, do have myocardial sinusoids in their primitive hearts. However as the fetus grows, the coronary arterial system takes over, and the sinusoids disappear in a process known as "compaction." In certain congenital anomalies such as pulmonary arterial stenosis without a ventricular septal defect, high intraventricular pressure may cause the direct channel between the right heart cavity to the sinusoids to persist, which could be demonstrated by contrast cardiac ventriculography. There are reports of failure of compaction persisting to adulthood of some patients, where the sinusoidal space can clearly be demonstrated by angiography. These patients suffer from impaired ventricular function and heart failure, presumably due to inefficient perfusion to maintain myocardial function. In the absence of such pathological conditions, the sinusoidal system cannot be found in postnatal mammalian hearts, or occasionally at most as minimal remnants.

In the report[14] on our "chicken blood study" in 1973, we concluded that even though the Vineberg operation could have merit, the underlying anatomical rationale was not valid. Instead, we suggested that angiogenesis stimulated by the implant procedure could provide a more likely explanation for the vascular anastomosis demonstrable between the implant and the native coronary arterial system. However, with the Vineberg implant procedure rapidly losing ground to the emerging CABG at that time, this matter was not pursued further and was largely forgotten.

Cardiac Acupuncture and TMR

Before we challenged the sinusoidal theory, P. K. Sen et al.[15] from India attempted another "snake heart operation" in 1965, by performing transmyocardial acupuncture using needles. His idea was to bring blood from the ventricular cavity through the puncture channel into the myocardial sinusoidal system. Soon it was found that these needle puncture channels rapidly became obliterated by scar formation. Following this, the idea of a "snake heart operation" remained dormant until 1982 when M. Mirhoseini[16] resurrected it by claiming that transmyocardial puncture created by laser could produce patent channels without fibrotic obliteration. A number of clinical trials, which were randomized but not blinded, showed favorable clinical outcomes, and this procedure was approved by the U.S. Food and Drug Administration for clinical use. Again, the original underlying concept was the existence of a spongelike myocardium with an extensive sinusoidal system, allowing myocardial perfusion to take place by blood flowing through the laser channels from the ventricular cavity.

Because of our earlier experience as described above, we were doubtful on the physiologic concept underlying this "transmyocardial laser revascularization" (TMR) procedure. First we did not believe the laser channels will remain patent, which was soon confirmed in animal and patient specimens. We postulated instead that since laser punctures, like the myocardial tunnels created for Vineberg implants, would produce myocardial tissue damage, subsequent inflammatory response to injury could induce angiogenesis as part of the healing process. Preliminary studies by our residents Mark Pelletier,[17] Victor Chu[18, 19] and others, confirmed that myocardial puncture by needle or laser could indeed elicit an inflammatory response, expression of angiogenic factors, and angiogenesis at the puncture sites with increased capillary density. Although for these works our young investigators were awarded with Resident Research Prizes from the U.S. Thoracic Surgery Directors Association, the validity of both the efficacy of laser TMR and the hypothesis that laser puncture-induced angiogenesis could provide effective reversal of myocardial ischemia, remains controversial to date. Some studies have reported results suggesting that the clinical efficacy of laser TMR could largely be accounted for by placebo effect. The angiogenesis we and others have reported has not been followed with convincing evidence that these newly developed capillary networks can persist without regression, or can mature into larger vessels to improve myocardial tissue perfusion. Nevertheless, the idea of inducing angiogenesis to treat ischemic myocardium not amenable to standard revascularization procedures has gained great interest in recent years.

Dawn of Therapeutic Angiogenesis

As it turned out, McGill investigators also played a pioneering role in the emerging field of angiogenetic therapy by means of delivering angiogenic factors. In the early 1990s, a team led by James F. Symes, then director of cardiothoracic surgery at the Royal Victoria Hospital, together with his colleague Alan Graham and graduate student Li-Qun Pu, published a series of papers demonstrating that local administration of endothelial cell growth factor (ECGF) purified from bovine retina could induce increased collateral circulation in the ischemic hind limb of the rabbit.[20, 21] ECGF is an acidic fibroblast growth factor (FGF) and had been shown to stimulate angiogenesis in the chick chorioallanoic membrane and corneal bio-assays. Their study was one of the earliest to examine the efficacy of FGF in inducing angiogenesis in a clinically relevant animal model.

In 1994, this team collaborated with Jeffrey Isner at St. Elizabeth Medical Center, Tufts University in Boston where Symes had relocated to become chief of cardiothoracic surgery, and published their experimental work on the efficacy of vascular endothelial growth factor (VEGF), which later led to clinical trials.[22] Studies on angiogenesis using adult stem cells derived from bone marrow are continuing at McGill, led by Kevin Lachapelle who was a member of Symes's team when still a resident.

Veins, Large And Small

Spiral Vein Graft

For many reasons, veins seem to be less amenable to surgical intervention than the arteries. Although autologous saphenous veins have been widely used to bypass coronary and popliteal arteries, outcomes of using venous substitutes to replace damaged veins have been rather unsatisfactory. This poses a particular problem for large caliber veins such as the vena cava.

Shortly after I went on staff at the Montreal General Hospital in 1973, I saw a patient operated upon several months earlier by Peter Blundell, a skilled senior associate of mine who trained in Wilfred Bigelow's department at the University of Toronto. Blundell operated on this woman for a malignant thymoma. This was in the days when CT and MRI were still not available. His dissection had progressed to a point of no return when he realized that the tumor had invaded the superior vena cava (SVC) such that he had to resect much of her cava. To prevent inevitable SVC syndrome as the result, he replaced it with a matching sized Dacron graft. She did well initially but by the time I saw her it had clotted, which was not a surprising outcome. Although prosthetic vascular grafts have been highly successful in the aorta, they have had dismal patency rate in the vena cava.

At a lunch break, I mentioned this case to Bill Mersereau and bemoaned the absence of a larger caliber autologous vein that can be used to replace the resected vena cava in such cases. Since Mersereau was a lab scientist and not a surgeon, I explained to him Virchow's triad as the risk factors for venous thrombosis, and my thought that a caliber matched autologous vein graft should be an ideal substitute. I wondered how best one could convert a smaller caliber donor vein, such as a saphenous vein, into a large caliber conduit, matching closely to the diameter of the vena cava to avoid flow stasis and turbulence, and yet retaining intact endothelium. The existing technique to provide such a composite vein graft was to sew together several parallel panels of vein segments

opened longitudinally, which I found to be technically
cumbersome and not elegant. Mersereau, who happened
to be an experienced Boy Scout master, suggested that
I could open the saphenous vein longitudinally, wrap it
around a chest tube in a spiral fashion like a bandage,
and sew it together to construct a larger vein.

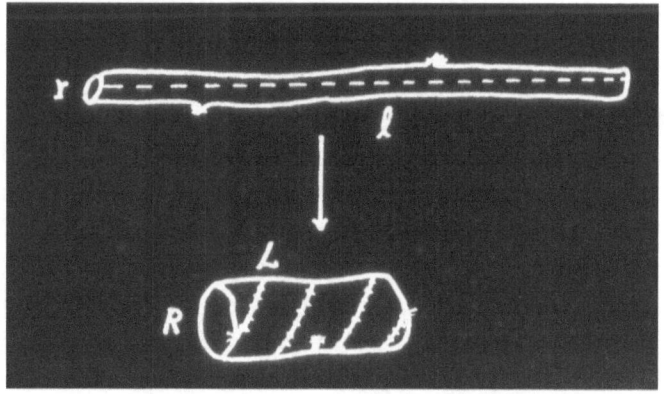

Fig 7:4 Technique for constructing "Spiral Vein Graft"

By selecting an appropriately sized chest tube as the
temporary in vitro stent, precise matching of the caliber
of the donor vein graft with the recipient site could be
achieved easily. Within a week, I replaced much of the
SVC with such a "spiral vein graft" in ten dogs, observed
them for a year with intermittent venography, and
found that if technical errors such as kinking due to the
mismatch of the length of the graft were avoided, the
patency rate was 100 percent at one year without any
anticoagulation.[23] This was indeed a very inexpensive,
simple solution to a difficult problem. Much of the
credit for clinically popularizing this procedure later,
however, goes to Donald Doty[24] in Iowa, who palliated
many patients with malignant SVC obstruction with this
technique.

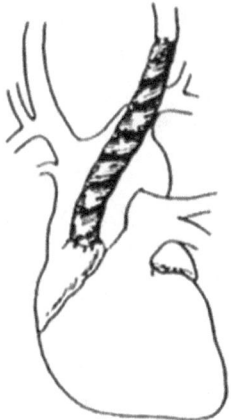

Fig. 7:5 Spiral vein graft for superior vena cava replacement

In subsequent years, many more patients have been treated with this technique for benign SVC occlusions, such as those caused by sclerosing mediastinitis, and by thrombosis associated with central venous catheters. The technique of spiral vein graft had been also applied to other anatomical sites, such as for internal jugular vein and femoral vein replacements. One of the advantages of using autologous grafts as compared to using prosthetic substitutes is in grafting an already or potentially infected site.[25] Today few realize that this surgical innovation originated from the intuition of a scout master having a lunch with a frustrated surgeon![26]

Retrograde Cardioplegia

It is often said that the surgical investigator is "a bridge tender taking the clinical problems to the laboratory and back again." In the early 1970s surgeons were still on the learning curve for CABG, and many used electromagnetic flow probes to measure the bypass blood flow, in part to assure the quality of the distal anastomosis. It became apparent that even with a good and patent anastomosis, some patients showed less than optimal bypass flow due to poor run-off associated with diffuse coronary arteriosclerosis. Several investigators independently advanced the idea of arteriolizing the coronary vein by placing a bypass graft distal to the ligated vein accompanying the diffusely occluded coronary artery. This is anatomically feasible because there are no valves in coronary veins, thus allowing unhindered retrograde perfusion. The rationale was that since atherosclerosis does not affect the venous system, one can always be assured of excellent run-off. Thus we took this clinical problem to the lab, seeking a solution.

In a sheep model, we bypassed the internal mammary arteries to the LAD or to its accompanying vein, ligating the bypassed vessels cephalad to the anastomotic sites. As mentioned above we had been measuring bypass blood flow using electromagnetic flow probes in patients undergoing routine CABG. Therefore we decided to also look at blood flow when a coronary vein was arteriolized and perfused retrograde. Quickly we found that the flow through the graft into the coronary vein was much higher than that into the LAD despite lack of distal occlusive lesions in either of these vessels. Furthermore from clinical experience, we knew that if during surgery we inadvertently damaged an accompanying vein, we could simply ligate or electrocoagulate the bleeding vein to achieve hemostasis, and there would be no appreciable harm with this maneuver.

The obvious conclusion from such observations is that there must exist a rich network of veno-venous anastomoses for shunting, in constrast to the coronary arteries, an end-artery system such that occlusion produces myocardial infarction. If extensive shunting exists in the venous system, then it is likely that the retrograde flow we establish would be shunted through the lower resistance vein-to-vein connections, bypassing the vital capillary bed required for tissue oxygenation and metabolism.

To test this hypothesis, we injected radioactive microspheres 15 microns in diameter, which would embolize to the capillaries and become entrapped within the myocardial tissue, while microspheres passing through the larger caliber venous shunts would be lost into the systemic circulation. Our data readily confirmed this hypothesis, as more than 90 percent of microspheres were lodged in the capillary bed of the myocardium when they were delivered through the LAD. When delivered retrograde into the accompanying vein, only less than a third were trapped in the myocardium. We followed this up by using vinyl-acetate casts to determine the escape route of the blood perfused retrograde into the vein. We found a significant portion drained into the ventricular cavity through the Thebesian venous system, although some also escaped through the greater cardiac vein and exited from the coronary sinus.[27]

These findings led to two interesting conclusions. Firstly, lack of nutritional capillary flow can explain the limited efficacy of the coronary sinus retrograde perfusion for an ischemic myocardium, known as Beck's procedure. Secondly, the retrograde venous perfusion can be highly efficient for cooling the myocardium because of the high flow through the widespread network of venules. Thus, retrograde coronary sinus perfusion should be an efficient way to cool the heart during cold cardioplegia.

In the mid-to-late-1970s, as hypothermic cardioplegia became increasingly popular, we were concerned about how to assure that effective myocardial protection had been achieved and maintained following the initial delivery of the cold cardioplegic solution. Since cooling of the myocardium played an important role in the protection afforded, the degree of cooling achieved is an important index of the adequacy of protection. In experimental animal models of cold cardioplegia in normal hearts, the interventricular septal "core" temperature was generally monitored to guide myocardial cooling. In patients undergoing coronary bypass, however, it appeared to us that core temperature would not necessarily reflect the protection afforded to the myocardium with occluded coronary arteries. Cold cardioplegic solution injected into the aortic root could be expected to go preferentially to the patent coronary arteries, while delivery to the territory supplied by the occluded coronary artery would be impaired.

To test this hypothesis, we had been clinically monitoring different regions of myocardial temperature following antegrade delivery of cold cardioplegic solution through the aortic root. As suspected, the territory supplied by the occluded coronary artery did not cool as efficiently as in the nonoccluded segments, with a temperature gradient in the same heart of up to 8°C, which was quite significant. Not only did the cold cardioplegic solution distribute heterogeneously in diseased hearts, but inadvertent rewarming took place even with moderate systemic hypothermia, at approximately 1°C per hour rise in myocardial temperature. The latter finding led to our recommendation for the use of "multiple cardioplegia," a practice not widely employed in those days.

Since the coronary venous system is not involved by the arteriosclerotic process, we theorized that retrograde delivery of cardioplegia would not encounter the same difficulty as antegrade cardioplegia in a heart with severe coronary arterial occlusions requiring bypass surgery. Furthermore, we reasoned that during aortic root operations, one would not have to interrupt the surgical procedures to recannulate the coronary ostia in order to deliver multiple cardioplegia if one delivered the cardioplegic solution retrograde through the coronary sinus.

This idea soon led to our first experimental paper entitled "Retrograde Coronary Sinus Perfusion for Myocardial Protection During Cardiopulmonary Bypass Surgery,"[28] published in 1978, and later on our first clinical experience in 1984.[29] It would be years before this procedure became accepted by centers worldwide. Unlike earlier attempts to nourish a beating normothermic heart by retrograde coronary sinus perfusion, when the heart is arrested and cooled during cardioplegia, the metabolic rate is markedly reduced so that the relatively limited capillary perfusion achieved with this technique is still adequate.

Looking back years later, it is ironic that the original idea of coronary venous arterialization as a treatment for patients with diffuse coronary arteriosclerosis failed, but retrograde coronary sinus cardioplegia, an offshoot of the former study, survived.

The Long March: From "Wrapping" and "Capping" to "Regenerating" The Myocardium

Dynamic Cardiomyoplasty

I always had an open door policy for my residents, so when Dennis Modry walked into my lab office one afternoon in 1975, I was not surprised. He said, "I think I have a good idea," as he seated himself in the chair beside me. "I think I can raise a muscle flap from the diaphragm, use it to replace damaged myocardium, and stimulate it with a pacemaker to contract with the rest of the heart." He was a surgical resident rotating through my lab, doing research on an unrelated subject for his Master of Science in Experimental Surgery. Later, after his training at McGill, he would initiate the first highly successful heart transplantation program in Western Canada. In any case, he was then a young man with what many of us thought to be a "crazy idea."[30]

Modry showed this procedure was technically feasible in a canine model, although no functional studies were carried out. In retrospect, we committed a cardinal sin in research since this experiment was carried out ad hoc, without a prior thorough literature search. If I had asked him to do so, we would have learned much, but then this project may have never started. The idea of using skeletal muscle to repair or assist the heart in fact goes back to René Leriche[31] in Paris in 1933, and in 1959 Adrian Kantrowitz[32] in New York electrically stimulated a muscle flap with the goal of providing cardiac assist. Since we were oblivious to such earlier efforts, we did not fully appreciate the difficulties associated with rapid development of muscle fatigue, as well as the need for a new stimulator to generate contractile force suitable for cardiac assist. We soon learned that even with maximum voltage available in an external cardiac pacemaker, a single pulse stimulation of the muscle flap failed to generate strong and sustained contractions seen in normal myocardium. This is a reflection of differences in the anatomical structure between cardiac and skeletal muscles. Cardiac muscle is a syncytium so that a single pulse electrical stimulation generates a synchronous all-or-none contraction, while skeletal muscle is composed of numerous individual motor units which respond to a train of impulses, thus both the contractile force and duration can be modulated.

In order to recruit sufficient motor units in the muscle flap for cardiac assist, I decided that we needed a new adjustable and synchronizable burst stimulator such that strong muscle contraction could be induced during a selected segment of the cardiac cycle. Using a homemade prototype stimulator, another McGill resident, Davis Drinkwater, demonstrated its feasibility and presented his findings at the Surgical Forum of the American College of Surgeons[33] in 1980. This was just the beginning of Drinkwater's successful academic career, as he would eventually rise to his current position as chairman of the department of cardiac and thoracic surgery at Vanderbilt University in Nashville, Tennessee.

This prototype stimulator caught the interest of the engineers at Medtronic Company, who then collaborated with us to develop the first "cardiomyostimulator." This device was used by another McGill resident passing through my lab, Michael Dewar who later joined the faculty of Yale University, to demonstrate in a canine model the feasibility of using skeletal muscle for cardiac assist. His paper was published as a lead article in the *Journal of Thoracic and Cardiovascular Surgery* in 1984, and raised much interest with subsequent input from many other investigators.[34] Notable among them were Larry Stephenson[35] at the University of Pennsylvania, whose team introduced the concept of muscle fiber transformation by chronic electrical stimulation to induce fatigue tolerance; and Alain Carpentier[36] of Paris, who identified the latissimus dorsi muscle as the optimal source for the muscle flap, refined the surgical procedure of muscle wrap around the failing ventricles, and brought it to an early clinical trial.

From 1986 to the mid-1990s, this operation, known as "dynamic cardiomyoplasty,"

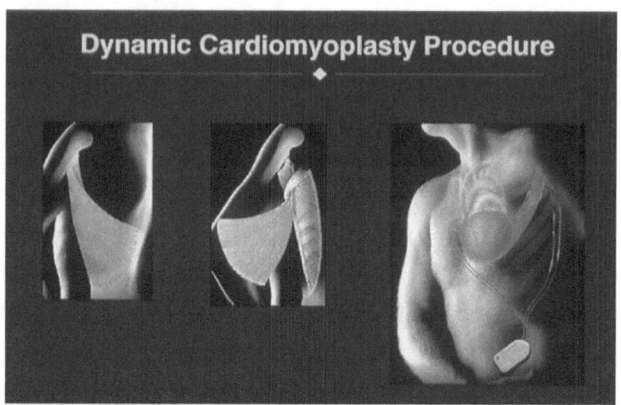

Fig 7:6 Dynamic cardiomyoplasty

underwent international multicenter Phase I and Phase II trials. Nearly a thousand patients underwent this procedure worldwide.[37] As experience increased, the operative mortality decreased from over 20 percent to below 4 percent.

In 1994, an FDA approved prospective randomized study to compare the safety and efficacy of dynamic cardiomyoplasty versus optimal medical therapy for heart failure was carried out under the sponsorship of the Medtronic Company. Unfortunately three years later, the Medtronic Company terminated the trial, primarily due to slow recruitment of cases into the study. There were two reasons for the slow enrollment. The first was the dilemma that this invasive procedure for very high-risk patients in New York Heart Association (NYHA) Functional Class IV was associated with prohibitive operative mortality; while in patients with good risks in Functional Class II were responding to advances in medical therapy for heart failure. Secondly, although the cardiomyoplasty patients showed improvements in exercise tolerance and subjective quality of life scores, the changes in systolic functional indices such as ejection fraction were not consistent. The benefit in survival rate did not reach statistical significance after one year, with a sample size of just over a hundred when the trial was terminated, which was only about one third of what was originally planned. Nevertheless a subgroup of patients showed remarkable improvement in quality of life in spite of marginal changes in systolic functions, so that although the placebo effect could not be completely ruled out, other factors might be at play for this observation, as will be discussed further below.

Throughout this trial period, cardiomyoplasty was carried out in Canada only at McGill University and the University of Western Ontario. Three of our eight patients, all with ejection fractions between 8 to 15 percent, survived for over five years, and most showed significant improvement in functional class before succumbing, often to intractable arrhythmias. The premature termination of this randomized trial represented the demise of cardiomyoplasty as we knew it, at least in North America. However, as it happens, this led to a couple of interesting new developments.

Ventricular Remodeling

During the trials for cardiomyoplasty, an unexpected finding in a patient operated on at Johns Hopkins Hospital in Baltimore gave us a clue to a novel insight. A young patient with dilated cardiomyopathy underwent ventricular functional study pre-op and postdynamic cardiomyoplasty, using pressure volume loops obtained with a conductance catheter. For some technical reasons, the latissimus dorsi flap of this patient was never effectively stimulated by the cardiomyostimulator. Amazingly, however, even without such stimulation, the presence of a passive muscle flap around the heart by itself appeared to reduce the progression of cardiac dilatation, and the pressure volume loop obtained one year post-op showed significant improvement. This phenomenon was described as "reverse remodeling"[38] of the ventricle, and it was postulated that the presence of a passive muscle wrap *per se* could modulate the deleterious progressive dilatation known as "ventricular remodeling" in heart failure.

This observation led to the first of two interesting offshoots of dynamic cardiomyoplasty research. As a result of the discovery of this "reverse remodeling phenomenon," we initiated a new study. Joong-Hwa Oh, our visiting research fellow who is now a professor of cardiac surgery at Yonsei University in Korea, tested a procedure which we called the "cardiac binding operation." Dilated cardiomyopathy was induced using a canine rapid pacing model, and the effects of wrapping the heart either with a skeletal muscle flap or with a Dacron sheet were observed. The results indicated that wrapping the heart with a muscle flap without dynamic stimulation, and to a slightly lesser extent, simply wrapping it with a prosthetic sheet, reduced the progressive ventricular dilatation that occurs as the result of rapid pacing. This modulating effect on the remodeling process appeared to preserve cardiac function. This idea evolved into the development of the "Acorn®" device, a polymer cup that can be fitted around both ventricles. This device is undergoing multicenter clinical trials at present. Together with the Battista's ventricular reduction operation and Buckberg's ventricular restoration procedures, use of this new device is aimed at preventing or reversing the deleterious ventricular remodeling process seen in heart failure.

Regenerative Stem Cell Therapy

The second spin-off of the dynamic cardiomyoplasty investigation was the discovery of the "cellular cardiomyoplasty" approach. In the course of our study using a stimulated skeletal muscle flap to assist the failing ventricle, we noted that the skeletal muscle fibers could sometimes be damaged by ischemia or by over-stimulation for contraction, but histologically they were able to repair themselves by regenerating damaged muscle fibers. We learned that this was due to the presence of so called "satellite cells" in close proximity to these fibers, which are in fact skeletal myoblasts capable of responding to injury to proliferate, migrate and differentiate, in order to repair the damaged muscle fibers.

In collaboration with Race Kao, then at Allegheny General Hospital in Pittsburgh, we studied the hypothesis that skeletal myoblasts implanted into a damaged myocardium might also undergo proliferation and differentiation to repair or compensate for damaged myocardium. This procedure, first reported by us in 1992,[39] later named "cellular cardiomyoplasty,"[40] ushered in the concept of cellular therapy for myocardial injury. Subsequent studies by us and others show that autologous skeletal myoblasts implanted into a myocardial scar were indeed able to differentiate into striated muscle fibers, and improve ventricular functions in various animal models. This approach reached Phase I clinical trials[41] in the year 2000, and is currently undergoing prospective randomized studies in Europe and the United States. In 1999, however, we shifted our focus to use autologous adult stem cells derived from bone marrow as the donor source for cell therapy, since these adult stem cells are pluripotent and capable not only of differentiating into neocardiomyocytes when implanted into the

myocardium,[42] but may also become endothelial cells
and smooth muscle cells to contribute to vasculogenesis
associated with myocardial ischemia.

Our first publication to confirm such findings was
published in the year 2000,

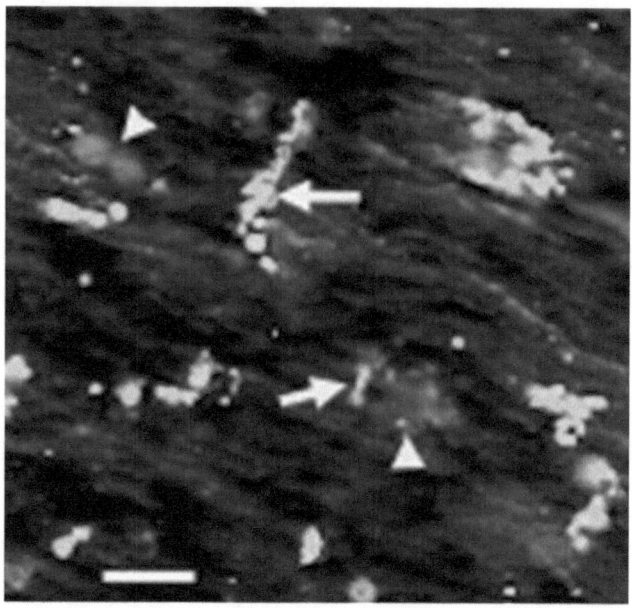

Fig 7:7 Cellular cardiomyoplasty. The arrows show
"intercalated discs" shown with immunohistochemistry
for Connexin 43; and the arrow heads show labeled
nuclei of neocardiomyocytes derived from the implanted
marrow stem cells.

and in subsequent studies we explored the
pathophysiological roles of patients' own bone marrow
stem cells in the repair process following myocardial
infarction. We found that upon myocardial injury, signals
are sent out to recruit adult stem cells from bone marrow,
which traffic through the circulation to reach the damaged

myocardium, where they undergo differentiation to participate in myogenesis and angiogenesis. These cells can be delivered therapeutically to help repair a damaged myocardium by local implantation or in acute myocardial infarction by systemic or intracoronary administration, as they are capable of homing to the injured site.

More recently, we demonstrated the ability for self-assembly by these neocardiomyocytes,[43] integrating themselves into the preexisting cardiomyofiber scaffold.

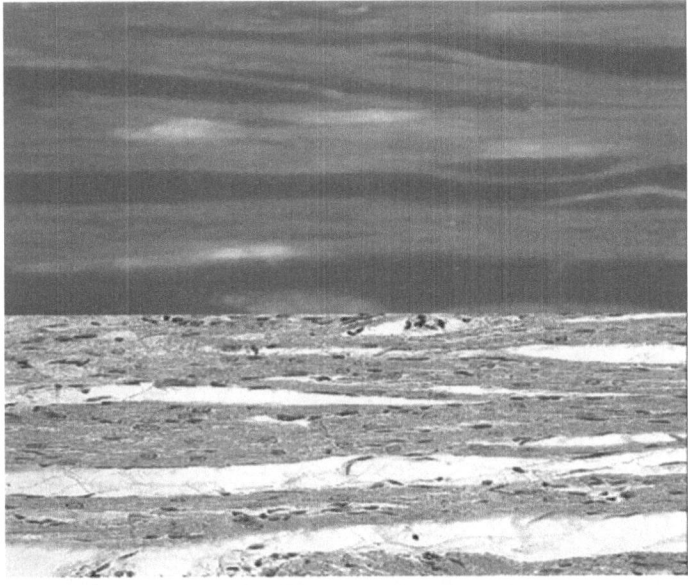

Fig 7:8 Self-assembly of neocardiomyocytes. Top: Fluorescent microscopic picture of a rat myocardial tissue, showing the neocardiomyocytes derived from implanted marrow stem cells labeled with fluorescent dye integrated into host myofibers. Bottom: same section stained with H&E, which shows normal appearing cardiac myofibers, indicating the self-assembly of the neocardiomyocytes.

Such cellular therapy is being shown to improve cardiac function impaired by myocardial infarction. One unexpected and potentially highly important finding is that these adult stem cells seem to induce immunological tolerance, capable of surviving and differentiating in allogeneic or xenogenic transplant recipients without immunosuppression.[44] At the time of this writing, we are focusing our research in confirming such findings, and exploring the possible immunological mechanisms to explain this phenomenon. The clinical importance of this observation, if confirmed, is the fascinating possibility of using such cells as "universal donors," opening a new era in the emerging field of regenerative medicine, not only for cardiac injury repair, but also for treatment of damage in other organs.

Epilogue

It is noteworthy that most of the works described above have been carried out by our residents and students under the supervision of the faculty members at McGill, which often shaped these trainees. This close integration of research and teaching at McGill can be seen as a continuation of our Oslerian legacy. Many international presentations of the research findings described above were first rehearsed by our residents in the Osler Amphitheatre at the Montreal General Hospital, with a large portrait of Sir William Osler gazing down upon the audience. One imagines that this great teacher of medicine, who taught and inspired many at this institution, would be gratified to see these young, inquisitive minds at work nearly a century later, and continuing into the future.

Acknowledgement

The author appreciates the valuable suggestions of Wendy S. W. Chiu, MD, CM, FRCPC, in the preparation of this chapter.

Notes:

1. E. H. Bensley, *McGill Medical Luminaries: Maude Elizabeth Seymour Abbott* (Montreal: Osler Library, McGill University, 1990), pp. 78-82.
2. E. H. Bensley, *McGill Medical Luminaries: William Osler* (Montreal: Osler Library, McGill University, 1990), pp. 42-45.
3. A. R. C. Dobell, "Maude Abbott: Portrait of a pioneer," *Second Clinical Conference on Congenital Heart Disease*, B. L. Tucker, G. G. Lindesmith, and M. Takahashi, eds. (Grune & Stratton Inc., 1982), p. 237-63.
4. A. R. C. Dobell and J. H. Gibbon Jr., "Part II: Personal reminiscences," *Ann Thorac Surg* (1982), 34: 342-44.
5. J. H. Gibbon et al., "The closure of interventricular septal defects in dogs during open cardiotomy with the maintenance of the cardiorespiratory functions by a pump oxygenator," *J. Thorac Surg* (1964), 28: 235.
6. A. R. C. Dobell et al., "Biologic evaluation of blood after prolonged recirculation through film and membrane oxygenators," *Ann Surg* (1965), 161: 617-22.
7. C. I. Tchervenkov et al., "Neonatal aortic arch reconstruction avoiding circulatory arrest and direct arch vessel cannulation," *Ann Thorac Surg* (2001), 72: 1615-20.

8. C. I. Tchervenkov et al., "Biventricular repair in neonates with hypoplastic left heart complex," *Ann Thorac Surg* (1998), 66: 1350-57.

9. C. I. Tchervenkov and S. Korkola, "Transposition complexes with systemic obstruction," *Ped Card Surg*, Annual Seminars in *Thorac Cardiovasc Surg* (2001), 4: 71-82.

10. A. M. Vineberg, "Development of an anastomosis between the coronary vessels and a transplanted internal mammary artery," *Can Med Assoc J* (1946), 106: 763-69.

11. J. T. Wearn et al., "The nature of the vascular communications between the coronary arteries and the chambers of the heart," *Am Heart J* (1933), 9: 143-64.

12. D. B. Effler et al., "Increase myocardial perfusion of the internal mammary artery implantation: Vineberg's operation," *Ann Surg* (1963), 158: 526-34.

13. J. B. Shrager, "The Vineberg procedure: the immediate fore-runner of coronary artery bypass grafting," *Ann Thorac Surg* (1994), 57: 1354-56.

14. R. C. J. Chiu and H. J. Scott, "The nature of early run-off in myocardial arterial implants," *J Thorac Cardiovasc Surg* (1973), 65: 768-77.

15. P. K. Sen et al., "Transmyocardial acupuncture: a new approach to myocardial revascularization," *J Thorac Cardiovasc Surg* (1965), 50: 181-89.

16. M. Mirhoseini, M. Muckerheide, and M. M. Cayton, "Transventricular revascularization by laser," *Lasers Surg Med* (1982), 2: 187-98.

17. M. P. Pelletier et al., "Angiogenesis and growth factor expression in a model of transmyocardial revascularization," *Ann Thorac Surg* (1998), 66: 12-18.

18. V. Chu et al., "Angiogenic response induced by mechanical transmyocardial revascularization," *JTCVS* (1999), 118: 849-56.

19. V. F. Chu et al., "Angiogenesis in transmyocardial revascularization: Comparison of laser versus mechanical punctures," *Ann Thorac Surg* (1999), 68: 301-8.

20. L. Q. Pu et al., "Angiogenic stimulation: A new approach for severe chronic limb ischemia," *Surg Forum* (1991), XLII: 365-67.

21. L. Q. Pu et al., "Enhanced revascularization of the ischemic limb by angiogenic therapy," *Circulation* (1993), 88: 208-15.

22. S. Takeshita et al., "Intramuscular administration of vascular endothelial growth factor induces dose-dependent collateral artery augmentation in a rabbit model of chronic limb ischemia," *Circulation* (1994), 90: II-228-34.

23. C. J. Chiu, J. Terzis, and M. L. MacRae, "Replacement of superior vena cava with the spiral composite vein graft: A versatile technique," *Ann Thorac Surg* (1974), 17: 555-560.

24. D. B. Doty and W. H. Baker, "Bypass of superior vena cava with spiral vein graft," *Ann Thorac Surg* (1976), 22: 490-93.

25. R. J. Fowl et al., "Use of autologous spiral vein grafts for vascular reconstructions in contaminated fields" *J Vasc Surg* (1988), 8: 442-46.

26. R. C. J. Chiu, "Spiral vein graft: a historical vignette," *Canadian J Surg* (1998), 41: 8-9.

27. C. J. Chiu and D. S. Mulder, "Selective arterialization of coronary veins for diffuse coronary occlusion— An experimental evaluation," *J Thorac Cardiovasc Surg* (1975), 70: 177-82.

28. J. Solorzano, G. Taitelbaum, and C. J. Chiu, "Retrograde coronary sinus perfusion for myocardial protection during cardiopulmonary bypass," *Ann Thorac Surg* (1978), 25: 201-8.

29. R. C. J. Chiu, "Cold cardioplegia via retrograde coronary sinus (RCS) infusion for myocardial protection," in *The Coronary Sinus*, W. Mohl, E. Wolner, and D. Glogar, eds., (New York: Springer-Verlag, 1984), pp. 275-283

30. R. C. J. Chiu, "Dynamic cardiomyoplasty: personal reflections on how it began," *Medtronic Science and Technology* (1996), 4: 2-6.

31. R. Leriche, "Essai expérimentale de traitement de certains infarctus du myocarde et de l'anévrisme du coeur par une greffe de muscle strié," *Bull Soc Natl Chir* (1933), 59: 229.

32. A. Kantrowitz and W. McKinnon, "The experimental use of the diaphragm as an auxiliary myocardium," *Surg Forum* (1959), 9: 266.

33. D. Drinkwater, R. C. J. Chiu, and D. Modry, "Cardiac assist and myocardial repair with synchronously stimulated skeletal muscle," *Surg Forum* (1980), 31: 271.

34. M. L. Dewar et al., "Synchronously stimulated skeletal muscle graft for myocardial repair: An experimental study," *J Thorac Cardiovasc Surg* (1984), 87: 325-31.

35. J. A. Macoviak et al., "Electrical conditioning of in situ skeletal muscle for replacement of myocardium," *J Surg Res* (1982), 32: 429.

36. A. Carpentier and J. C. Chachques, "Myocardial substitution with a stimulated skeletal muscle: first successful clinical case," *Lancet* (1985), 8440: 1267.

37. R. C. J. Chiu, "Cardiomyoplasty," in *Cardiac Surgery in the Adult*, L. H. Edmunds Jr., ed. (New York: McGraw-Hill, 1997), pp. 1491-1504.

38. D. Kass et al., "Reverse remodeling from cardiomyoplasty in human heart failure: external

constraint versus active assist," *Circulation* (1995), 91: 2314.

39. D. Marelli et al., "Cell transplantation for myocardial repair: an experimental approach," *Cell Transplantation* (1992), 1(6): 383-390.

40. R. C. J. Chiu, A. Zibaitis, and R. L. Kao, "Cellular cardiomyoplasty: myocardial regeneration with satellite cell implantation," *Ann Thorac Surg* (1995), 60: 12-18.

41. P. Menasche et al., "Myoblast transplantation for myocardial infarction," *Lancet* (2001), 357: 279-80.

42. J. S. Wang et al., "Marrow Stromal Cells for Cellular Cardiomyoplasty: Feasibility and Clinical Advantages," *J Thorac Cardiovasc Surg* (2000), 120: 999-1006.

43. E. G. Chedrawy et al., "Incorporation and integration of implanted myogenic and stem cells into native myocardial fibers: Anatomical basis for functional improvement," *JTCVS* (2002), 124: 584-590.

44. T. Saito et al., "Xenotransplant cardiac chimera: Immune tolerance of adult stem cells," *Ann Thorac Surg* (2002), 74: 19-24.

CHAPTER 8

MANITOBA

THE HISTORY OF

CARDIAC SURGERY IN WINNIPEG

Jaroslaw Barwinsky

The evolution of cardiac surgery in Winnipeg is closely linked to the enhancement of academic, scientific and professional interest in the subject by the University of Manitoba's Faculty of Medicine at the beginning of the 1950s. Historically, this period also followed the first successful surgical treatment of mitral stenosis as well as congenital heart anomalies. These developments led to better local teaching thanks to an improved understanding of rheumatic fever, acquired cardiac diseases, and congenital heart anomalies, including applied basic sciences.

The driving force in this process was Dr. Joe Doupe, Professor and Head of the Department of Physiology, who was responsible for the introduction of its new curriculum. Beyond a doubt, its implementation had a positive impact not only on the knowledge developed by medical students, including their clinical exposure, but also on their subsequent professional and academic choices. Hence, the Faculty of Medicine at the University of Manitoba deserves credit for providing the educational and intellectual stimulus for the evolution of cardiac surgery in Winnipeg.

Further Developments

Recruitment of Manpower

Dr. Lennox Bell was an excellent Dean of Medicine at the University of Manitoba, who responded positively to dramatic achievements in medical sciences and in various branches of surgery and medicine. At the beginning of the 1950s and thereafter, there was an obvious need to expand the professional academic manpower of the faculty as well as the medical specialists in the community at large.

In light of this, Dr. Colin Ferguson was appointed as the first full-time Professor of Surgery at the University of Manitoba on July 1, 1953 at the young age of 32 years. Dr. Ferguson graduated from the Medical Faculty at the University of Manitoba in 1945 and served with the Royal Canadian Navy. After the war, he undertook postgraduate studies in surgery at McGill University in Montreal, followed by surgical research at the University of Pennsylvania. He then spent 3 1/2 years at Boston Children's Hospital under Dr. Robert Gross in pediatric general surgery and cardiac surgery. While in Boston, he was also a Teaching Fellow in surgery at Harvard. Dr. Ferguson's appointment as Professor and Head of the Department of Surgery at the University of Manitoba brought much needed expertise in pediatric and cardiac surgery to Winnipeg as well as strong academic skills. Along with his academic appointment, he was granted surgical privileges at Children's Hospital as Surgeon-in-Chief and at St. Boniface General Hospital. For purely medical-political reasons, he encountered difficulties at Winnipeg General Hospital as appointments to its staff were fully controlled by the two private groups of doctors.

Following his arrival, Dr. Ferguson established a pediatric general surgical unit at Children's Hospital followed by a cardiac surgical unit. In addition, he performed some adult heart surgery such as mitral commissurotomies at St. Boniface General Hospital.

With the help of Dr. Joe Doupe, the Head of Physiology, and with private financial assistance, Ferguson established an experimental surgical laboratory at the Medical College to conduct animal research with the pump oxygenators in preparation for open heart surgery. In these efforts, he was assisted by Drs. Walter Zingg and Lawrence Whythead. This work eventually led to the first successful open heart procedure at Children's Hospital in October 1959.

Dr. Morley Cohen graduated from medical school at the University of Manitoba in 1948. He then took his residency training in surgery in Minneapolis at the University of Minnesota under Drs. Owen Wangensteen, Richard Varco and Walton Lillehei. During his training he was involved in surgical research related to extracorporeal circulation for which he received his Ph.D. Subsequently, he was involved with problems of cross-circulation in the first open-heart procedures for congenital anomalies performed at the University of Minnesota Hospital. For his research accomplishments Cohen received the Albert Lasker Award from the American Public Health Association for advances in cardiac surgery.

In 1955, he returned to Winnipeg and was appointed to the Department of Surgery at the University of

Manitoba and to the surgical staff at St. Boniface General Hospital. In performing these duties, Dr. Cohen was an exemplary teacher and an excellent surgeon, gaining respect and support throughout the city. In addition, he gained full support from the Order of Grey Nuns, the owners of the hospital, Dr. R.O. Burrell, the Surgeon-in-Chief, and prominent members of the Department. Cohen's aim was to develop a cardiac surgical unit at St. Boniface. With additional financial assistance from granting agencies and private sources in Winnipeg, he developed a surgical research laboratory at the hospital to conduct animal experiments dealing with problems of extracorporeal circulation and related innovative technological advances. This effort resulted in Winnipeg's first successful open heart pediatric procedure for repair of congenital heart problems, which was done at St. Boniface General Hospital in April 1959. That first patient is still alive and doing well at the time of this writing.

After the sudden death in 1962 of Dr. Maitland B. Perrin, who had been associated with the Winnipeg Clinic and the thoracic surgeons at Winnipeg General Hospital, Dr. Cohen was appointed by Dr. Colin Ferguson in 1967 as Head of Thoracic and Cardiovascular Surgery at the University of Manitoba. At the same time he was appointed Director of the Cardiovascular and Thoracic Unit at St. Boniface, to which the hospital authorities assigned 38 beds devoted to cardiovascular and thoracic surgical patients.

Dr. Cohen was also promoted to the rank of Associate Professor in Surgery of the University of Manitoba and appointed Director of the Postgraduate Training Program in Thoracic and Cardiovascular Surgery. In 1974, he received the University of Manitoba Alumni

Jubilee Award and in January 1987 was awarded the University of Manitoba Certificate in recognition and appreciation of long and loyal services. Dr. Cohen retired from practice in cardiac surgery in the summer of 1987. He died on August 18, 2005.

Dr. Jaroslaw Barwinsky graduated in medicine from the University of Manitoba in 1955. While still in medical school he developed a special interest in cardiovascular and respiratory physiology and subsequently in cardiology and respiratory diseases, as influenced by Dr. J. D. Adamson, Professor of Medicine, and cardiologist Dr. Robert Beamish. The developments in cardiac surgery were just on the horizon. As a result, Dr. Ferguson's lectures and group seminars had a decisive impact on his career path. Following his graduation Dr. Barwinsky was among the first group of four accepted into Dr. Ferguson's Surgical-Diploma Postgraduate Course in Surgery.

Dr. Hugh Sanderson, President of the University of Manitoba at the time, used his influence in helping Dr. Ferguson bring the postgraduate curriculum entirely under the university's control. The program was approved by the Royal College of Physicians and Surgeons of Canada and by the American Boards of Surgery.

During three years of surgical training and rotating through services at the St. Boniface, Winnipeg, and Children's hospitals, Dr. Barwinsky decided to continue his training in thoracic surgery. With Dr. Ferguson's approval, he accepted the opening at the Case-Western Reserve University in Cleveland, Ohio. During his additional three years of training under Dr. Fiorindo Simeoni and Dr. George Clowes, he spent one year in research, studying alterations of cardiac output following various types of surgery and various physiological aspects of extracorporeal circulation and hypothermia, especially relating to lung structure and function in the postoperative period. In addition, Dr. Clowes introduced a new method for repairing mitral valve insufficiency using the Merendino technique of mitral valve annuloplasty which was developed and practiced at that time and which Dr. Barwinsky brought with him to Winnipeg in 1961.

With advice from Dr. Wilfred Bigelow and a recommendation from Dr. Frederick G. Kergin of the University of Toronto, Dr. Barwinsky returned to Winnipeg in July 1961 and was appointed as a Lecturer in Surgery at the University of Manitoba. He was granted surgical privileges at St. Boniface General Hospital, Winnipeg General Hospital and Children's Hospital, but concentrated primarily at St. Boniface, working as an independent thoracic and cardiac surgeon. He was successful in passing the required examinations for Fellowship of the Royal College for General Surgery and the Royal College Certification in Thoracic Surgery as well as the American Boards of Surgery Examinations in both general and thoracic surgery. Shortly thereafter, he was appointed by the University of Manitoba to be in charge of the fourth year Undergraduate Surgical Teaching Program at St. Boniface General Hospital. In addition, he received research grants to continue his investigative studies. Drs. Morley Cohen and Richard R. Burrell were very supportive of these efforts.

In 1963, Dr. Barwinsky was appointed Director of the Surgical Research Laboratory at St. Boniface originally established by Dr. Cohen. He continued in this position until the end of 1973. During that time, he advanced through the usual academic promotion process and in 1983 he was promoted to full Professor of Surgery at the University of Manitoba. Subsequently, he was appointed as Director of the Provincial Program of Cardiac Surgery, Head of Cardiovascular and Thoracic Surgery and Director of Post Graduate Program in Cardiovascular and Thoracic Surgery. Along with these academic appointments he served as Head of CVT Surgery at St. Boniface General Hospital and the Health Sciences Centre.

During the academic year 1997-98 Dr. Barwinsky took a sabbatical leave of absence to study Medical Ethics at the University of Chicago and received an additional Fellowship Degree in Medical Ethics from that university. Upon his return to Winnipeg he continued to practice cardiac surgery for an additional six months and retired on January 1, 1999 at the age of 72.

In January 1987 Barwinsky received the University of Manitoba Certificate in appreciation of long and loyal services. In May 2001 he was awarded the status of Professor Emeritus of the University of Manitoba in recognition of Distinguished Services. In October of that same year, he received the Distinguished Alumni Award from the university's Alumni Association. On May 24, 2005, he was officially recognized by the Legislative Assembly of the Province of Manitoba by probate bill which was passed unanimously for his contribution to cardiac surgery in Winnipeg and for his cardiac care to the people of Manitoba.

Highly significant contributions were made to the development of heart surgery in the early period by investigative or invasive cardiologists Drs. Gordon Cummings, David Mymin and Anthony Miller.

Dr. Gordon Cummings was strictly devoted to pediatric cardiology at Children's Hospital. He was trained at the Cleveland Clinic, and upon his return to Winnipeg he developed a cardiac catheterization laboratory at Children's Hospital with the full support of Dr. Colin Ferguson.

At St. Boniface General Hospital, Drs. David Mymin and Anthony Miller also organized a catheterization laboratory during the early 1960s, including coronary angiography. They were instrumental in introducing angiographic transseptal left atrial methodology to assess the structure and function of mitral valve disease, which had a great impact on the selection of patients for valve surgery.

Cardiac Anaesthesia as a subspecialty did not exist at the beginning of this evolutionary period and each case had to be individualized. During the second half of the 1960s, cardiac anaesthesia was established at St. Boniface with the late Dr. Jack Culligan as its leading force. This eventually led to the development of this subspecialty at the Heath Sciences Centre and within the Department of Anaesthesia of the Faculty of Medicine.

Similar developments also occurred in intensive care units and professional skills of nursing personnel. These evolved gradually during the 1960s to the level of excellence in post-operative care to which we are accustomed today.

In addition, in the early 1980s we developed a special educational program for nurse clinicians with specialized curriculum contents followed by employment. This program became very productive and rewarding in dealing with patients during admission, postoperative care and follow-up.

Heart Surgery in Winnipeg During the 1950s

At the beginning of this period the occasional heart surgery performed was closed commissurotomy. These procedures were done in three different hospitals: St. Boniface General Hospital, Winnipeg General Hospital and Grace Hospital. Surgeons involved were usually certified general surgeons who developed a special interest in surgery of the lungs and heart. The first mitral commissurotomy was performed by Dr. Art Lerner in 1953 at the Grace Hospital. This first patient did very well but later on developed mitral valve insufficiency. Consequently in March 1962 the patient underwent open-heart mitral valve annuloplasty, performed by Dr. Barwinsky at St. Boniface using the Merendino technique, which he had learned during his residency training with Dr. George Clowes. In addition to being the first mitral commissurotomy, this was the first successful mitral valve annuloplasty performed in Winnipeg. The patient survived for over 13 years and died in California from non-cardiac causes.

From a 1961 review of mitral commissurotomies done in Winnipeg between 1953 and 1960 on over 200 patients, we learned that in all cases the indications for surgery were based entirely on clinical history, physical examination, PA, and lateral chest film and routine EKG. According to the quality standards of these days the outcomes were satisfactory and encouraging, but the majority of surviving patients required open-heart procedures at a later date.

With the arrival of Drs. Colin Ferguson and Morley Cohen the spectrum of cardiac surgery expanded to include congenital heart lesions and research related to cardiopulmonary bypass. This led to the first open heart procedures at the St. Boniface General Hospital in April 1959 and at the Children's Hospital in October 1959. Between then and the beginning of 1960 each institution performed approximately 20 open-heart procedures. All open-heart surgeries at St. Boniface were performed by Dr. Morley Cohen at that time. After the appointment of Dr. Jaroslaw Barwinsky in 1961, cardiac procedures were performed by the two surgeons.

Heart Surgery in Winnipeg During the 1960s

After the successful initiation of open-heart surgery in two teaching hospitals, cardiac surgery in Winnipeg continued to expand. This included not only increasing patient volumes but also a variety of operative procedures, basic research and related academic obligations. At the Children's Hospital, Dr. Colin Ferguson increased the volume and varieties of congenital heart lesions. In a written report of 1965, he outlined his experience in over 168 patients operated on between 1959 and January 1, 1965. The overall survival rate at that time was 89.6%. He continued his efforts until 1977 at which time he retired from clinical practice. By then he had performed over 860 pediatric open-heart procedures with gratifying outcomes. Prior to Dr. Ferguson's retirement and after the departure of Dr. Walter Zingg to Toronto, the animal-research laboratory at the Medical College ceased to exist.

At St. Boniface General Hospital the caseload of acquired heart disease continued to expand but the number of congenital heart problems started to decline towards the end of the decade due to a decrease of backlogged cases. Throughout this period we devoted our time to clinical cardiac surgery, surgical research and medical education. In early 1960, we were also receiving referrals of patients with cardiac arrhythmias and Stokes-Adam attacks. In light of this, on Monday, February 12, 1962, Dr. Barwinsky performed the first permanent pacemaker implantation for complete heart block using a Medtronics pacemaker. At that time this was done via left thoracotomy with both electrodes implanted into the left ventricular muscle. The original battery was good for only two years, although it improved thereafter. The patient survived for over 16 years and required numerous changes of pacemaker battery units.

The initial cost of the pacemaker unit in 1962 was $330.00. Since the hospital did not have a budget for this purpose, the funding had to be obtained from outside grants and charitable organizations. As the pacemaker technology evolved, transthoracic implantation was discontinued and the basic procedure was frequently transferred to cardiologists.

In the field of valvular heart disease there were also noticeable changes. Due to better and more detailed assessment of mitral valves by our invasive cardiologists, as previously mentioned, closed mitral commissurotomy gradually faded away and was replaced by open heart procedures: either repair of the mitral valve, known as annuloplasty-valvuloplastry, or mitral valve replacement. One of the last cases of closed mitral commissurotomy was done in May 1966. Following closed mitral commissurotomy the female patient developed severe mitral insufficiency. Consequently on May 26, 1966 at the age of 36, she underwent emergency mitral valve replacement performed by Dr. Barwinsky using a Starr Edward Silastic Ball Valve prosthesis. She did well and survived until December 2005 at which time she died at Brandon General Hospital at the age of 75.

The first elective mitral valve replacement at St. Boniface General Hospital was done by Dr. Morley Cohen in August 1962.

It is of interest to recall the scientific sessions of the Annual Meeting of the Royal College of Physicians and Surgeons of Canada held in Edmonton in January 1964. Our surgical colleague from Edmonton, the late Dr. John Callaghan, presented a paper reporting three successful cases of mitral valve replacement using Starr Edwards Silastic Ball Valve prostheses. During the discussion period, the participants included cardiac surgeons from Montreal reporting two cases, from Toronto reporting three cases and from Winnipeg also three cases. This was an historic moment for most of us.

Our caseload of cardiac valve replacements both mitral and aortic was increasing annually with very good immediate and long-term outcomes. Initially we used the Starr Edwards prosthesis almost routinely. However, towards the end of 1960, we experienced approximately 7 cases of sudden death following aortic valve replacement with this device. Autopsy examinations revealed Silastic Ball valve damage or ball variance in all cases. All damaged silicone balls were recovered and analyzed, confirming that the Silastic Ball damage was due to a manufacturing defect in the silicone material. Our findings were presented at the annual American Heart Association Meeting in Florida.

In view of this problem, we changed to the hollow metal ball valve, and as of 1969-1970 to the Björk-Shiley valve, which was also more beneficial for aortic valve replacement with narrow aortic root.

Myocardial Revascularization Procedures

Following the introduction of coronary angiograms at St. Boniface General Hospital we focused our efforts on the problems of myocardial revascularization. Coronary bypass grafting was as yet unknown but the Vineberg procedure was widely discussed and used. Consequently, during the second half of 1960 Drs. Cohen and Barwinsky operated on approximately 96 patients using the Vineberg procedure of intramyocardial implantation of internal mammary arteries. Some patients received a single implant of the left internal mammary artery to the anterior aspect of the left ventricular muscle and some received double mammary implants—left mammary to posterior left ventricle and the right mammary across the mediastinum to anterior left ventricle. Our immediate postoperative mortality rate was around 5% but the long-term outlook was very difficult to assess. Eventually, practically all long-term survivors underwent coronary bypass grafting surgery at a later date. We were also concerned with myocardial blood flow following the Vineberg procedure in spite of angiographic demonstration of patency of the internal mammary implants.

In response to this issue Dr. Barwinsky received a research grant from the Medical Research Council of Canada to study the myocardial blood flow and metabolism following the Vineberg procedure. From the experimental animals in our surgical research laboratory, we learned that among long term survivors (which were very few), the contribution of blood flow to ischemic myocardium via patent left mammary artery pedicle implant was less than 40% of original blood flow in previously patent LAD. This study was presented at the STS Meeting in Atlanta, Georgia in January of 1970 and was published in the *Annals of Thoracic Surgery*.

In the meantime at the national level the use of the Vineberg procedure declined due to the success of the coronary bypass grafting procedure, which was developed and introduced by Favaloro in 1967 and then by Johnson. In view of this, we discontinued our Vineberg procedure. The first coronary bypass graft at St. Boniface General Hospital using reverse vein graft to LAD was performed in August of 1969 by Dr. Morley Cohen.

Prior to that, during the 1960s we performed right coronary angioplasty using cardiopulmonary bypass in over 20 patients with coronary artery stenosis with either saphenous vein patch or pericardial patch graft. There was no operative mortality. Although the immediate results were good, they all occluded within two years and required coronary bypass graft surgery at a later date.

Heart Surgery in Winnipeg During the 1970s and Thereafter

This was the beginning of the most productive period of growth in open-heart surgery in Winnipeg. Our caseload of cardiac surgery continued to grow and the waiting lists were getting longer. Following the retirement of Dr. Colin Ferguson in 1977, and from 1978 until early 1980, some pediatric surgery at Children's Hospital was performed by Dr. Alberto G. Dela Rocha who was trained in Toronto. However his clinical practice was more focused on general thoracic surgery at the Health Sciences Centre, which in itself had a negative effect on the pediatric cardiac surgery at Children's Hospital. With the establishment of the Provincial Program in Cardiac Surgery practically all cases were done by Dr. Barwinsky, initially at St. Boniface General Hospital and then at Children's Hospital with very satisfactory final outcomes. More complex cases such as transposition of the great vessel were referred to Toronto and the Manitoba Health Services covered all expenses. A total of more than 250 pediatric cardiac procedures were performed in Winnipeg during this period. During the late 1980s, pediatric cardiac surgery was performed at Children's Hospital by Dr. Kim Duncan, originally from Edmonton. He was trained in Edmonton and then in London, England, followed by fellowship training in Toronto. After a relatively short period of practice in Winnipeg he moved to the U.S.A. The Departments of Cardiology and Surgery at Children's Hospital then appointed Dr. Jonah Odim to the surgical staff. His performance resulted in very high mortality and became the subject of a judicial inquiry. Subsequently he departed to the U.S.A. As a result of these events, pediatric cardiac surgery was completely discontinued at Children's Hospital and all patients in need of surgical treatment were referred to Edmonton.

During the early 1970s, attempts were made by some surgeons, such as Dr. Whythead and Dr. Graham to establish an adult cardiac surgical unit at the Health Sciences Centre. However after a short trial, this effort was discontinued when Dr. Alan Downs became the head of the Department of Surgery.

At St. Boniface General Hospital cardiac surgical services continued to grow and expand. In our research activities, we included educational aspects for undergraduate medical students and for postgraduates including surgical residents. We participated in the Bachelor of Science Medicine Program for medical undergraduates involved in animal experiments in cardiovascular physiology related to cardiac surgery. This allowed them to obtain an additional Bachelor of Science in Medicine Degree with their M.D. at the time of their graduation. One of these students became a prominent cardiologist in Canada. In addition three postgraduate students received their Masters of Science Degree in Medicine after working in our laboratory. One resident in cardiac surgery obtained his Ph.D. in cardiac sciences while working at St. Boniface Research Institute under Dr. N. Dhalla, and another obtained his Master of Science degree while working with Dr. E. Pascoe.

With increased demand for technological manpower in cardiac surgery, we were also involved in training pump technicians as a part of the National Program. Some of them are still employed in Winnipeg at the time of this writing.

Our postgraduate training program in cardiovascular and thoracic surgery was approved by the Royal College of Physicians and Surgeons of Canada in 1969. The program was located entirely at St. Boniface General Hospital. Dr. Morley Cohen as the Section Head of CVT Surgery was appointed as Program Director at that time, followed by Dr. Barwinsky in 1984. During the late 1980s the program was expanded to include the Health Sciences Centre. Beginning in 1970 and throughout the 1980s our program trained 21 CVT surgeons. There were four residents from the U.S.A., one from Spain and two from India. The others were Canadians. All of our Canadian residents and some of the Americans successfully passed the Royal College Examination. Only one of our Canadian residents moved to practice in the U.S.A. All of the others are practicing in Canada, of whom six stayed in Winnipeg.

One of the first female CVT surgeons was our resident Dr. Dorothy Thomson who also served as Head of CVT surgery at the University of Saskatoon. A total of four

Canadian graduates from our program have served as CVT Surgery Department Heads in Canada. The program continues to be approved and remains active with Dr. A. Menkis and Dr. J. Lee in charge.

Towards the end of the 1970s and in the early 1980s, our annual caseload of open-heart surgery was over 360 operations. At the same time our waiting list increased to more than 160 patients. Some individuals were waiting for over a year. The majority of patients required coronary bypass grafts or valve surgery. In addition we were involved in surgery of the thoracic aorta. In the majority of our patients, we used Björk-Shiley and St. Jude mechanical valves, and some bioprosthetic valves. In the bioprosthetic valve spectrum,we started with Ionescu-Shiley valves but due to unfavourable reports, we changed to porcine bioprostheses and other bovine pericardial valves.

In the initial series of Björk-Shiley valves we experienced five fatal failures. Three additional patients with aortic valve failure came to the hospital on time, were re-operated upon, survived and did very well.

During this period we encountered very interesting experiences with our female patients. Some young women who needed valve replacement were also determined to have a family. Consequently we used bioprosthetic valves. After they regained sinus rhythm postoperatively, the oral anticoagulants were discontinued, which allowed them to proceed with their pregnancy and family planning. All of these patients had two to three children, and all required redo surgery for valve replacement at 4 to 5 year intervals either after or between pregnancies. They all survived and were still alive at the end of the 1990s, and their children were also normal. One patient underwent valve replacement three times. In the same category of patients, we had a teenage girl who arrived in Winnipeg from the Far East in severe congestive heart failure and pulmonary edema due to severe mitral valve incompetence. She underwent urgent surgery and mitral valve replacement with Starr Edwards Silastic Ball valve prosthesis. The patient did well and married several years afterwards. She had a very strong desire to have her own family, but due to being on oral anticoagulants, she suffered multiple miscarriages. When the patient was around 30 years old, her cardiologist decided to substitute well-controlled daily heparin injections. This permitted her to maintain a healthy pregnancy until approximately 35 to 36 weeks. At that point, her mitral valve suddenly thrombosed, and she was admitted to maternity hospital in a moribund state. The patient was immediately transferred to our cardiac unit at St. Boniface General Hospital under the care of Dr. Barwinsky. The fetal heart sounds were still present. She was placed immediately on cardiopulmonary bypass and caesarian section was done on the pump by the obstetrician. She then underwent redo replacement of her mitral valve with porcine bioprosthesis. Both the mother and her child, a son, survived and did well. The son is a prominent businessman in Winnipeg at the time of this writing, while the patient went on to have another uneventful pregnancy and delivery.

In dealing with thoracic aorta, we experienced another challenging problem. A young woman in her late teens became pregnant. During her last trimester, she developed eclampsia and was hospitalized for several months to receive appropriate treatment. During that period, she also experienced several episodes of severe chest pain. Her delivery was uneventful and her child has grown into a healthy adult. Subsequent investigation revealed extensive dissection of the thoracic aorta starting at the orifice of the left subclavian artery and extending to aortoiliac bifurcation. In less than two years, the patient developed thoracoabdominal aneurysm extending to the aortoiliac region. Consequently she was referred to our surgical unit under the care of Dr. Barwinsky. At surgery, the entire aorta was replaced with tubular graft starting at the transverse aortic arch and extending to aortoiliac bifurcation. Special care was taken to implant major intercostal branches and all branches of the thoracoabdominal aorta. The patient did well and is leading a normal life approximately 28 years after surgery. Follow up studies at around 20 years after surgery revealed normal configuration of the graft and full patency of all implanted vessels.

With the increased caseload and commitments during the mid 1970s it became obvious that there was a need to increase our surgical manpower. Our preference was to offer these positions to our own residents after completion of their training.

Consequently during the mid to late 1970s, Drs. Sung-Whan Kim and Samir Bhattacharya joined the CVT surgical staff as full members. Dr. Kim was involved in pacemaker implantation in addition to other cardiac surgical procedures. This was followed by the appointment of Dr. John Teskey in 1978 who spent an additional year of training in Toronto. Dr. Keith Warrian spent an additional year in training with Dr. Denton Cooley in Texas during the academic year of 1980-81 before joining the staff.

During the 1980s our CVT surgery section developed an interest in cardiac transplantation. At the same time our resident Dr. Ed Pascoe was very keen to pursue this challenge. Therefore after completing his formal residency training, and with grant support from the

Graduate Studies Department of the University of Manitoba and the Heart and Stroke Foundation, he spent one full year in Richmond, Virginia under Dr. Richard Lower in Cardiac Transplantation Program. Upon his return to Winnipeg in 1986, he was also appointed to the staff of CVT surgery at St. Boniface General Hospital and the University of Manitoba, becoming an enthusiastic surgeon and a very good teacher.

With time Dr. John Teskey moved to the U.S. and Drs. Kim and Dr. Bhattacharya retired. Drs. Warrian and Pascoe continue to enjoy their duties.

As previously mentioned, the number of operative cases at St. Boniface General Hospital was increasing and our waiting list for surgery was also growing longer. In addition, our operative mortality for elective coronary bypass surgery during 1980-81 was between 1.8 and 2.1%, but the mortality among patients waiting for coronary surgery was around 6%. At the same time, as documented by medical records, the referral rate from the Health Sciences Centre to the St. Boniface Cardiac Unit over a 5-year period was between 25 and 27%. This figure became well known to everyone in the community. Nevertheless, the Chief Executive Officer at the hospital was not very enthusiastic about increasing its open-heart facilities. This policy persisted in spite of several meetings with the cardiac surgeons, the provincial Minister of Health and the Premier of Manitoba. As a result of this impasse another open-heart unit was established at the Health Sciences Centre during Dr. Alan Downs' tenure as head of the Department of Surgery and Dr. Jim Parrott was appointed to the surgical staff.

In the subsequent provincial election, a new government was elected and the new Minister of Health decided to review the wait-list problem. A special committee was established and discussions were held at the Manitoba Legislative Assembly. As a result of these efforts a Provincial Program in Cardiac Surgery was established in 1983, similar to the present Cardiac Science Program. This initiative was approved by the Faculty of Medicine at the University of Manitoba, the boards of both teaching hospitals, Manitoba Health Services, and the Minister of Health. After a rather extensive review and search process, Dr. Barwinsky was appointed as Director of the Provincial Program in Cardiac Surgery, in addition to his other academic duties. The basic aim of the Provincial Program was to coordinate and manage cardiac surgery problems in both centres, including quality assurance. The office of the Provincial Program was located at St. Boniface General Hospital.

For a short period thereafter, the provincial government increased funding for heart surgery at St. Boniface and the Health Sciences Centre. This helped to increase the volume of surgeries and improve facilities in both hospitals, as well as improving pediatric cardiac surgery at Children's Hospital.

In 1987, the Provincial Program in Cardiac Surgery initiated a statistical review and analysis of the number of open-heart cases that needed to be done in Winnipeg. On the basis of this study it was estimated that there would be an ongoing need for approximately 1,250 to 1,270 surgeries in the province annually.

Efforts were also made to establish cardiac transplant services in Winnipeg, especially since Dr. Ed Pascoe had been trained for that purpose. Numerous discussions were held at all levels. Initially, in the early1980s the number of patients from Manitoba referred to other centres for heart transplants was between 20 and 22 cases per year. In time, this number decreased dramatically by more than 50%, as a result of different and improved management of heart failure. As a result of this change, the governing bodies were less interested in proceeding with the cardiac transplantation program, bearing in mind the quality of patient care with such a small caseload. Consequently, the heart transplant program did not become a reality during the 1980s.

At the end of 1989, when Dr. Barwinsky's position as Director of the Provincial Program was due for renewal after six years of service, he decided not to continue in this position any longer and the program ceased to exist. However, the operative caseload remained the same as before and was increasing in both institutions.

Dr. Parrott left Winnipeg shortly thereafter. During the 1990s, various cardiac surgeons were appointed to the Health Sciences staff in CVT surgery, some Canadians and some from the U.S.A., but they stayed for only short periods of time. After completing his training in our CVT Program, Dr. Michael Raabe was appointed to the staff, and he continues to work there to this day.

Since that time there have been several external reviews of our cardiac programs in Winnipeg. The most recent of these was done by Dr. Koshal from Edmonton in April 2003. This review recommended a single cardiac surgery unit for Winnipeg located at St. Boniface General Hospital. After a lengthy search process, Dr. Alan Menkis was appointed as Director of the Cardiac Sciences Program and Head of Cardiovascular Surgery at the University of Manitoba. I am also hopeful that this will lead to the establishment of the Winnipeg Heart Institute.

CHAPTER 9

HEART SURGERY IN SASKATCHEWAN

Ed Busse

This chapter is written with the advantage of having reviewed the first edition of Dr. Goldman's book *Heart Surgery in Canada*. Also, it is written from augmented memory rather than diligent research.

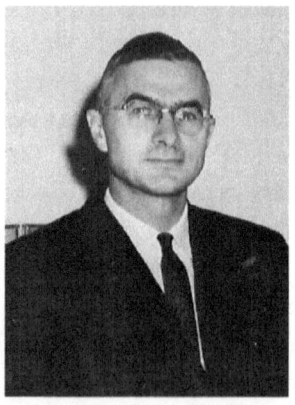

Fig. 9:1 Art Boyd (1921-1990)
Saskatchewan's First Heart Surgeon

Those who introduced heart surgery to Saskatchewan acted out much the same events as elsewhere in Canada; the cast of characters was different but the stages and performances much the same. In the four western provinces programs were developed by each of the four medical school university hospitals, and in each province by private practice counterparts: St. Boniface, Regina, Calgary, and Victoria. If one wished to explore the nuances of town-gown issues in the development of subspecialties in medicine one could well start here.

The cast of characters in this saga included brave souls, many of them WWII veterans with experiences in broad aspects of surgery and anaesthesia including a good dollop of thoracoabdominal and vascular trauma. They had acquired a military concept of duty and of comradeship. Their ambitions were spawned by post war euphoria; they were recruited widely within the British Empire and had received their cardiac training particularly in London and New England. Their broadly-based training experiences made it natural for them to attend international congresses, particularly the meetings of the American College of Surgeons. Their repertoire was broad and most often included general surgery, vascular surgery, and thoracic surgery for carcinoma and for tuberculosis—the last of which likely required the most demanding delicate surgical techniques. They fed their surgical urges regularly on a diet of late night ruptured abdominal aneurysms, pre-seatbelt chest trauma, acute abdomens and pulmonary resections.

As a reader of these historical accounts one has a tendency to think of these individuals as the eminent figures they became in their later years and as they appear in their photographs in our hallways. One needs be reminded that when these events were occurring the participants were young thirty-something individuals bearing the burdens of introducing new and dangerous procedures for the relief of a large group of otherwise incurable patients. The support they received from the senior members of their profession who were well aware of the good work they were attempting was profound. Today these procedures attract little attention from our colleagues, and when they do it is more often about our expanding resource needs than about the value to patient care.

These pioneers worked as a team developing a new service, and were motivated by the large population of end-stage cardiac patients with conditions for which, finally, surgical repair had become available. Smaller centres such as our two in Saskatchewan developed in response to this large patient load, the lack of insurance provisions for the referral of patients to larger centres, and the presence of most of the medical and surgical skills necessary to get started. All that was required for implementating these procedures was a heart-lung machine, some cardiac catheters and a pressure monitor. Add to that a motivated radiologist and/or young cardiologist and a surgeon that knew how to run the pump and to train a technician to do it and the team was up and running.

In Saskatoon the surgical team at the University Hospital was organized by Eric Nanson and run by Bev Lynn and Clayton Robinson, both of whom were trained primarily as thoracic surgeons. Cardiologist Lou Horlick organized the diagnostic side, which was managed and expanded by Jose Lopez from Chicago.

In Regina services were developed by members of the Medical Arts Clinic working with the Grey Nuns and Regina General Hospitals. "Surgeon-unencumbered-by-doubt" Clayton Crosby, recently of the Montreal General surgical unit in Europe, got things started by recruiting Art Boyd as the lead surgeon. "Cold Steel" Doug McAlpine and cool headed Mel Bowering provided the level of anaesthesia required for these ambitions

projects, while Gene Rodko in Radiology and Gerald
Ewing in Cardiology introduced diagnostic imaging and
CCU management. Ed Busse, your raconteur, joined the
Regina team in 1969 just after Firor and Bharadwaj had
joined Saskatoon.

Outwardly the two centres appeared dissimilar: the
town-gown thing again. Differences in funding resources
and administrative support, generally favoured the
University on the justifiable argument of supporting
medical training. The academic referral and teaching
centre in Saskatoon differed from the Comprehensive
Group Practice model in Regina and these differences
encouraged rivalry and sometimes distrust: maybe the
military influence again.

Internally, however, things played themselves out much
the same in the two centres. The Medical Arts Clinic
held its academically oriented in-house clinical meetings
and participated in the Hospitals'; teaching and audit
rounds. Similar rounds and events were probably more
frequently scheduled and more impressively named in
the Saskatoon teaching hospitals. The levels of clinical
assessment, management, and research in both centres
were judged to be quite parallel by Cardiac Surgeon
Dwight McGoon of the Mayo Clinic when he was
commissioned to evaluate them in 1967. This opinion
allowed the Saskatchewan Department of Health to
commit support to both centres and precipitated the
recruitment of the next generation of recently trained
CVT surgeons Bharadwaj and Firor from Toronto to
Saskatoon and Busse from McGill to Regina.

In this early phase of cardiac surgery congenital anomalies
were a major part of the surgical volumes; transpositions
and tetralogies were as much a part of the schedule as

closed mitral commisurotomies. Aortic and mitral valve replacements increased toward the end of the first era, which was marked by the introduction of aortocoronary bypass procedures.

A brief chronology of events in Saskatchewan paralells, in time, events in other provinces. Closed mitral commisurotomies began at the Regina Grey Nuns Hospital by Boyd, Crosby and McAlpine in 1957 and in Saskatoon by Nanson in 1958. Open heart procedures were begun at the Regina General Hospital by Art Boyd in 1959 and Saskatoon by Nanson and Bev Lynn the same year. Ed Busse (your author) with Art Boyd marked the end of the first era of cardiac surgery with a LIMA to LAD bypass in early 1971. By that time a full list of congenital procedures and valve replacements had been established and diagnostic procedures were being performed by the cardiologists rather than the surgeons which had been the earlier arrangement.

The second era of cardiac surgery, likely the Golden Era, began with increasing volumes of surgery for coronary artery disease and the addition of more surgical staff. In Saskatoon Jean Lemaire stayed for a few years before going to Long Beach, California; Lloyd Black followed the same course; following Black, Stuart Nutting ended up in the New Orleans area; Dorothy Thomson remained and was eventually joined by Taras Mycyk and more recently Greggory Dalshaug. Art Boyd and Ed Busse in Regina were joined in turn by John Burgess, Andrew Maitland (both now in Calgary), Rand Forgie (now in Saint John, NB), and John Ofish (now in Victoria). Leith Dewar (from UBC), John Tsang (McGill), Steve Korkola (McGill), and Amhad Moustapha (University of Alberta) comprise the current (2007) Regina cardiac surgical team. Your author, Busse, retired from clinical surgery in 2005 and spends his time writing stuff like this.

Brief Biographies of the Major Surgical Players of the First Era:

Art Boyd (1921-1990) Born in China to missionary parents, fluent in Mandarin. MD U of T, 1944, surgical training in England and at the Mass. General in Boston, recruited to the Medical Arts Clinic, 1957

Baikunth Bharadwaj, Toronto. Trained in CVT Surgery and backbone of the Saskatoon program. Recruited to the Foothills in Calgary as chief of their Cardiac Surgery Program in 1988.

Ed Busse, Saskatchewan born and raised, MD from Johns Hopkins, 1961, and CVT surgery training in the McGill Program, arrived Regina 1969 and still here (2007).

Whit Firor, MD from Hopkins and CVT training in Toronto. Switched from surgery to cardiac rehabilitation. Whit died of pancreatic carcinoma in his early 50s.

Bev Lynn, Queen's grad. British trained, co-author of textbook on vascular surgery with Ian Aird. Arrived in Saskatoon 1957 and after several years returned to Queen's as Chief of CVT Surgery, retired in the 1980s into the antiques business. Died in a motor vehicle accident, 2007.

Eric Nanson, Kind and caring New Zealander. Spent time at Hopkins in the '50s, Professor of Surgery at the University of Saskatchewan Medical School, 1957-68, returned to New Zealand as Professor of Surgery there.

CHAPTER 10

CARDIAC SURGERY IN ALBERTA:
A TALE OF TWO CITIES

EDMONTON

Zlatko I. Pozeg and Arvind Koshal

Thoracic surgery began in Edmonton in the mid-1940s. At that time there were three hospitals equipped to carry out such procedures: the University of Alberta Hospital (established in 1922), the Royal Alexandra (which opened its doors in 1910), and the Edmonton General Hospital (which opened in 1895). A Faculty of Medicine had also been established at the University of Alberta, and graduated its first class in 1925. The early pioneers of closed cardiac surgery in Edmonton were Drs. Carleton Whiteside, Herb Meltzer, Colin Ross and Colin Dafoe.

Dr. W. Carleton Whiteside (1900-1967) graduated from the University of Alberta medical school in 1928. The following year was spent as an intern in Pennsylvania, after which he did an externship in Edmonton for two years. Whiteside qualified as a fellow of the Royal College of Physicians and Surgeons of Canada in 1931 and began a general surgery practice in Edmonton after spending time abroad with various surgeons. Between 1941 and 1945 he served in the Royal Canadian Army Medical

Corps, and upon his return to Edmonton commenced the practice of thoracic surgery in 1946. Dr. Whiteside was stimulated by the exciting new field of cardiac surgery and carefully studied progress in the field by traveling to various centres, including a visit to Dr. Clarence Crafoord in Sweden.

Edmonton cardiologist Robert S. Fraser has compiled a detailed study of Dr. Whiteside's early cases with the assistance of the surgeon's son, Dr. Carl Whiteside of Victoria, and Miss B. Schultz, former record librarian at the University of Alberta Hospital. The first recorded cardiac surgery in Edmonton was performed at the University Hospital on a sixteen-year-old girl, who on September 22, 1948, had a patent ductus ligated with two #3 silk sutures by Dr. Whiteside.

The first Blalock-Taussig procedure performed there took place on April 28, 1949, on a sixteen-year-old boy who was severely cyanotic. In his note, Dr. Whiteside stated that, "For historic purposes this is the first Blalock operation performed at the University Hospital, there being four others done in the city previously by me." This patient was well for twelve years when he presented with heart failure in 1962 and died two weeks after an attempted repair under cardiopulmonary bypass as a result of a right ventricular infarct. The details of this case are well delineated in Dr. Fraser's book.

On August 16, 1948, Dr. Whiteside had performed a Blalock shunt at the Royal Alexandra Hospital, with Dr. Leslie Willox as assistant. This was likely the first such operation in the province. Whiteside then performed two more shunt procedures there in early 1949, the first of these on January 29, on a nine-year-old girl.

During 1949, Dr. Whiteside also ligated two ductuses. The following year he performed a Pott's shunt, a Blalock shunt, and a mitral split. An attempt to do a second Blalock procedure was unsuccessful, as the patient died of cardiac arrest in the operating room.

In 1951 he performed a coarctation repair at the Misericordia Hospital, in addition to two ductuses, and another mitral split, and in 1952 carried out a second coarctation repair (again using the left subclavian artery), as well as five mitral splits and two ductal ligations.

Nineteen fifty-three saw an increase in the number of cardiac procedures carried out by Dr. Whiteside, with twelve operations in the first seven months. These included seven operations on the mitral valve (two of them unsuccessful), three ductuses, and two pulmonary valvotomies. Throughout this seven-year period, Dr. Whiteside maintained a busy thoracic and vascular practice in all of the Edmonton hospitals.

In August 1956 Dr. Whiteside moved to Victoria, British Columbia, where he continued to practice thoracic and cardiac surgery. He died suddenly of cardiac arrest on January 19, 1967, while discussing a paper at the Royal College of Physicians and Surgeons meeting in Ottawa.

Carleton Whiteside should be regarded as one of the true pioneers of cardiac surgery in Canada. He had the determination, skill, and perseverance to proceed in a specialty still in its infancy, performing many "firsts" in Alberta during the pre-heart-lung machine era.

The only other individual who had performed a cardiac operation prior to 1953 in Edmonton was thoracic surgeon Herbert Meltzer, who performed a pericardiectomy on a twenty-eight-year-old woman diagnosed with constrictive pericarditis. This is the only cardiac procedure performed by Dr. Meltzer on record.

Dr. Colin Dafoe began practicing thoracic surgery in Edmonton in August 1950, but apparently did not begin doing cardiac procedures until 1953. Between 1940 and 1946, Dr. Dafoe had served with the (British) Royal Army Medical Corps in various overseas postings, including seven months in Yugoslavia, where he had an indelible influence while operating on the wounded, and is still revered for his efforts. Dafoe's partner at the Royal Alexandra Hospital was Dr. Colin Ross. Together they performed a variety of closed-heart procedures including valvular cases, ligation of the patent ductus and coarctation corrections. In addition, Dafoe spent time with Dr. Charles Bailey in 1956 in Philadelphia, to develop his skills in valvular surgery. Both surgeons continued to perform an increasing volume of pulmonary and esophageal procedures, but did not continue in the field of cardiac surgery when the era of extracorporeal circulation began.

Colin Dafoe unfortunately disappeared under mysterious circumstances while hiking in Waterton National Park in 1969. His body was found three years later. Dr. Ross continued a successful career in thoracic surgery and surgical research until his premature death in 1980 at the age of sixty-one.

These four—Drs. Whiteside, Meltzer, Dafoe and Ross— were the pioneers of cardiac surgery in Alberta. The operations they performed are considered "closed" procedures, that is, not requiring extracorporeal circulation, and were thereby essentially limited to closure of the ductus, coarctation repair, Blalock-Taussig shunts, and mitral and pulmonary valvotomies. Nevertheless, their bravery, persistence and sincere dedication laid the substrate and foundation for the development of open-heart surgery in the province.

As a result of postwar advances in the field of cardiology, the importance of establishing a diagnostic cardiologic unit was recognized by the administrators at the University of Alberta. The inception of cardiology, as a department dedicated to the diagnosis and treatment of heart disease, began at the University Hospital in 1953, in the form of a cardiovascular unit. The advent of cardiac catheterization allowed for the accurate diagnosis and subsequent initiation of therapy for many types of cardiac disease, both congenital and acquired. The cardiovascular unit was directed by Drs. Robert S. Fraser and Joseph Dvorkin, and approximately ninety catheterizations were performed in 1956; the first having been performed in November 1953 by Dr. Dvorkin.

The chairman of the department of surgery during the 1950s was Dr. Walter C. Mackenzie. He was a visionary and was aware of the exciting new developments in surgery on the heart. Realizing that a leading department of surgery would require individuals who could provide skill and knowledge in both the clinical and research aspects of this new discipline, he recruited Dr. John Carter Callaghan (1923-2004) to establish a program in open-heart surgery at the University Hospital.

Dr. Callaghan was born in Hamilton, Ontario in October 1923. He graduated from the University of Toronto medical school in 1946 and spent the following year as a junior rotating intern at the Toronto General Hospital. After spending a year working as a demonstrator in anatomy as well as a medical officer for the Lyndhurst

Lodge paraplegic rehabilitation centre, the adventurous Dr. Callaghan went to Aklavik in the Northwest Territories (now Nunavut) as a medical officer with the Indian Health Services. Upon returning to Toronto in 1949-50 at the age of twenty-seven to continue his postgraduate education, Callaghan was appointed Research Fellow at the Banting Institute. It was here that he began his seminal work on hypothermia and cardiac pacing with Dr. Wilfred G. Bigelow

Between 1950 and 1953, Callaghan continued his training in cardiac surgery as a resident and fellow at the University of Toronto. In 1953, he was awarded a McLaughlin Travelling Fellowship and acted as assistant to Lord Russell Brock at Guy's Hospital in London and fellow to Dr. Frank Gerbode at Stanford University. In August 1955, at the end of his surgical training, Callaghan took up an appointment as Lecturer in Surgery at the University of Alberta. In 1958 he was promoted to assistant clinical professor, and two years later became professor of surgery and head of the division of thoracic and cardiovascular surgery.

Upon his arrival in Edmonton, Dr. Callaghan was charged with the task of developing a cardiac surgical program. Many individuals contributed to this monumental endeavour. Certainly, the whole process would not have been possible without the support of Walter Mackenzie, surgeon in chief at the university hospital. The cardiologists, Robert Fraser and Joseph Dvorkin, worked closely with the cardiac surgeons in the diagnosis, treatment (both medical and surgical), and postoperative care of heart patients; they were pillars of the surgical program.

Prior to attempting the first open-heart case a significant amount of preparatory work and research was required.

Dr. Callaghan became involved in the development of a large research infrastructure at the university's Surgical Medical Research Institute (SMRI). Here Callaghan conducted experimental surgery and along with Drs. Fraser and Dvorkin developed the techniques necessary to attempt their first open-heart procedure.

Dr. Callaghan was given a room at the SMRI to prepare the circuit and pump oxygenator. In this capacity he had the help of Drs. Morris Friedman and Eric Elliot from the General Surgery group, who were instrumental in building the first heart-lung machine used at the University of Alberta.

Anita Wilde, a nurse, was given the task of running the pump oxygenator for the first case as well as ensuring complete sterility. The prototype that Callaghan decided to use was the Lillehei-DeWall pump. He and the team traveled to the University of Minnesota several times and studied every detail of the pump and oxygenator with Drs. Lillehei and DeWall.

With the preparatory work completed, the cardiac surgical team was now ready to perform its first clinical procedure, scheduled for September 18, 1956, with Dr. Ted Gain as anaesthetist for the first case, Anita Wilde as pump technician, and Lois Eiffert as the scrub nurse. Dr. Leslie Willox, a veteran cardiovascular surgeon who had assisted Carleton Whiteside in his first shunt operation, was Dr. Callaghan's assistant. Drs. Dvorkin and Fraser were also present and responsible for monitoring the electrocardiogram, arterial and venous pressures, and oxygen saturation.

The candidate selected for the first open cardiac surgical procedure was a patient of Dr. Adam Little, an internist in the department of medicine. The patient was thirty-year-old James Harmon, who was diagnosed with symptomatic pulmonary stenosis, and underwent an uneventful operation.

Dr. Callaghan has confirmed that the team had deliberately chosen a case involving a familiar procedure that did not necessarily require a pump oxygenator, so that in the event of an equipment failure, Mr. Harmon could still undergo a successful repair. However, the heart-lung machine was used successfully that day, albeit for a short period of time.

For the next case, the pump oxygenator was absolutely necessary. This is regarded by Dr. Callaghan and his team as the first procedure in Canada involving a heart-lung machine. The event occurred on October 24, 1956, after two unsuccessful attempts at repair of tetralogy of Fallot. Ten-year-old Suzanne Beattie underwent repair of an atrial septal defect. In December of the same year the team successfully operated on two-year-old Sherry Anderson who had pulmonary stenosis and a VSD, and early in 1957 they performed the first complex tetralogy of Fallot repair in Canada on Dolly Ann Morrow. Both went on to live long and happy lives. A total of thirty-five operations were performed within the first year.

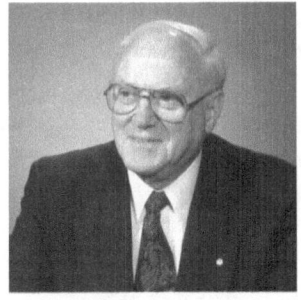

Fig. 10:1 John C. Callaghan

Another Canadian milestone occurred at the University of Alberta Hospital in 1962, when Dr. Callaghan implanted the first Starr-Edwards prosthesis in the mitral position. On June 7, 1967, the team performed its one thousandth open-heart procedure on five-year-old Monica McAllister, a pulmonary stenosis patient, and the same week carried out its first coronary bypass operation. In March 1986, Dominico Marano's coronary bypass became the University Hospital's seven thousandth open-heart procedure.

John C. Callaghan was the leader of the cardiac surgery movement in Edmonton. He continued a very busy practice until his retirement in 1990, as well as continuing to oversee the evolution of Edmonton's cardiac surgery program. Throughout his illustrious career, Dr. Callaghan received innumerable awards and merits, including the Order of Canada in 1985 and the Queen Elizabeth II Golden Jubilee Medal in 2002. In 1996, at the fortieth anniversary of the first open-heart operation, the University of Alberta Hospital dedicated and announced the opening of the Dr. John C. Callaghan Surgery Intensive Care Unit.

Dr. Callaghan can be counted among the true giants of cardiac surgery such as Cooley, Lillehei, Kirklin, and Bigelow. However, his surgical colleagues and successors, Drs. Cec Couves and Larry Stearns, also played significant roles in maintaining and further developing the department.

Dr. Cecil Melville Couves (1919-1991) was born in Lang, Saskatchewan, in December 1919. He graduated from the University of Manitoba Faculty of Medicine in 1945, and received surgical training at the University of Edinburgh and the Sheffield Royal Infirmary. Couves then spent two years with Dr. Michael E. DeBakey at Baylor University, from 1954 to 1956, and the following year was appointed as research fellow in cardiovascular and thoracic surgery at the University of Alberta. In 1958 he was admitted as staff cardiac surgeon. Couves had a busy practice in cardiac, vascular and thoracic surgery, in addition to being a prolific researcher and supervising several graduate degrees in cardiac surgery research. In 1974, Dr. Couves moved St. John's to become chairman of the department of surgery at the Memorial University of Newfoundland.

Dr. Lawrence Perrin Stearns was born in Ottawa in 1930. He graduated from the faculty of medicine at Queen's University in 1955, and proceeded with internship and a year of residency at the Montreal General Hospital. Sterns spent two years at the University of Minnesota as an assistant resident, followed by another two-year stint as senior assistant resident at the Montreal General. He then returned to the University of Minnesota for four years, and in 1965 was awarded a PhD for his thesis on "Selective Cardiac Hypothermia." In 1966 he began his career in Edmonton as a lecturer in the division of cardiovascular surgery, University of Alberta. Dr. Stearns retired after a long and successful career of pediatric and adult cardiac surgery in 1990.

Dr. Elliott Gelfand joined the team of surgeons in 1974. He graduated from the University of Alberta in 1965, and interned at the University Hospital. Upon the direction of Dr. Couves, Dr. Gelfand undertook his surgical training in Milwaukee at Marquette University and the Medical College of Wisconsin, in general surgery and cardiovascular and thoracic surgery, respectively. There he trained with coronary bypass surgery pioneer Dr. Dudley Johnson. After spending two years on staff at the Montreal General Hospital, 1972-1974, Gelfand was recruited to the University of Alberta, where he has ever since been a valuable member. He has held the positions of chief of the division and program director.

Dr. Patricia Penkoske was hired in 1984 and began a practice in congenital heart surgery. A graduate of the Washington University Medical School in St. Louis, she completed a two-year cardiothoracic residency program in Boston, including six months' training in pediatric cardiac surgery with Dr. Aldo Castaneda at Boston Children's Hospital, followed by a one-year fellowship in this subspecialty at Toronto's Hospital for Sick Children under Drs. George Trusler and Bill Williams.

An important addition to the department occurred in 1991 with the arrival of Dr. Arvind Koshal from Ottawa. After training with Dr. Wilbert Keon and at Harvard with Dr. Lawrence Cohn, Koshal spent several years on the staff of the University of Ottawa Heart Institute before his appointment as chief of cardiac surgery at the University of Alberta Hospital. A visionary akin to Drs. Callaghan and Keon, Koshal has brought about significant advances in the Edmonton cardiac surgery program. His chief ambition was to develop the first Heart Institute in Western Canada, on the Ottawa model established by Dr. Keon.

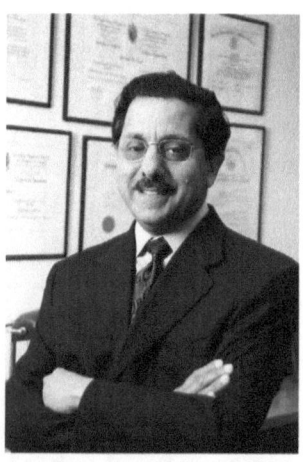

Fig. 10:2 Arvind Koshal

Toward this goal, Dr. Koshal focused on developing a team approach in the treatment of heart disease. This required the involvement of surgeons, cardiologists, allied health care workers, hospital administration, government and the community. In 1995, under his leadership, the Cardiac Sciences Program was established. Its overall mission was to develop a coordinated and integrated patient-centered program, which would allow for excellence in the prevention and treatment of heart disease, prompt and equal access to diagnostic, treatment and rehabilitation modalities, and leadership in education and research.

In order for this vision to be realized, several spheres of cardiovascular and thoracic surgery were developed. First, the clinical cardiac surgery program was expanded, with the number of adult cases increasing from 571 in 1991 to 1,350 in 2002, along with a commensurate drop in the mortality rate from 6.2 percent to 2.9 percent over the same period.

Secondly, a thoracic transplant program was launched, with Dr. Dennis L. Modry as director. A 1973 graduate of the University of Alberta, he completed his training in general and cardiovascular and his thoracic surgical training at McGill University. Dr. Modry then had the opportunity to obtain a fellowship with the pioneer of thoracic transplantation, Dr. Norman Shumway of Stanford University. Upon his return to Edmonton in 1984 he took on the responsibility of developing a thoracic transplant service at the University of Alberta Hospital. Dr. Modry was the sole transplant surgeon in Edmonton until 1991, when he was joined by Arvind Koshal, and the subsequent arrival of Dr. John C. Mullen from Toronto, who performed Alberta's first (and Canada's third) living-related donor lung transplant in

February 2001. The first heart transplant in Edmonton took place on July 28, 1985, followed by the first heart-lung the following year, and the first lung transplant in December 1989; all with Dr. Modry as surgeon.

Drs. ShaoHua Wang and David B. Ross has since joined the surgical staff and also perform heart transplants. Dr. Wang completed his medical degree in China, and surgical training in Edmonton, and continues a busy general adult cardiac surgery practice. Dr. Ross arrived from Halifax, where he was on staff, in 2001. He trained in both adult and congenital cardiac surgery in Toronto and then in London at the Royal Brompton Hospital with Mr. Chris Lincoln. He continues to be the only surgeon in Alberta whose practice encompasses the whole of cardiac surgery, including adult, complex congenital, and cardiac transplant. The transplantation program continues to be very successful with eighty-five thoracic transplants being performed in the year 2002, the greatest number in Canada, with excellent results.

The third sphere of development was in the field of pediatric cardiac surgery. In the 1980s and early 1990s pediatric cardiac surgery struggled in Edmonton. In 1991, Dr. Koshal enlisted a former trainee, Dr. Zohair al-Halees from Saudia Arabia, to become an itinerant pediatric surgeon. The pediatric program was solidified with the addition of Dr. Ivan Rebeyka.

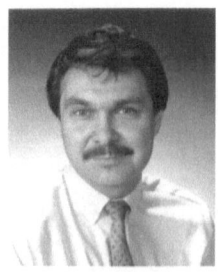

Fig. 10:3 Ivan Rebeyka

Dr. Rebeyka completed his general surgery training in Saskatchewan in 1984, and then went on to Toronto where he completed adult and pediatric cardiac surgery training under Drs. Tirone David and George Trusler in 1988. Rebeyka then went on to Virginia to do research with Dr. Andrew Wechsler prior to returning to a Toronto staff position in 1989. In 1996 he was appointed head of pediatric cardiac surgery at the University of Alberta, and was joined by Dr. David Ross in 2001.

The University of Alberta has become the major center for congenital heart surgery in Western Canada, with significant consolidation of care after the closure of programs in both Winnipeg and Saskatchewan. As a result, the case-load of pediatric open-heart surgery has increased from thirty in 1991 to 312 in 2002. The overall mortality of 1 percent is the lowest in North America, despite a large case-load of complex congenital heart defects.

The fourth sphere of the Cardiac Sciences Program was resident educational development, which evolved to include an organized teaching program and the involvement of residents in research. Residents went on to complete research projects and obtain graduate degrees. Dr. Rizwan A. Manji completed a doctor of philosophy in xenotransplantation. Several residents also received Master of Science degrees, including Drs. Gurmeet Singh, Roderick MacArthur, Zlatko Pozeg, and Steven R. Meyer. Residents continued to publish and present in international forums. Dr. John Mullen became program director of cardiac surgery after the departure of Dr. Penkoske in 2000.

Research has continued at the SMRI under the leadership of Dr. Ray V. Rajotte. Extensive collaborative investigations are done with Dr. Gary Lopaschuk in myocardial metabolism, and Drs. Stephen Archer and Evangelos Michelakis of the Vascular Biology Group. In addition, an extensive clinical and research fellowship program has been established in both adult and pediatric cardiac surgery, which has attracted individuals from all over the world including Japan, South Africa, Australia, Korea, and Saudi Arabia.

Therefore, in the year 2000, with all of these elements in place, Dr. Koshal was able to proceed with the planning of the Alberta Heart Institute. With the full support of medical and surgical colleagues, hospital administration, and government, the Cardiac Sciences Program became a high priority. In January 2001, Premier Ralph Klein announced the allocation of a $125 million grant for the development of a Cardiac Center of Excellence in Edmonton with the planned opening in 2005.

In the fifty years from the first open-heart case in 1956 to the opening of the Alberta Heart Institute in 2005, cardiac surgery in Edmonton has seen tremendous progress in the treatment of heart disease as a result of the coordinated and dedicated effort of many individuals who worked together as a team and built on the achievements of their predecessors. Cardiac surgery continues strongly into the twenty-first century in Edmonton, and continues to develop as a premiere facility for the surgical treatment of people with heart disease, and for the training of future cardiac surgeons.

References:

Cairney, Richard. 1997. "Pioneering Alberta cardiac surgeons walked into uncharted territory 40 years ago." *Can Med Assoc J* 56: 549-51.

Callaghan, John C. 1986. *Thirty years of open-heart surgery at the University of Alberta Hospitals.* Edmonton: University of Alberta Hospitals.

—. 2003. Personal communication, September 7, 2003.

Corbet, Elise A. 1990. *Frontiers of medicine: A history of medical education and research at the University of Alberta.* Edmonton: University of Alberta Press.

Fraser, Robert S. 1992. *Cardiology at the University of Alberta, 1922-1969.* Edmonton: University of Alberta.

Jamieson, Heber C. 1947. *Early medicine in Alberta: The first 75 years.* Edmonton: Canadian Medical Association, Alberta Division.

Shumacker, Harris B., Jr. 1992. *The evolution of Cardiac Surgery.* Bloomington and Indianapolis: Indiana University Press.

Street, Brian J. 1987. *The parachute ward: A Canadian surgeon's wartime adventures in Yugoslavia.* Toronto: T. H. Best.

428   Heart Surgery in Canada

CALGARY—HOLY CROSS HOSPITAL

Victor Aldrete

The first open-heart operation at the Holy Cross Hospital was carried out on October 17, 1962, on nine-year-old Marilyn Wren, ten short years after Floyd John Lewis, inspired by Wilfred G. Bigelow's experimental work on hypothermia had performed the first direct vision repair of an atrial septal defect. The founders of cardiac surgery in Calgary were Dr. George E. Miller, University of Alberta graduate class of 1945, and Dr. John C. Morgan, Queen's University graduate class of 1950.

Dr. Miller interned at the Holy Cross Hospital in 1945. Over the next five years, he spent time in the army, worked as a general practitioner with his father in Elkpoint, Alberta, helping in the control of a diphtheria epidemic, and for a time studied pathology in Saskatoon. The latter would be of great use to him later on in his surgical career. During this same period Dr. Miller joined the Calgary Associate Clinic for a couple of years as a general practitioner, before going on to the Mayo Clinic where, between 1950 and 1954, he trained in surgery under Dr. John Kirklin, followed by two more years in Minneapolis where he formed part of the first generation of formally trained cardiac surgeons.

Miller returned to Calgary in April 1956 to rejoin the Calgary Associate Clinic (the oldest group of physicians in the city) with the specific goal of starting a program in cardiac surgery and, in association with Dr. John C. Morgan, a cardiologist, began the development of a cardiac service in earnest.

Morgan had interned at the Toronto General Hospital, where he was exposed to the teachings of Drs. Gordon Murray and Wilfred G. Bigelow. As an American Heart Association Fellow in cardiology he went to Johns Hopkins and worked with Helen Taussig and Alfred Blalock. Dr. Morgan arrived in Calgary in September 1956, thus forming a medical-surgical team that was to endure through several decades of progress and improvement, overcoming a variety of obstacles along the way.

Between 1957 and 1962, the team was involved in the management of congenital heart conditions requiring surgical treatment, beginning with patent ductus arteriosus and coarctations of the aorta, and evolving to the closure of atrial septal defects, using systemic hypothermia and the inflow occlusion technique. At this time, the more complex cases were referred to Vancouver or to the Mayo Clinic, as a planned safety policy had been implemented to allow the program to grow on solid foundations of treatment excellence. These young pioneers had the vision to understand their limitations and acted accordingly. During the same period, after hours and with no pay, the team established an animal laboratory for the training of all associated personnel: scrub and circulating nurses, anaesthesiologists and cardiopulmonary technicians, thus putting into practice a team approach within the operating room.

The first open-heart case at Holy Cross Hospital was performed using a Pemco cardiopulmonary bypass machine with a Kay-Cross Disc Oxygenator purchased by the Calgary Associate Clinic. Then, between 1963 and 1964, the hospital administration made possible the design and construction of a new cardiac catheterization laboratory, with the full support of Dr. Douglas

Florendine, head of the department of radiology. Further consolidation of the program was achieved by the vision of Dr. Raymond G. "Paddy" Magner, medical director of Holy Cross, who in 1967, fused the divisions of cardiology and cardiovascular surgery into a single department with all the advantages that such an administrative structure is now well known to provide.

During these early years the Calgary program also had the invaluable support of Dr. John C. Callaghan, head of cardiac surgery at the University of Alberta and the university hospital in Edmonton, reiterating the importance of specialization in this groundbreaking discipline. From the treatment of congenital cardiac problems, the team moved on to the performance of closed cardiac surgical operations, such as mitral valve commissurotomies. This then led to myocardial revascularization with a few attempts at the Beck procedures, followed with Vineberg's operations in the mid-1960s

Drs. Morgan and Miller also undertook an unpublished trial of a treatment for the underdeveloped limbs of children stricken with poliomyelitis. This procedure involved the creation of an arterio-venous fistula in the femoral arteries of the affected limb in an attempt to enhance its growth without triggering cardiac failure. The follow-up lasted five years, and the growth of the limbs and the cardiac effects of the A-V fistulae were carefully documented. Although not strictly a cardiac intervention, this trial demonstrates the ingenuity of these physicians at a time when little could be done to help children affected by this condition.

Dr. A. Stanley Goldstein, who had trained in England, Winnipeg, and Houston, arrived on the scene in 1967 to join Dr. Miller as Holy Cross's second cardiovascular and thoracic surgeon. He brought with him new ideas, such as the use of bloodless prime for the cardiopulmonary bypass, and a wealth of surgical abilities. Dr. Robert H. Walker followed him in 1969 after training in Edmonton and at the Cleveland Clinic, bringing with him personal experience in the newly developed technique of direct coronary artery revascularization. Following his arrival, coronary artery bypass cases grew steadily and were in line with the caseload at the University of Alberta Hospital in Edmonton.

During the early years cardiac surgery was performed only at Holy Cross, a community general hospital without interns or residents, and the surgeons were so busy in clinical practice that there were essentially no academic activities. All heart operations were done with two cardiac surgeons present, leading not only to great cohesion between the surgeons but also to a rapid dissemination of new ideas and techniques between them. The postoperative care also fell on their shoulders, as the independent work of intensivists was not commonplace at that time.

This team of three surgeons remained unchanged until 1985, a sixteen-year period during which clinical work in Calgary became exhausting. The operative schedule was filled with cardiac, pulmonary and peripheral vascular procedures, as well as the lighter task of implanting pacemakers. As time passed, cardiovascular and thoracic procedures were carried out by one or another of these surgeons at a growing number of Calgary hospitals: Rockyview General, Foothills General, Colonel Belcher, and finally the Alberta Children's Hospital. This extensive clinical practice allowed for the development of great expertise, and the technical skill that each of these surgeons already possessed became even more honed.

Dr. Miller developed a subspecialty in congenital surgery and pacemaker implantation, while Dr. Goldstein expanded his expertise in pulmonary and abdominal aortic surgery. Dr. Walker, meanwhile, operated on every heart patient who had any possible chance of benefiting from his surgical skill. Some of these patients, whom more conservative surgeons would consider inoperable, he was able to help with his great skill and an ever positive attitude founded on his strong religious beliefs, which helped him face his own death in 1998 with a calm and tranquility that many of us would wish to acquire during our lives.

In January of 1985 Dr. Victor Aldrete joined the team and in July of the same year Dr. Alexander J. "Alec" Bayes became the fifth partner of the surgical group. The former had trained in Toronto and the latter in Montreal, bringing with them variations in surgical techniques that were quickly integrated into the daily practice at the Holy Cross Hospital. Blood cardioplegia was initiated with the arrival of Aldrete, a strong proponent of this myocardial preservation technique. The other surgeons quickly recognized its benefits, and it was universally accepted and implemented within months, thus making the perfusionists' lives far less complicated.

Yet the introduction of blood cardioplegia to the open-heart team brought with it the challenge of delivering it to the patient, since the disposables available for the mixture of the blood and potassium solution available at the time were crude and had little flexibility. This problem was solved with the use of two small pump heads that could be run at different speeds, allowing the blood to cardioplegia ratio to be adjusted with greater ease and based on the patient's serum potassium level. Mr. Peter Fortini, chief perfusionist at the Holy Cross, introduced this system. His ideas and communication with Sorin Biomedical led to the development of the integrated module later known as the Blood Cardioplegia Console, which later became commercially available, thus facilitating the delivery of blood cardioplegia in a more flexible manner.

The addition of Drs. Aldrete and Bayes to the surgical team in 1985 allowed for expansion of the program. The number of open-heart operations jumped by nearly a hundred cases that year and continued to increase over the following years, to a maximum of 499 cases in 1994. As Dr. Miller retired from cardiac surgery and demand continued to increase, new surgeons were recruited to join this group in private practice. Dr. Gregory D. Prystai arrived following his training in Edmonton, and Dr. William T. Kidd joined the group after completing his cardiac surgical training in Montreal.

Academic medicine arrived in southern Alberta following the opening of the University of Calgary's Faculty of Medicine in 1970, with the Foothills Hospital (FHH) as its main teaching facility. A decade later, Dr. Eldon R. Smith was recruited from Halifax to head the division of cardiology at both institutions and opened an up-to-date cardiovascular diagnostic laboratory in late 1980. As the university's cardiology program became more influential within the city, the lack of cardiac surgical services at FHH triggered a major disagreement between the clinical and academic practitioners, which became so severe by 1984 that it reached the local news media with provincial political implications. Despite this dispute, the cardiac surgical program at Holy Cross continued for over ten years, with continued expansion of its facilities and in the number of cardiologists and surgeons on staff. In the mid-1990s, however, in an effort to curtail provincial debt, Premier Ralph Klein's government undertook a major revamping of the health system and instituted substantial cutbacks to health care. The Holy Cross and General hospitals were closed in March 1996 and the whole cardiac program moved to FHH, which was renamed the Foothills Medical Centre.

The Foothills Hospital had in the meantime been very active in the creation of a separate cardiac surgical program, which eventually came to fruition in 1988 with the arrival of Dr. Teresa Kieser, a recent graduate of the Ottawa training program, and Dr. Andrew Maitland, who had trained in Toronto. Dr. Kieser became the acting director of the division of cardiac surgery at the FHH until September 1990, when Dr. Baikunth B. Bharadwaj arrived on the scene as chief of the division.

An external review of cardiac surgery at Holy Cross and FHH released just prior to the merger of the two programs in March 1996 revealed that the surgical results at Foothills were out of line with those at other sites, with an operative mortality rate over the past four years of 7.5 percent, compared with rates of 3 percent at Holy Cross and a national average of between 3 and 5 percent. At this time, the political tune had reached its highest pitch, and was compounded by the need for expanded facilities at the FHH in the wake of the merger.

A yearly volume of three hundred open-heart operations grew to eight hundred, almost triple the caseload. A team of three cardiovascular surgeons changed to six, and soon a seventh, in addition to two thoracic and three vascular surgeons, while there was a similar increase in the number of cardiologists, technologists and nursing staff, all of whom had somewhat different working habits as a result of having come from two different "cultures."

At the same time, Dr. Maitland replaced Dr. Bharadwaj as divisional chief.

The move to the FHH was accompanied by many other changes, some of them in a dramatic fashion and others more gradually. The practice of having two cardiac surgeons in the operating room was specifically removed by the administration, while the cardiovascular and thoracic surgery service was divided into three separate disciplines, with vascular surgery being moved to a separate hospital, and thoracic procedures placed in the hands of two thoracic surgeons.

The volume and acuity of heart surgery cases continued to increase, creating greater demands on the cardiac surgeons, although early postoperative care had now been transferred to the intensivists, who were under a separate division and department. At this period cardiac surgery was a division of the department of surgery, while cardiology was a division of the Department of Medicine. Not until several years later were the two divisions reunited into a dedicated department of cardiac health.

In 2001, Dr. John Burgess arrived in Calgary after spending a number of years in Regina. At present, there are six cardiac surgeons in the city, all working out of the Foothills Medical Centre, and doing exclusively cardiac surgery and the occasional pacemaker implant. The caseload has continued to increase both in numbers and acuity, as has the associated workload of the interventional cardiologists.

BEGINNING OF CARDIAC SURGERY AT FOOTHILLS HOSPITAL, CALGARY

Terry Kieser

Cardiovascular and thoracic surgery was already well established in Calgary at the Holy Cross Hospital with Drs. George Miller, Robert Walker, Stanley Goldstein, Victor Aldrete, and Alex Bayes. Dr. George Miller had performed the first heart surgery at Holy Cross Hospital—an atrial septal defect repair in March 1962. Now that we are all one big happy family (Holy Cross and Foothills joined forces April 1996 at Foothills), we can more easily go back and look at those difficult beginnings. To put it mildly, there was great opposition to opening a unit of cardiac surgery at Foothills Hospital. There were financial reasons and political agendas; but knowing human nature, probably the biggest reason for this opposition was simply natural resistance to change. Two independent commissions at a total cost of more than $300,000 to Albertan taxpayers, one the "Education Health Environment Study of Open Heart and Cardiovascular Services in Alberta," concluded that there should be a cardiac surgery unit at Foothills Hospital. The cardiac surgery physical plant (at a cost of $13 million) was actually in place by December 1986. However it wasn't until September 12, 1988, that the first cardiac surgical procedure was performed at Foothills Hospital; it had taken at least eight years of lobbying before 1986 to get to this stage. Newspaper clippings of the day were replete with titles such as "Holy Cross Renews Heart Surgery Fight," "Foothills Cardiac Unit—Wise Decision," "Heart Unit will Cut Waiting List," "Moore admits hospital dilemma," (Marvin Moore was the current hospital's minister for Alberta) and "Foothills is left in state of shock" (still). Even more to the point was the article in the *Calgary Herald*, February 14, 1987

(Valentine's Day—no less), "Irate doctors slam cardiac surgery plan—Surgeons tried to mothball unit," and this was just after the writer was hired to start the Unit along with Dr. Brad Bush of Hamilton. In this article of February 14, 1987, it states, "The cardiac unit should have been opened already, but its opening was delayed when twenty heart surgeons across Canada and the United States turned down positions with it. Two recently qualified heart surgeons finally accepted. The unit will open only when an operating budget has been assured." I am not sure why they had such a tough time hiring a heart surgeon to open this, at that time, state-of-the-art cardiac surgery unit. Two things again come to mind, money and politics. Probably no surgeon in their right mind would accept this position with such political history and potential resulting difficulties. This is probably why they settled on a newly minted female arrhythmia cardiac surgeon in October 1986. One of the carrots/rationale for the government opening a second heart surgery unit in Calgary was the need for arrhythmia surgery. Foothills was replete with electrophysiology cardiologists—Drs. George Wyse, Hank Duff, Anne Gillis and Brent Mitchell—with no surgeon for their arrhythmia patients. This is quite ironic, given the total takeover of arrhythmia surgery by catheter ablation today.

The first surgeon (your humble scribe) arrived on January 1, 1988. Dr. Bush was to have started at the same time however with such a delay in start up, accepted a job in Hamilton. They weren't too impressed when their "cardiac surgery coordinator" (for some reason they found it difficult to call a just graduated surgeon "chief" or even "acting chief") was twenty weeks pregnant with her first child. You could hear them saying, "I knew we shouldn't have hired a woman!" However, everything worked out just fine: in those days the Foothills Cardiac

Surgery Unit was all about new birth. While days were spent planning, organizing, training staff, and personal waddling, the operating budget took a long time to materialize. Even when finalized ("Heart unit gets go ahead"—17 May 1988, *Calgary Herald*) it took several more months. The due date for opening the unit was 1 July 1988 and the EDC for our new unit (Alexandra) was the twenty-third of June 1988. As things often do work out for the best, the writer's first child was born on 23 June and the cardiac surgery unit's first case took place September 12, 1988.

The following is a small article written for the hospital newsletter *Quest* by the author just before the unit opened.

CARDIAC SURGERY AT FOOTHILLS
July 1988

The advent of cardiac surgery at Foothills Hospital has had all the characteristics of the coming "Messiah." Many have awaited its coming, skeptics have doubted its ever existing, some have steadfastly believed in its eventuality and most have continued to hope for a long time—1973: Dr. I. Belenki (first GFT cardiologist) and Dr. A. White joined Dr. A. Kahn to manage cardiology patients at Foothills. Thereafter Drs. G. Wyse, J. Cohen, H. Duff, A. Gilles, W. Giles, M. Knudtson, D Manyari, B. Mitchell, P. Russell, H. ter Keurs, J. Tyberg and W. Warnica came on board, establishing one of the most productive teams of cardiologists in the country under the leadership of firstly Dr. E. Smith in 1980 and subsequently Dr. G. Wyse in 1986; 1982: Opening of cardiovascular labs with state-of-the-art echocardiography, nuclear cardiology, electrocardiography, exercise testing, invasive electrophysiology, vascular and cardiac catheterization. Mid-1980s: Critical and chronic patient care enhanced with expansion of the CCU and ward unit #92. However, without cardiac surgery, these services were still incomplete: all patients had to be transferred from their *hospital to a different one for their surgery; high risk patients (i.e., those requiring renal dialysis) also faced the same shuttling. Arrhythmia patients, investigated and diagnosed at Foothills, were sent to Eastern Canada for their requisite surgery. Patients awaiting angioplasty have been and still are spending days on Heparin drips awaiting transfer to Holy Cross. Physical evidence of the new unit became resoundingly clear as the ninth floor walls came crashing down to make way for a cardiovascular "Ne Plus Ultra"—all of cardiovascular endeavor occupying the same floor. "Lest we forget"—here lie the victims of office relocation to accommodate these plans: ninth floor Audiology and Ophthalmology moved to the main floor; main floor Respiratory Technology, Doctors' Lounge and the Business Department moved to the ground floor, main floor and South Tower respectively. Ninth floor Neurophysiology Labs moved to the eleventh floor and ninth floor Cardiology offices migrated to the eighth floor. Eighth floor OBGYN and Medicine offices moved to the second floor and second floor Finance and Histopathology moved to the South Tower and eleventh floor; finally ground floor Physical Plan Services and Material Management moved to Hawaii.*

Several million dollars later and finally *upon Marvin Moore's go-ahead, we are now in final stages of preparation for cardiac surgery. Your team presently comprises: G. Wagner—cardiac OR nurse;*

A. Scott-Douglas—perfusionist; M. Lebo—CV-ICU head nurse; K. Dayah—cardiac surgery RT; Drs. L. Strunin, C. Eagle, J. Haigh, C. Moir and D. Towns—cardiac anaesthetists; Dr. W. Lester— cardiac pathologist; and Drs. A. Maitland and T. Kieser—cardiac surgeons. This team, just finishing spring training, is poised for full service cardiac surgery this fall.

On the research front, weekly meetings are taking place with Heritage scientists (Drs. J. Tyberg, H. ter Keurs, and W. Giles), cardiologists and surgeons to plan clinical and laboratory research projects. The Cardiovascular Research Group has been steadily growing—from six academic faculty members producing seven papers in 1980 to nineteen members producing sixty-nine papers in 1987. The addition of cardiac surgical research will advance the already high profile of the University of Calgary in this field, providing an unsurpassed learning opportunity for the surgeons and physicians of the future. It is the mandate of this division not only to deliver excellent health care, but also to provide the teaching and research that will assure excellence in the health care of tomorrow.

The "Spring Training" referred to in this article was somewhat unique. We were concerned that the brand new equipment had yet to be broken in, and the team had never worked together before (some of us had not operated for several months). We therefore decided to have a "wet" run. It was a little difficult to get Dr. Clarence Guenther, vice president of development and affairs to agree, but when we asked him, "Would you rather a real human be the guinea pig or a pig be the guinea pig?" he finally consented to our request. So early one morning through the ground floor of Foothills Hospital, we wheeled a covered gurney with a rather large (but actually quite short!) body from the Medical Sciences building. Unfortunately our anaesthetic technique was somewhat inadequate and there were some startled patients as the "body" started to squeal and grunt. However, all of the equipment worked and the team had a good run as we put "pig on pump." We did discover three things that was either not working or hooked up incorrectly; nothing life threatening but we certainly felt more comfortable with our first case.

Early in the summer Dr. Andrew Maitland was hired as a second surgeon, trained in Toronto and having worked the previous two years in Regina. It was one-in-two call for the first two and a half years. Also for the first nine months the two surgeons (author and Dr. Maitland) assisted each other, so "off call" wasn't all that off. Fortunately with both of us being Monty Python fans someone would get us going and we would regale the OR team (when things were stable of course) with the well known skits of: the "Dead Parrot," the "Cheese Shop" (without any cheese) the "Spanish Inquisition" with its "two—no, three!—methods of torture," and of course we could almost never get through a case without breaking into "I'm a lumberjack and I'm okay . . . just like my dear mama!" Having nearly killed Andrew and I in the first years, a decision was made to hire a third surgeon, Dr. Baikunth Bharadwaj from Saskatoon. Never was there a more gentle or relaxed chief. I can still remember him ambling down the office hallway early in the morning; he had been a surgeon for so long and had had so much experience that nothing made him anxious or hurried. Dr. Bharadwaj was one of the fastest surgeons in the operating room, but to watch him it looked as if he was moving quite slowly. His gift for speed was simply due to no wasted time or movements. When finished the distals and proximals he would "walk about" the operating room waiting for the patient to come off pump. There is no truth to the rumor that one day he forgot to do the proximals. His assistant gently reminded him and he came over and did them. "Proximals are anti-climatic anyway!" The pediatric cardiologists greatly appreciated his skill and ready availability for coarctation repair, shunts and PDA ligation of newborns and infants. Now these children, with the exception of newborns needing PDA ligation are all sent to Edmonton for surgery. Dr. Bharadwaj was also the main bridge over troubled waters for the merging of the Foothills and Holy Cross Cardiac Surgery Programmes in 1996; an amazingly smooth union, given the political background history of the two centres. Dr. "B" (as he was fondly called) retired in 1996 after a surgical career of thirty years and selectively audible pagers not withstanding, his fatherly ways in the OR, on the ward, and as chief have been missed. Our current chief Dr. Andrew Maitland along with Dr. Brent Mitchell, head of cardiac sciences have shepherded us through the development of an independent department of cardiac sciences and toward our next iteration: the Libin Cardiovascular Institute of Alberta, incepted January 27, 2004.

Foothills has come a long way from the beginning of cardiology in 1973, the start up of angiography in 1981, the start of heart surgery in 1988 and subsequent amalgamation with the Holy Cross Hospital in April 1996. Town and gown have merged very successfully and at present the physical plant is still for the most part contained on the ninth floor of Foothills Hospital. There is a unit for day patients waiting for cardiac cath or PTCA, noninvasive testing, stress echo, nuclear studies, a postoperative cardiac surgical ward with thirty-six beds, invasive angiography, PTCA and five cath labs, two electrophysiology cath labs, two cardiac ORs (with windows looking to the mountains) and a new fourteen bed cardiovascular ICU (and a partridge in a pear tree). This ninth floor space each year performs ten thousand heart caths, three thousand angioplasties and twelve hundred heart surgeries in distinct contrast with our first year two thousand heart caths, 270 angioplasties (plus 634 angioplasties at Holy Cross Hospital) and 261 heart surgeries. "All beginnings are tough." Although certainly true for the beginning of cardiac surgery at Foothills, those of us who are still going strong today have the new birth of the Libin Cardiovascular Institute of Alberta to be proud of and well worth the struggles of those early days.

CHAPTER 11

THE DEVELOPMENT OF CARDIAC
SURGERY IN BRITISH COLUMBIA

Lawrence H. Burr

"What kind of men are these thoracic surgeons?
Problem solvers and decision makers by nature and tradition."

It has been said that cardiac surgery was the last surgical frontier. In British Columbia, as elsewhere, cardiac surgery started with operations progressively closer to the heart prior to direct cardiac procedures themselves. Until the latter part of the 19th century the medical profession thought the heart to be surgically untouchable; however a number of conditions existed whose nature suggested the possibility of surgical treatment and a few intrepid surgeons were prepared to proceed into the unknown These pioneering surgeons were an interesting group. They tended to be powerful individuals, accustomed to success, aggressive and often egocentric. "Often wrong, but never in doubt" might be an overstatement, but a pithy one.

The Early Years in Vancouver

In the 1930s the heart was regarded as foreign territory; few surgeons dared to approach it. In 1933 at Shaughnessy Military Hospital, Dr Shinbein bravely performed the first known heart operation in BC, a pericardiectomy (probably partial).

The 1940s was a more aggressive decade. In 1947, experienced Vancouver General Hospital (VGH) surgeon Ross Robertson returned from visiting Bailey, Harken, Blalock, Gross, and other North American surgeons. His surgical background was in both orthopedic and thoracic surgery, but he had developed a strong interest in palliative and corrective surgery for cardiovascular abnormalities. In a four-week period at VGH he performed a Blalock shunt, pericardiectomy, patent ductus arteriosus, and coarctation of aorta, all successfully. Ross Robertson was a major force in developing cardiovascular surgery in Vancouver.

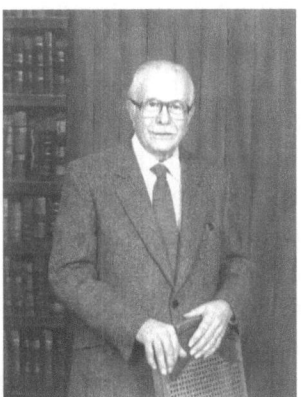

Fig. 11:1 Ross Robertson

Now the heart itself was being approached directly. During 1948 Charles Bailey in Philadelphia and Russell Brock in England demonstrated closed mitral commisurotomy. Just one year later, in 1949, Ross Robertson did the first closed mitral commisurotomy at the VGH, effectively launching the closed heart surgery program in BC.

The 1950s saw the development of true open heart surgery, or what C. Walton Lillehei of Minneapolis refered to as "Surgery under Direct Vision." In 1953 Gibbon in Philadelphia successfully closed an atrial septal defect (ASD) with the heart lung machine, using 28 minutes of cardiopulmonary bypass. Progress came quickly. During 1954 Lillehei closed a VSD and corrected AV canal and a Tetralogy. In 1956, John Callaghan of Edmonton performed the first open heart procedures in Canada, closing an ASD in October 1956, and a VSD in December.

In British Columbia, during the 1940s and 1950s, circumstances coincided that made it possible to undertake and develop various aspects of cardiac surgery. The Province had grown and there were hospitals large enough to support sophisticated surgical programs. There were a number of high profile physicians with specialized training in cardiology who recognized the need for new treatment methods. These included Drs. Fritz Strong, Don Munroe, Max Walters, Victor Hertzman, Hugh Stansfield and John Osborne. The latter had been added to the staff at VGH to set up a cardiac investigation laboratory. In pediatric cardiology were pioneers Maurice Young and later Dennis Vince. The Medical School at the University of British Columbia was established in 1950, and research facilities were available at Vancouver hospitals. The continued development of anaesthesia had made intrathoracic surgery possible and some primitive electronic equipment was available for monitoring cardiac function during surgery. In addition, there were several surgeons in the Province who had the background, experience and recent training to initiate and develop cardiac surgery.

Peter Allen had trained at the University of Toronto (MD 1946), and during that year confirmed his Toronto links by marrying Mary, daughter of Dr. Roscoe Graham. He then did a year of surgery in Amsterdam and a year in a rural Ontario general practice before entering the Gallie Course in Surgery in Toronto in 1949. After obtaining his FRCS(C) in 1953, Allen moved to Vancouver to a General Surgery staff position at VGH, with an emphasis on vascular surgery, and a research appointment at the BC Medical Research Institute. The BCMRI Director, Kenneth Evelyn, was delighted to encourage academic surgeons, especially those working on cardiovascular disease, and stimulated Allen and others to pursue concepts germane to cardiac surgery. Allen continued to perform surgery at VGH until his retirement, and was Acting Head of Cardiovascular and Thoracic Surgery at VGH and UBC from 1974-1977, and 1978-1979.

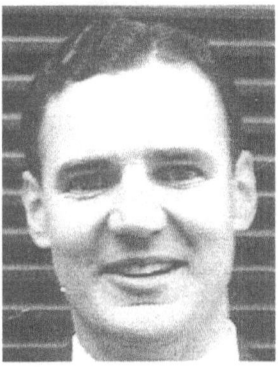

Fig. 11:2 Peter Allen

Phillip Ashmore was raised in Bralorne, BC, and did pre-med at UBC. He transferred to Toronto and graduated MD in 1948. Following his internship at Toronto General Hospital his skills were developed by residency training at the Hospital for Sick Children. In 1955, he won an R.S. McLaughlin Travelling Clinical Fellowship and spent a year in London at Guy's Hospital with Sir Russell Brock and the Hospital for Sick Children Great Ormond Street with David Waterston. Upon returning to Vancouver Ashmore was appointed Pediatric Surgeon at VGH, based in the Health Centre for Children, a new building on the VGH campus specifically designed for and dedicated to infants, children and adolescents.

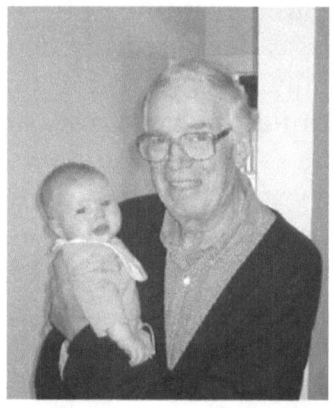

Fig. 11:3 Phil Ashmore

William G. (Bill) Trapp was born in New Westminster, BC, studied at UBC and graduated MD in 1939 from McGill. During his internship, he contracted tuberculosis from a patient and was confined to Tranquille Sanatorium in rural BC. While at Tranquille he practised medicine, including some surgery; in 1950 he returned to surgery studies with FRCS(C) in 1954. His expertise in thoracic surgery was invaluable in the early days of cardiac surgery. He was a natural inventor, and in 1975 published and patented a myocardial stabilizer device for off-pump coronary surgery, a procedure that he had pioneered in 1970. With John Masterson, he developed a tissue valve holder for intraoperative use. Electrophysiology fascinated him as well and he was an early adopter of new technologies such as the lithium-iodide (CPI) pacer.

Now the stage was set for further development. Under the direction of Dr. Rocke Robertson, Head of the Department of Surgery at UBC and at Vancouver General Hospital, the surgical colleagues set to work to develop a pump-oxygenator. A fortuitous circumstance at VGH was the interest taken by the Department of Anaesthesia. W.A. (Bill) Dodds became an integral member of the team during the preclinical development of open heart techniques, and subsequently led the anaesthesia component of the clinical work, sharing responsibility with the surgeons for developing "heart-lung bypass" technology. This later became known as the "perfusionist" department. Dodds was given free time from his clinical work to allow him to join the surgical group in their work in the BCMRI laboratory, and was instrumental in recruiting and training staff to assemble the necessary equipment for the bypass machine and to operate it during the surgical procedures.

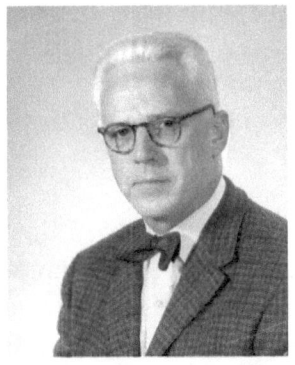
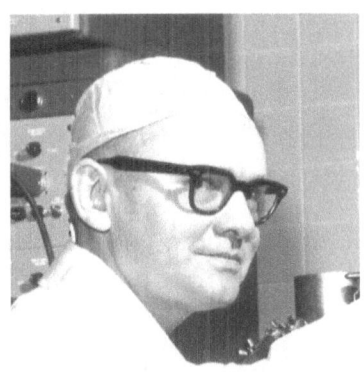

Fig. 11:4 Bill Trapp   Fig. 11:5 Bill Dodds

In 1956 Allen was awarded a McLaughlin Fellowship and travelled to Minneapolis to study with C. Walton Lillehei, enjoying pioneering heart surgery experiences with colleagues Norman Shumway, Christiaan Barnard and Matt Paneth. He also briefly visited Denton Cooley, Al Meredino and others, gleaning information about their surgical units. In July 1957, Allen returned from the United States with the essential parts for a heart-lung machine. The component parts had been offered to him by Lillihei on the completion of Allen's year. After discussion with Rocke Robertson, the team was assembled: surgeons Allen, Ashmore, Trapp and Robertson; perfusionist John Basaraba; and anaesthetists Bill Dodds and Jack Nixon.

During the summer the machine was assembled and successfully tested in Ken Evelyn's BCMRI dog lab, the surgeons operating and Bill Dodds providing anaesthesia and recovery skills. However, Rocke Robertson would not allow the program to continue until open heart operations were performed on twenty dogs, of which sixteen must survive. Consequently, the team members very quickly became post operative care specialists, sitting through the operative night and subsequent days with the dogs. In those simpler days, the dogs were obtained from the Vancouver Dog Pound in exchange for offerings of Scotch whisky. Many of the post-op dogs were adopted by nurses and staff of the BCMRI.

One unexpected complication occurred when Lillehei sent Allen an invoice for the pump parts, which had been originally assumed to be a gift. To raise the money an evening of Bingo was held at a nearby Legion Hall, courtesy of a Mr. McDonald. In 1957 Bingo was illegal in Vancouver but the evening's profits were sufficient to pay for the pump. A commotion was heard at the front door—it was the police raiding the Legion Hall! Mr.McDonald escaped with the cash through the back door and brought it safely to the Department of Surgery the next day.

By late September 1957, sixteen of twenty dogs had survived and Rocke Robertson authorized the program to begin. Terry Stout of the Red Cross solved the blood donor challenges. Miss Pinchin (Head Nurse VGH ORs) masterfully assembled her best nurses and the essential equipment. The search was on for a suitable first patient. John Evans (age 8) was admitted to the Health Centre for Children at VGH with an inguinal hernia. A cardiac murmur was detected and he was diagnosed by Maurice Young with atrial septal defect.

The open heart surgery era was ready to begin in Vancouver. On October 29, 1957 the ASD was repaired in VGH Heather OR #3 using 23 minutes of cardio-pulmonary bypass. The surgeons were led by Allen, with anaesthesia administered by Bill Dodds and Jack Nixon, perfusion by Basaraba running the Lillehei-deWall pump-oxygenator, and the OR nursing by Joan Burnett, June David, Elsie Muir and Daphne Clough. Postoperatively, the patients were recovered in the far corner of an old "Nightingale Ward" that had been converted into a PAR. The early cases were nursed by Bev Wilson, Bernice Moore and Jeannette Binkley; Binkley invented a device to clear the chest tubes of clots—the Binkley Stripper—which is in use to this day.

The cardiac surgery program initially consisted solely of congenital heart disease cases. Numerous glitches and amusing incidents occurred whilst building the program. One morning, there was no perfusionist—he was in jail! John had been the projectionist in the union hall the previous evening, but unfortunately they were showing a 'blue' movie when the police arrived and arrested him. The entire heart team filed into Magistrate's Court to vouch for his character, and to inform the judge that he was the lone perfusionist in the program. After a stern lecture, John was released and heart surgery began again. Shortly thereafter, VGH appointed John Ward as John's assistant; later, Ted Flegel and Ted Bush were added. On another occasion, when it was planned to increase from three to four surgeries per week, the VP Medicine refused permission. His arguments of insufficient OR staff, availability of blood, and lack of beds were easily refuted. Then—his trump card: the laundry couldn't handle the extra load! After a firm reminder that the VP himself had stated that VGH had the most modern hospital laundry in Canada, his interference crumbled, and four cases per week were performed.

Large quantities of heparinized blood were used for priming the pump; often at the end of the procedure, the keen gardeners on the OR staff would take bottles of the spent blood home to use as rose food! The cardiac OR had been designed for general surgery; the extra equipment made the room crowded and warm. The OR orderly (this author one summer) was despatched to the cafeteria at 10:30 each morning to fetch ice cold chocolate milk for the surgeons and scrub nurses, delivered via straws to the thirsty crew. And speaking of ice, some of the early cases were surface-cooled prior to surgery by packing the patient in ice in the nearby neurosurgery scrub sink.

One of the many challenges in the early years of heart surgery was arterial thromboembolism. To mitigate this problem, Phil Ashmore, working in the BCMRI during the 1960s, developed an in-line arterial line filter to reduce the amount of incipient thrombotic material reaching the patient's circulation. It was commercially produced and successfully marketed for some years, until improved models became available.

In 1959, adult cases were added, with mitral regurgitation repair and open correction of mitral and aortic stenosis. During early 1962, aortic valve stenosis was treated by implantation of Hufnagel cusps made of Teflon. In some cases, the hypertrophied left ventricles of these end-stage patients failed post-operatively, stimulating increased attention to improving intraoperative coronary perfusion techniques.

Surgical indications grew rapidly as intracardiac access made acquired valve lesions surgically accessible. The mitral valve was repaired, but if necessary was replaced (as was the aortic valve) with Starr-Edwards prostheses. In early May 1963, Robertson did the first Starr-Edwards AVR at VGH, and in June 1963 the first MVR; neither patient survived hospital stay. In August 1963, Allen did successful AVR with excellent long-term success, setting the stage for our continuing interests in conservative and replacement valve surgery and the long-term follow-up of cardiac valve patients. As newer and better valves evolved, Smeloff, Magovern, Bjork-Shiley, Lillehei, Hall-Kaster and others were used. During 1966, cardiac homografts were surgically harvested, then prepared by a laboratory technician for freeze-drying. Twelve homograft aortic valve implants were done in 1966-67; most failed within six years, and by 1978 the last had been explanted. Discontent with complications from mechanical valves led to the introduction of porcine bioprostheses in 1974. Favourable early results from the implants permitted wide acceptance of these devices to the present day, although valve repair has remained the cornerstone for mitral and tricuspid valve surgery.

The Pioneers at St. Paul's Hospital

In 1955 St. Paul's Hospital recruited a physiologist, Harold Rice, MD PhD, from Edmonton. He developed the St. Paul's screen pump-oxygenator, the only such device designed and built in Canada. It was a stainless steel apparatus modeled after, but vastly superior to, the Mayo-Gibbon device. The machine was used for over 1,000 open heart cases, and was retired when disposable equipment became available in the early 1970s. Supporting Rice was perfusion technician Tom Osborne, and later, Encole Leona.

The Clinical Investigation Unit was founded in 1956 and Rice was appointed Director. It was totally funded by contributions from the Internal Medicine staff. An inventive man, Rice created blood pressure monitors and magnetic blood flow meters for the heart lung machine (all reusable and autoclavable), a rapid blood gas analyser, and a blood pH meter for intraoperative and postoperative use. His pioneering research at St. Paul's and the BCMRI accelerated the cumulative effort towards open heart surgery. Rice's wife, Dorothy, age 43, was the first open heart patient at the Mayo Clinic (1953), and had the fourth ASD closure in the world. She was a keen golfer until age 76.

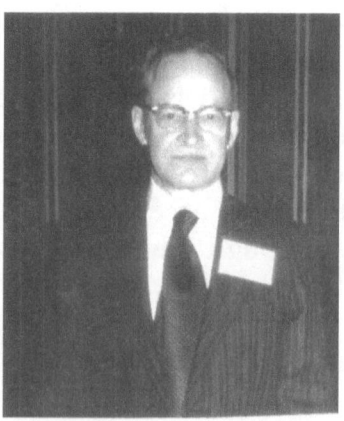

Fig. 11:6 Harold Rice

Robert Gourlay, Chief Surgeon 1958-78, obtained his MD from McGill in 1942, much to the pleasure of his father, a surgeon at St. Paul's, and his mother, a graduate of the first Nursing class from the same hospital. Post graduate training resulted in an MSc in Experimental Surgery in 1951, and he returned to Vancouver to practice.

Ted Musgrove trained at the Mayo Clinic in general and thoracic surgery. He came to St. Paul's in 1952 and developed vascular surgery there. Gerald Coursley was also trained in general and thoracic surgery, an essential requirement for the early cardiac surgeon. He, too, had a strong interest in peripheral vascular surgery and concentrated on that for most of his professional life. The three surgeons teamed up with Harold Rice to design and build the pump-oxygenator, and test it on dogs prior to clinical usage.

On May 22,1960, Gourlay, Musgrove, and Courlsey made history at St. Paul's by closing an ASD in OR 14 of the old hospital. The patient was Elizabeth Laverty, age 12, cute and freckled; the heart-lung machine was run by Harold Rice and Tom Osborne. Norman McMillen and J. O'Donnell were the anesthesiologists. Osborne would join the group to become the first perfusionist at St. Paul's. Gloria Stephens, R. Stringer, G. Webb and B. Polvi were the scrub nurses. The patient made an uneventful recovery and still enjoys full health.

Cardiologic support was crucial. Doris Kavanagh Gray had trained at the Henry Ford Hospital in Detroit in both pediatric and adult cardiology. In 1959, she was immediately hired by Bill Hurlburt (Head, Department of Medicine) as the first cardiologist at St. Paul's. Kavanagh Gray was primarily responsible for developing a cardiac investigation program, including the nascent cardiac catheterization laboratory. She took special interest in the surgical activities, and was very active in postoperative management of the patients. Six years later Dwight Peretz joined the staff; his training at McGill and the Royal Victoria Hospital was immediately put to full use when he developed the Intensive Care Unit and the Coronary Care Unit in what had been the Sisters of Providence's common room.

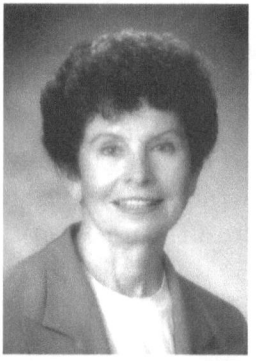
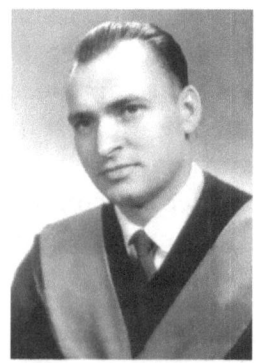

Fig. 11:7 Doris Kavanagh Gray   Fig. 11:8 Al Gerein

Alfred Gerein joined the St. Paul's cardiac team in 1962. He had graduated with the first UBC Medical School class in 1954, trained in general surgery in Detroit, and completed his cardiac surgical training with Fred Cross and Earl Kay in Cleveland. His life-long interest in heart valve surgery significantly added to the expertise at St. Paul's. The first mitral valve replacement at St. Paul's was done by Gerein on May 26, 1963 using a Starr-Edwards valve. He performed Canada's first double valve replacement on February 26, 1964 and a triple valve replacement shortly afterwards. The first permanent pacer implant at St. Paul's occurred in 1964, and coronary bypass surgery was introduced there by Gerein in 1969, after he had performed many successful

Vineberg implants. after academic divisional status was granted by UBC in 1969, Gerein became the hospital's Head of Cardiovascular and Thoracic Surgery until 1991, smoothly guiding the Unit through expansions and the changing complexities of modern surgical practice.

Victoria—The Start of Cardiac Surgery on Vancouver Island

In Victoria, Jack Stenstrom made a remarkable contribution to the early development of cardiac surgery in BC. He had graduated from McGill in 1938 and took his early surgical training at the Montreal General Hospital. He served in the Armed Forces in Europe from 1942 to 1946; on his return he added to his surgical experience at the Johns Hopkins Hospital in Baltimore. There he assisted with cardiac and vascular surgery and became thoroughly familiar with Blalock's shunt procedure. He relocated to Victoria in 1948.

Initially a large proportion of his work was in general surgery, but included thoracic surgery, and from the beginning of his practice he conducted a series of experiments in the animal laboratory to study the potential for myocardial revascularization. He also successfully performed ligation of the patent ductus in a number of children, and Blalock shunts in children with tetralogy of Fallot.

In 1952 Stenstrom was joined in his practice by Hugh Ford, and they continued to practice closed heart surgery, including mitral commisurotomy and the Vineberg procedure to stimulate revascularization of the myocardium. Their referral base was not confined to Vancouver Island; they also treated many patients referred from the northwestern United States.

Carleton Whiteside moved from Edmonton to Victoria in 1956. He had graduated MD from the University of Alberta, trained in Pennsylvania and Edmonton, and began general surgery in 1931. World War II service stimulated his surgical interest, especially in cardiovascular procedures. He continued his busy practice in Vctoria until his premature death by cardiac arrest at a Royal College meeting in 1967.

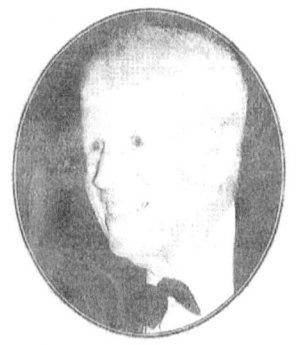   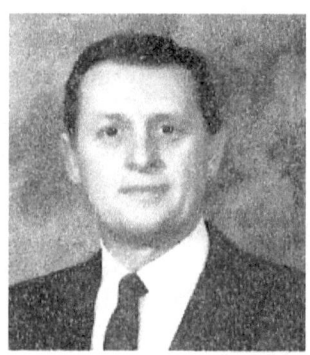

Fig. 11:9 Jack Stenstrom   Fig. 11:10 Ralph Smith

Surgeon Ralph Smith moved to Victoria and started practice in January 1961, coinciding with the arrival of cardiologist George Woodwark. Smith graduated MD in 1949 from the University of Western Ontario, and after interneship entered the McGill Diploma course in General Surgery. A research year with Vineberg in 1952 was spent studying stress and coronary circulation, followed by a year at Children's Memorial in Montreal. The next three years were spent with Richard Overholt in Boston and Charlie Bailey in Philadelphia. Smith bounced back to Canada for a year in Montreal, and then back to the US in private practice in Cleveland for two years. He finally settled in Victoria in 1961 with the promise (ah, promises !) of starting an open heart unit, as postulated by Woodwark.

The two doctors were keen to start a unit in Victoria, but immediately became embroiled in controversy, as each of the two large hospitals, Saint Joseph's and Royal Jubilee, wanted the program sited at its institution. Finally, the Ministry of Health became involved, and settled the dilemma in a typically bureacratic manner: a committee! Three doctors from Vancouver met in June 1961, to interview interested parties, and in September produced their recommendations: two felt that Royal Jubilee should have a unit, but one (the Chairman, the Professor and Head of Dermatology at UBC), felt that *no* unit should be established, and that all patients should be sent to VGH in Vancouver. His political clout outweighed the others, and the status quo prevailed. Smith continued to practise thoracic, esophageal, closed heart and peripheral vascular surgery, and the idea of a cardiac surgical unit languished for almost a decade.

The Next Generation—Expansion in the Coronary Bypass Era

Vancouver General Hospital

An important step in the progress of cardiac surgery in BC was made in 1967 when VGH took over the 2nd and 3rd floors of the Willow Chest Centre, the tuberculosis facility on the VGH Campus. This provided dedicated surgical space, including two large ORs with overhead viewing galleries, a third regular sized OR, space for an 10 bed ICU, a cardiac laboratory, and a step-down unit, with pre- and post-operative ward space upstairs. The laboratory was managed by Isabel Connon who had been with the team since 1958; in 1967 Evelyn Rapanos, a homograft technician, was added when the new laboratory was opened, and later Sue Calvert when Connon was further promoted. The first pump case in the new OR suite was an ASD.

The timing was fortuitous. Myocardial revascularization had been limited to the successful but incomplete Vineberg procedure; in 1965, Peter Allen presented photographs of two-colour latex infusion experiments, demonstrating connection between Vineberg implants and dog coronary circulation. Direct coronary surgery included localized endarterectomy, patch coronary angioplasty, or interposition vein grafts. In 1960, Boetz in New York had anastomosed an IMA to a human coronary artery; in 1964 Garrett first used saphenous vein in desperation. General clinical use of coronary bypass began during 1967 in Cleveland and quickly spread throughout North America. In June 1969 the first coronary bypass case was done in VGH by Allen, and by March 1971, 120 VGH cases had been collected for presentation by Allen at the 1972 meeting of the Society of Thoracic Surgeons of Great Britain and Ireland. Bill Trapp felt that patients might be harmed by the heart-lung machine, and by 1970 was performing most coronary cases off-pump, including use of the IMA. In late 1972, VGH Cardiac Surgery moved temporarily to Shaughnessy Hospital while Willow Chest was further renovated and modernized. The "new" Willow Chest was then used until 1987 when the Jim Pattison Pavillion was opened with contemporary Cardiac Surgery OR and ICU facilities. As per tradition, the first booked case was a secundum ASD.

Ian Munro graduated MBBS in 1955 from King's College Hospital, London, England, with postgraduate studies in Orthopedics, Emergency Surgery and Pediatrics (Great Ormond Street with David Waterston). He returned to King's for further surgical training, including Urology,

Thoracic, Cardiac and General Surgery. While working at the Brompton Hospital with Bill Cleland in 1963, he was attracted to cardiac surgery as a Senior Registrar to Matt Paneth and then Oz Tubbs at St. Bartholomew's. An opportunity to be a BC Heart Foundation Fellow in Vancouver for one year in 1966 resulted in a staff appointment in 1967, and he practised Cardiothoracic Surgery at VGH for 30 years. A meticulous, well organized surgeon with a superb knowledge of anatomy, Munro was an inspiration to a generation of trainees.

Lawrence H. Burr was born at VGH, trained at UBC (BA 1958, MSc 1961,MD 1964 with Silver Medal), and interned at the Hospital of the University of Pennsylvania. After five years of general practice in rural BC, he returned to UBC/VGH for CVT training, obtaining his FRCS(C) in 1974. Burr won the first of the "new" McLaughlin Fellowships, and spent 18 months at the Brompton Hospital with Matt Paneth and Christopher Lincoln, Great Ormond Street (Jarda Stark, Mark de Laval) and the National Heart Hospital (Donald Ross, Madgi Yacoub). Time spent in Paris with Alain Carpentier was an equally valuable learning experience. Burr joined the VGH staff in1977; his primary interests were mitral valve surgery (especially repair), cardiac pacing and adult congenital surgery. A founding member of the VGH Pacer Clinic, he was also active with the valve followup registry. Burr was always interested in transplantation, however, and even in 1971, as a BC Heart Fellow in the BCMRI, he had kept isolated dog hearts perfused for 24 hours, and successfully restored their cardiac function. Burr has been a member of the International Standards Organization valve and pacer committees since 1985, and since 2000 the founding Chair of ISO/TC150/ SC6—Active Implantable Medical Devices.

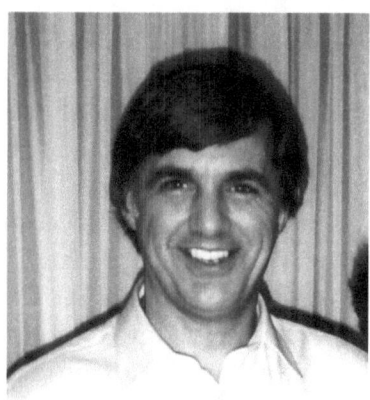

Fig. 11:11: Larry Burr

W.R. Eric Jamieson graduated MD from Dalhousie in 1966. After 5 years of general practice he did General Surgery at the University of Alberta, then Cardiovascular and Thoracic Surgery at U of A, VGH and University of Toronto. Jamieson joined VGH in 1978, and enjoyed a wide range of CVT surgical activities. Shortly after joining the staff, he reviewed the explanted homografts and the short follow-up information on the good and not-so-good mechanical valves of the 1960s and early 1970s. He felt that longitudinal study was the best method of cardiac valve follow-up, caught the 'Research Bug' and initiated and developed the Cardiac Valve Database for valve surgery outcome studies, as well as continuing his extensive basic and applied research in the animal laboratory. His principal focus now is research, and Jamieson is the Professor and Head, Clinical Cardiac Research, UBC. He travels the world extensively presenting results related to the followup of 7,000 valve replacement procedures, mostly porcine bioprostheses, basic laboratory research work, and currently participates in cardiac valve International Standards Organization activities.

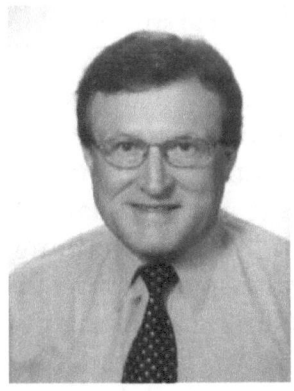

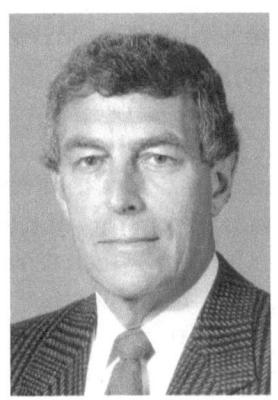

Fig. 11:12 Eric Jamieson   Fig. 11:13 Frank Tyers

G.Frank O. Tyers obtained his MD from UBC in 1962. He did General Surgery at the Hospital of the University of Pennsylvania (HUP) and CVT training at HUP, Children's Hospital of Philadelphia and in Toronto at TGH and the Hospital for Sick Children. By 1977 he was Professor and Chief, Division of Thoracic Surgery at the University of Texas, Galveston. In 1979 he returned to BC to be the UBC Professor and Head of the newly created Division of Cardiovascular and Thoracic Surgery, a position he held until 2000. Tyers had many surgical interests such as myocardial protection with crystalloid cardioplegia and computer-generated OR and Discharge Reports, but pacing was his real love. He did much research with pulse generators and leads, and established many patents regarding multi-programmability, rechargability of generators, real time telemetry, and polyurethane lead coatings. A true pacing aficionado, he was instrumental in supporting NASPE and in establishing the VGH Pacer Clinic. Lead extraction was a long-time interest, and Tyers acquired an international reputation for laser lead removal.

In 1984, Michael Janusz, a 1974 graduate of the University of Manitoba, joined the VGH staff after residency at

Baylor University. An excellent technical surgeon, Janusz has a special interest in thoracic aortic surgery, with both clinical and research aspects. Spinal cord protection in descending and thoraco-abdonminal aneurysms, monitoring of spinal column pressures, and intraaortic stents are concepts that were investigated in the laboratory and then brought into practice. The challenging surgeries of the aortic root with valve-sparing procedures, and post-infarction LV remodelling are handled with aplomb. James is now Head of the new Section of Aortic Surgery and coordinates a central referral system for aortic surgery and its follow-up assessment.

Guy Fradet graduated MD from Laval University in 1979, and after general surgery at the Montreal General Hospital did a CVT residency at VGH and St. Paul's. He joined the VGH staff in 1988, but immediately did a one-year Saxton Memorial Fellowship in thoracic surgery and heart/lung transplant at Harefield (Donald Ross), Papworth (Terence English, John Wallwork), Brompton Hospital (Magdi Yacoub, Margaret Hudson), and Great Ormond Street (Marc de Laval). An expert operator, facile with all procedures, and excelling in valve surgery, Fradet performs heart/lung and single/double lung transplants, and was long-time Director of the Solid Organ Transplant CPU. He is currently Divisional Associate Head at VGH and has a busy surgical schedule.

VGH surgeon Virginia Gudas graduated from Memorial University in St. John's in 1978, did general surgery in Ottawa, and succumbed to the lure of the West Coast by training in CVT Surgery at VGH/St. Paul's. After a one year Transplant Fellowship at Stanford University, she returned to VGH in 1988. Later that year, on December 6th, Gudas performed the first cardiac transplant in

BC, and went on to spearhead a successful city-wide program. She continues to be active in cardiac surgery and teaching.

St. Paul's Hospital

At St. Paul's, the new Catheterization Laboratory was established in 1968, and the demand for cardiac surgical procedures increased. On September 7, 1973, the Cardiac and Respiratory Unit was opened on the Third Floor of the Centre Wing, easing the strain on the physical facilities and the burgeoning waiting list. Leading research continues to be done in the multi-disciplinary iCapture Centre, established in 2000 to further research in heart, lung, and blood vessels diseases.

Robert Miyagishima graduated MD from UBC in 1960, interned at TGH, then did one year of General Surgery at VGH. The next year was spent in Toronto at the Banting Research Institute where he worked with Ron Baird on arterial gas embolism from perfusion cannulae, and lower limb vein replacement experimentation. He then returned to Vancouver in 1963 to complete his training in general surgery, followed by CVT training in Toronto at TGH and HSC, followed by additional work in thoracic surgery at the Frenchay Hospital in Bristol, England; the FRCS(C) for CVT Surgery was granted in 1967. Following a BC Heart Foundation Fellowship in mechanical circulatory support, Miyagishima joined the St. Paul's staff in October 1969, and maintained a very busy clinical practice of cardiac, thoracic, and vascular surgery until 2004. During this time he continued to pursue research interests, and was also Acting Head of UBC CVT Surgery for two years and St. Paul's CVT Divisional Head 1989-1993.

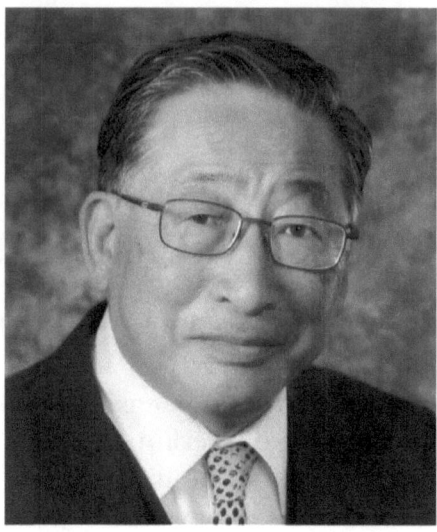

Fig. 11:14 Bob Miyagashima

Andy Tutassaura graduated MD from the National University in Bogota, Colombia in 1960, pursued general surgery at the University of New York, then started cardiac training with two years at the Hospital for Sick Children in Toronto, followed by full CVT studies at Toronto Western Hospital. After a year at the Karolinska Institute, Stockholm, he came to St. Paul's in 1971. His full cardiac, thoracic and vascular practice was interrupted for three years by hospital-acquired tuberculosis, but he retired in 1996 in good health.

Hilton Ling received his MB, MCh from the University of Witwatersrand in 1968 and proceeded to general surgery then CVT residency at VGH until his 1979 FRCS(C). After a BC Heart Fellowship he joined St. Paul's in 1980. Ling is a quick, accurate operator, skilled at all adult cardiovascular and thoracic surgery. His special interests include aortic root and aneurysm surgery (collaborating with Michael

Janusz on special cases as joint operators), cardiac transplantation, arrythmia surgery, and reoperative cases. Despite his hectic schedule, Ling continues his research interest in valvular surgery.

Sam Lichtenstein originally trained in Mechanical Engineering at the University of Toronto, then Biomedical Enineering at Johns Hopkins (PhD 1975). His MD was obtained from the University of Maryland in 1977, followed by general surgery (1982) and CVT surgery (1984) at U. of T. He lectured in Mathematics at Ryerson Polytechnical Institute in Toronto and the University of Baltimore, and in Physiology at U of T. Lichtenstein was on the CVT Surgery staff at St. Michael's Hospital in Toronto, becoming co-director of its Cardiovascular ICU. He came to St. Paul's in 1992 as Director of CVT Surgery. He was next appointed Program Medical Director for St. Paul's Hospital Heart Centre (1995), and Consultant CV Surgeon at VGH. Lichtenstein holds ross-appointments as Clinical Professor of Surgery and Physiology at UBC.

In 2000 Lichtenstein succeeded Frank Tyers as Head, UBC Division of Cardiovascular Surgery. His areas of special interest are based in both physiology and surgery, especially regarding leading research in warm blood cardioplegia, limitation of acute myocardial infarction size, long-term heart and lung preservation, and mitral valve repair. Lichtenstein has recently developed a sutureless technique for coronary vessel anastamosis, using matched magnets as vessel couplers. He is now going "back to the future" by performing closed heart trans-apical aortic valve replacements in high-risk patients. Definitely a free-thinking ideas man, but grounded in Physiology, he is now promoting minimally invasive surgeries, including robotics.

James Abel graduated BSc, MSc Pharm and finally MD in 1983 from U of T. The General Surgery FRCS(C) was granted in 1989, and CVT Surgery in 1991. He joined UBC/St.Paul's as Attending Staff Surgeon in July 1993 and immediately became known for surgical therapy of atrial fibrillation, VAD implantation, mitral repair, trans-apical aortic replacements and high risk surgery as an alternative to transplant. In 1995, he became the Co-Director of the Cardiac Sugery ICU, and in 1997 the Surgical Director of Transplantation at St. Paul's.

Kassam A. Ashe received MD from the University of Western Ontario in 1984, completed General Surgery at U of T with FRCS(C) in 1990, then earned a Vascular Surgery Fellowship and practiced at McMaster University for three years. He moved to Vancouver in 1997, completed his Cardiovascular and Thoracic FRSC(C) in 1997, and did a transplant year at the London Health Science Centre. An accomplished and technically superior surgeon, Ashe joined St. Paul's Hospital as CV Surgeon and UBC as Assistant Professor in 1998, leaving in 2003 to found the Cardiac Surgery program at St. Mary's Heart Centre, Kitchener.

Karin Humphries started in Biochemistry and Kinesiology at Simon Fraser University (1980) and then pursued Experimental Pathology at UBC with MSc in 1985. She continued her education with an MBA at SFU in 1991 and DSc from Erasmus University, Netherlands in 1999, focussing on Health Services Research and Epidemiology. Humphries was General Manager of the Canadian Lipoprotein Standardization Laboratory, Director of Research and Health Promotion for the Heart and Stroke Foundation of BC/Yukon, and since 1998 has been a Research Associate at Centre for Health Evaluation and

Outcomes Sciences (CHEOS) based at St. Paul's Hospital. She is currently Assistant Professor at UBC with many Principal and Co-Investigator research awards. Projects include cardiovascular epidemiology, women and CV disease health evaluation and outcomes, waiting times for cardiac interventions, secondary prevention and ethnicity differences in access to CV procedures.

Royal Jubilee Hospital, Victoria

By the late 1960s, the people of Victoria started to agitate for an open heart unit, as they were tired of travelling by ferry to Vancouver for surgery. In 1971, Minister of Health Ralph Loffmark bowed to public (and medical) pressure and granted permission for Royal Jubilee to create an open heart unit. Smith went to Toronto to work with Bill Bigelow for six months to refresh his surgical skills, and a search was made for a second cardiac surgeon.

Richard Brownlee was selected to join the team. He had trained at the University of Alberta in Edmonton, with MD in 1963, followed by interneship and a Medical Research Institute Fellowship until 1965. He then entered CVT training, obtaining an MSc in Experimental Surgery (lung transplantation) and FRCS(C) in 1969. He obtained one of the last of the "original" McLaughlin Fellowships and studied with Senning at the Cantonspital in Zurich, Björk at Karolinska in Stockholm, and Donald Ross at Guy's Hospital, London. Brownlee returned to Edmonton to practise CVT Surgery, and became Surgical Instructor at U of A, and Co-Director of the ICU in Edmonton. Brownlee arrived He arrived in Victoria in December 1972, and immediately he and Ralph Smith organized the nascent open heart program. They seconded hospital space for surgery, acquired and calibrated/tested the

heart-lung machine, and practiced surgical techniques.
Their chosen test animal was not the dog, the traditional
laboratory animal, but the pig. Dreams of roasts and
chops from their six large porcine subjects dissipated
when the hospital authorities mandated injection of
methylene blue into the animals at sacrifice.

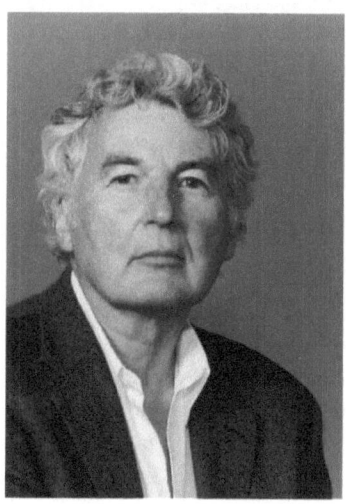

Fig. 11:15 Dick Brownlee

By this time, heart surgery was a "hot button" topic
around this political town, with strong emotions on all
sides; it actually became difficult to recruit ICU nurses
due to the intense media scrutiny, and the first case was
delayed for two weeks by lack of staff. Finally, in July 1973,
the first case was performed, a RCA coronary bypass
graft. Heart surgery then became a media "darling", with
daily reports in the newspaper on the patients' progress;
tour buses would pass the hospital and commentary re
the program and the progress of the latest heart surgery
patient would ensue. An information leak amongst the
hospital staff was discovered and the media frenzy settled
down shortly therafter.

James W. Dutton graduated with his MD in 1969 from the University of Alberta as Gold Medallist, moved to Montreal for interneship at the Montreal General and Children's hospitals and entered general practice in Penticton, BC, for one year. He then started general surgery training at MGH, and obtained FRCS(C) in 1976, which included a Fellowship year with the MRC in Montreal yielding a MSc in Experimental Surgery. Two years of cardiovascular and thoracic surgery training in the Montreal hospitals followed, with FRCS(C) in 1978. He immediately moved to Victoria to practise surgery, and in 1988 became Chief of Cardiac Surgery, Royal Jubilee Hospital. In 1999 he was made Program Director, Heart Health, for the Vancouver Island Health Authority based in Victoria. Active in many organizations, Dutton has been president of the Canadian Society of Cardiac Surgeons, and was Physician to Her Majesty, Queen Elizabeth II and Prince Philip during their three visits to Victoria during the past 20 years.

William A.Griswold obtained his MD in 1969 from the University of Alberta, interned and started Thoracic and Cardiovascular Surgery training there for four years, then completed CVT at Queen's University, Kingston, with FRCS(C) in 1977. He operated as Attending Staff at Kingston General Hospital for a year, and then came to Victoria to practice. Unfortunately his professional career has been truncated due to cardiac problems requiring several operative procedures; over the years, he has concentrated on pacemakers and electrophysiology, vascular surgery, and operative assisting. Griswold joined the Canadian Forces as a Navy Reservist in 1959, and during the 1960s was an Assistant Weapons Officer, and then Commanding Officer of both HMCS Scatari and HMCS Porte St. Jean. He is a charter member of the Bolitho Society of the Pacific Coast Squadron.

Barry Bjorgaard completed the BMedSc from the University of Alberta in 1982, and did his Rotating Interneship at the Victoria General Hospital in BC. He studied general surgery and cardiovascular and thoracic surgery in Saskatoon and London, Ontario, obtaining his FRCS(C) in CVT Surgery in 1989, and passing the written exams in general surgery in both Canada and the U.S. He joined the Active Staff at the Victoria Hospital in London, Ontario, then moved to Minot, North Dakota to practise. He then practised at the Royal Jubilee Hospital in Victoria, BC, from whence he moved back to Minot.

John G. Olfiesh attended McGill University, obtaining BSc (Honours) in 1975, studying Physiological Psychology. His MD,CM was earned in 1980, followed by FRCS(C) in general surgery in 1985 (University Hospital, London, Ontario) and cardiothoracic surgery (Edmonton) in 1992. He became Associate Staff Surgeon in Edmonton for six months, then did eight months as a transplant Fellow at Papworth Everard. He joined the CVT Surgery Section at the Plains Health Centre, Regina in 1993; three years later he moved to Victoria to continue his practise in CVT Surgery. Olfiesh's special interests include valve repair, off-pump surgery, and cardiac resynchronization therapy (ICD, bi-ventricular pacing, laser lead extraction, arrhythmia ablation surgery). He is the Head of Cardiovascular Surgery at the Royal Jubilee Hospital.

Michael J.Perchinsky graduated BMSc in 1987 from the University of Alberta, and MD in 1989. He interned in Phoenix, and from 1990-1995 did general surgery at Kaiser in Portland, Oregon. He finished cardiothoracic surgery training in Vancouver, obtained FRCS(C) in 1998, and is qualified in both countries. Perchinsky has been a busy, meticulous surgeon at Royal Jubilee Hospital, Victoria since 1998, perfroming the full spectrum of cardiac and aortic surgery on patients from all parts of British Columbia.

Royal Columbian Hospital, New Westminster

Robert I. Hayden received his MD,CM from McGill in June 1970, after BSc(Honours) in Biology from Mount Allison University. He moved to the University of Western Ontario for internship and general surgery training, with FRCS(C) in 1974. He practised as a general surgeon in New Brunswick for five years before moving to British Columbia in 1980 to begin a CVT Residency, obtaining a FRCS(C) in thoracic surgery in 1981 and a full FRCS(C) in cardiovascular and thoracic surgery in 1983. Hayden is also certified in the United States in all of these disciplines. Hayden joined VGH in 1983 as CVT Surgeon and became Associate Director of the Willow Chest Cardiac ICU and Ward Service Chief. In 1990 he transferred to the Royal Columbian Hospital in New Westminster, to organize and become the founding Chief Surgeon of the Cardiac Surgery program there. To inaugurate the new unit, the first case, done on February 21, 1991, was a triple coronary bypass graft.

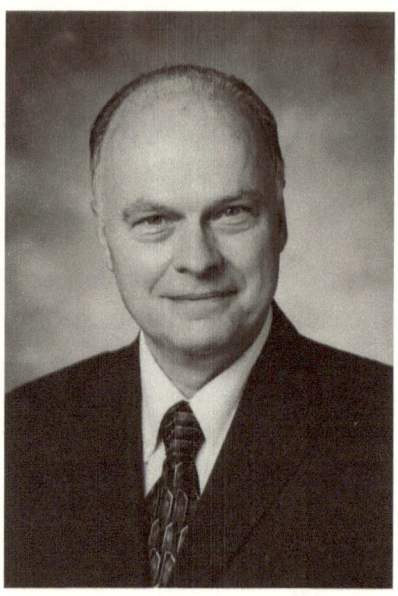

Fig.11:16 Bob Hayden

Keir Stewart received his MD from Dalhousie University, and after interneship there studied General Surgery at the Montreal General Hospital from 1981-1986, earning FRCS(C) that year. He then transferred to Vancouver to train in Cardiovascular and Thoracic Surgery at VGH and the other UBC Hospitals, with FRCS(C) in CVT Surgery awarded in 1989. He joined the Royal Columbian CVT Surgery Staff in January 1991, and performed the first 100 cases in the new unit with Hayden. After seven years in practice in New Westminster, he moved to Halifax, where he performs the full gamut of cardiac procedures, including aortic, transplant and electrophysiological cases.

Shahzad S. Karim studied Biochemistry at UBC with a BSc in 1985, then trained in Medicine, graduating MD in 1989. Internship at Toronto Western Hospital preceded

General Surgery residency at the UBC Affiliated Hospitals with FRCS(C) in 1996. He then entered the CVT program at UBC, completing his Fellowship in 1998. Karim immediately joined the Active Staff at Royal Columbian Hospital to perform all cardiac procedures, including aortic surgery. Over the next 18 months, he also preceptored with Frank Tyers learning laser lead extraction, and following Tyers' retiremenent became Surgical Director, UBC Lead Extraction Programme (based at VGH) and Co-Director of the VGH Pacemaker Clinic. In 2001 Karim was made Program Director of Post Graduate Education for the UBC Division of CV Surgery.

At Last, A Dedicated Children's Hospital

With the advent of cardiac catherization and cardiac ultrasound, pediatric cardiology became busier in the mid 1960s. Congenital lesions were diagnosed more accurately, and as surgery could be more precisely planned, there were fewer "nasty surprises" in the operating room. Young and Vince were augmented by Shirley Hazell, Basil Bolton and Kee Ho Wai; the latter left in 1972 and was replaced by Michael Patterson. In 1976 Marion Tipple and George Sandor joined the staff of the Health Centre for Children at VGH. These cardiologists, in conjunction with the cardiac surgeons and Victor Huckell, an adult cardiologist, formed the Pacific Adult Congenital Heart (PACH) clinic for systematic review of adult patients with congenital defects, both repaired and *de novo*.

During 1982, the new free-standing BC Children's Hospital was opened on the spacious grounds adjacent to the old Shaughnessy Hospital in Vancouver. All pediatric patients were transferred to the new site, with

Phil Ashmore as Head of Pediatric Surgery and also as the sole heart surgeon. The first open heart case: secundum ASD. The surgical volume rapidly increased to five cases of closed and open heart procedures weekly. Phil was fortunate to have a skilled pediatric General Surgeon, Dr. Graham Fraser, assist him for many years; he was a valuable asset to the program, and became *de facto* a part-time cardiovascular surgeon.

The Children's Hospital cardiac team now included cardiologists Vince, Hazell, Michael Patterson and George Sandor; anaesthesiologists Gerry O'Connor and Michael Smith; and a highly dedicated pediatric nursing staff. Both an Intensive Care Unit and a step-down unit were designed to maximize pediatric patient care. The cardiac sciences staff continue to be strong supporters of the Variety Club annual Telethon and the BC Heart Foundation annual campaign.

Jacques Le Blanc was awarded MD in 1976 from Laval University, and studied at the Hospital for Sick Children, Ochsner Clinic, St. Michael's and TGH, obtaining his FRCS(C) in 1983. After a year on staff at HSC, he joined BC Children's Hospital in 1984 performing the full range of pediatric cardiothoracic surgery. He was admitted to staff at VGH in 1991 and St. Paul's in 1994, to consult and operate on cardiac patients. Le Blanc became Head of the Division of Cardiovascular and Thoracic Surgery at Children's in 1992 following Phil Ashmore's retirement. He has been very active in professional organizations, as a Royal College examiner, Chair of the Children's Network Miracle Telethon, and a council member with the Canadian Cardiovascular Society. His special interests include computer-based teaching of teaching of congenital malformations, and database management; he has published extensively on the results of congenital heart, lung, and esophageal surgery. When Halifax's sole pediatric cardiac surgeon left the city in 2000, Le Blanc flew twice yearly from Vancouver until 2003 to operate and provide post-op care for a two-week period at the IWK Children's Hospital. Since 2003 he has also travelled twice yearly to Shanghai, China, along with a medical/surgical team from the BC Children's Hospital, performing surgery and training colleagues at the Fudan University Children Hospital in the surgical care of complex congenital cardiac diseases in infants and children. He is currently preparing a Cardiac Sciences Training Program for Fudan and considering teaching in India.

Suvro Sett graduated MD 1983 and FRCS(C) in General Surgery from the University of Saskatchewan, then took CVT training at UBC between 1988 and 1991. After two years at the Hospital for Sick Children, Toronto, he returned to BC to practise Pediatric Surgery at the BC Children's Hospital. In 2004, he moved to New York State, and is the Chief of Pediatric Surgery at The Maria Fareri Children's Hospital in Westchester.

Enter the Millenium—The 21st Century Surgeons

In late 2003, the UBC Division of Cardiovascular Surgery established a cross-site cardiac surgical group (VGH and St. Paul's Hospital) to provide integrated clinical coverage and teaching at both institutions. In 2004, the group established a joint wait list for inpatients awaiting urgent cardiac surgery, allowing for quick and efficient triage while maximizing the use of available clinical resources. This effort has contributed to the significant *decrease of the cardiac surgical wait list in BC.* A Provincial

Access and Triage initiative is currently underway with targeted benchmark objectives to be achieved by December 2007. This will require further coordination at the provincial level of all patients awaiting cardiac surgical revascularization as well as a new influx of surgical resources critically distributed across the region.

Vancouver General Hospital

Peter Skarsgard, brother and son of doctors, obtained his MD from UBC in 1992, followed by a PhD and FRSC(C) (General Surgery), also from UBC. Cardiothoracic Surgery training at Harvard Beth Israel Deaconess Hospital resulted in FRCS(C) in that specialty, and he joined the UBC Division of Cardiovascular Surgery at VGH in 2003. Skarsgard is a busy, confident surgeon, performs all adult surgeries and continues his interest in nitrous oxide and small vessel disease as a funded part-time researcher. Skarsgard and Richard Cook established a Minimally Invasive Valvular Surgery program in 2005.

Richard Cook completed his MD at the University of Alberta in 1992, and undertook CVT training at the UBC Hospitals, earning his FRCS(C) in 2004. A fellowship year was shared between Christopher Acar in Paris doing mitral valve repair, and Randolph Chitwood in Greenville, North Carolina learning MIS and robotic surgery. On February 11, 2008 Cook and Skarsgaard used the 4-arm da Vinci "S" robot at VGH on the first robotic case in British Columbia, a coronary bypass patient.

From Kiev comes Karim Qayami MD 1975. After many detours, he studied General and CVT Surgery at the UBC Hospitals, completing his studies in 2003. Qayumi is a consummate teacher of surgical technique, and is the founding Director of the Centre of Excellence for Surgical Education and Innovation (CESEI) at the Vancouver General Hospital. He is very active in undergraduate and post-graduate education for surgical and anaesthetic residents, and utilizes high-tech mannekin and computer simulated learning techniques.

Jian Ye obtained his MD from Wenzhou Medical College, China in 1983. After two years of General Surgery he studied Cardiovascular Surgery in Fujian and Zhejiang, obtaining MSc. In 1990 he went to the Cleveland Clinic as an International Scholar and then to Case Western University as a Post-Doctoral Fellow. He moved to Canada as a Surgical Technical Research Officer for the Institute of Biodiagnostics of the National Research Council and was also affiliated with the Departments of Biochemistry and Medical Genetics in Winnipeg. In July 1999 he refreshed his surgical training at the University of Manitoba and received FRCS(C) in 2004. Six months as a Clinical Fellow at St. Paul's led to a staff appointment in January 2005. As his overriding interest is in teaching, Ye is on staff at CESEI at VGH. He also performs a full range of cardiac procedures. His research intests include hypothermic cardiac arrest, and cerebral protection and myocardial injury during surgery, including the use of hyperbaric oxygenation.

St. Paul's Hospital

Anson W. Cheung joined St. Paul's as clinical Assistant Professor in 2000. He graduated BSc in 1988 and MD in 1992 from the University of Manitoba. After internship and General Surgery (MSc, 1995) he spent a year at Stanford University Medical Centre and two years at the University of Western Ontario in Cardiac Surgery residency, obtaining his FRCS(C) in 1999. Cheung then did transplant and ventricular assist device Fellowships for one year in Pittsburgh. Since July 2001 he has been the Surgical Director, Cardiac Transplantation for BC. In October 2005, Cheung (with Lichtenstein and Abel) did the first known catheter-based trans-apical aortic valve replacement, and they have now performed 60 cases. In 2007 Cheung and Lichenstein did the first known trans-apical catheter-based mitral replacement, into a failing bioprosthesis. The VAD program is active: there have been 15 short-term "Impella" implants, including North America's first, and over 50 Thoratec "Heartmate" I and II implants to date.

Ahmad Poostizadeh obtained his MD in Tehran during 1978, studied General Surgery at UBC, Thoracic Surgery at the Medical College of Virginia, and CVT Surgery at St. Paul's and the University Hospital of Cleveland. He is now on staff at St. Paul's and VGH doing cardiac surgery.

Jamil Bashir became BMedSc in 1989, and MD Summa cum Laude in 1991, both from the University of Alberta. After interneship, he did General Practice and surgical assisting for six years, then returned to study Internal Medicine in 1998/1999. After converting to surgery, he obtained the Royal College CVT Fellowship in 2004, then went to Goteborg Universitet, Sweden, for six months of arrhythmia and cardiac resynchronization therapy study. This was followed by a Fellowship at the Hermann Hospital, Houston for six months of aortic surgery. Bashir came on staff at St. Paul's in 2005, with special interests in resychronization therapy, pacer lead extraction and endovascular stenting for aortic aneurysm. In 2006 he was made Program Director for CVT Surgery Undergraduate Education.

Children's Hospital

Andrew Campbell graduated MD from the University of Ottawa in 1993, and completed a PhD from U of T in Molecular Biology. He studied CVT Surgery at Children's Hospital of New Jersey, and came to BC in 2006. His special research interest is angiogenesis in pulmonary hypertension. He primarily operates at BC Children's Hospital, but also does adult congenital cases at St. Paul's.

Royal Columbian Hospital

Timothy B. Latham graduated MD *Cum Laude* from the University of Western Ontario in 1992, and after internship at Western became a General Surgery Resident at the University of Alberta 1993-95. He then entered the Cardiac Surgery program there from 1995-98 with FRCS(C) in 1999. Following an 18-month Fellowship, split between Edmonton and the Toronto General Hospital, he came to BC to join the Royal Columbian Hopsital in New Westminster as Staff Cardiac Surgeon in July 2000. He has now completed his MSc in Experimental Surgery from Edmonton and is a busy clinical surgeon and teacher.

Derek Gunning graduated with BSc (Distinction) in Biochemistry and Microbiology from the University of Victoria, BC in 1995, and was awarded MD from the University of BC in 2000. After interneship, he trained in Cardiac Surgery at the University of Ottawa Heart Institute, with FRCS(C) in 2006. Gunning took further training at UBC, obtaining a second FRCS(C) in Critical Care Medicine in 2007. He then joined the Royal Columbian Hospital staff as a Cardiac Surgeon and Intensivist, and continues to pursue reseacrh interest in cytokines and inflammation, endothelial progenitor cell function and low-range anticoagulation for ON-X valve patients.

Royal Jubilee Hospital

John Peachell was briefly in Victoria, between July 2004 and 2006. He trained at the University of Manitoba, obtaining a BSc in 1991, University of Alberta (MD, 1995) and FRCS(C) in Cardiovascular and Thoracic Surgery in 2000. After a year at the Mayo Clinic (CVT Surgery) he moved to St. Boniface, Winnipeg, and then to Victoria. He has now settled in Alberta where he does cardiac surgery and enjoys life in the outdoors, especially the mountains.

Daniel R.Wong has recently joined the group in Victoria. His 1995 BSc from U of T was in Biochemistry, and he graduted MD (Honours) in 1999. He entered the Cardiac Surgery program at Dalhousie University, obtaining FRCS(C) in 2006. These years included a Master of Public Health from Harvard in 2003, and research time in Cardiac Surgery and Nutrition in Boston. An aortic surgery Fellowship with Coselli in Houston preceded his move to Victoria in 2007. He quickly established a full surgical practise at Royal Jubilee Hospital as a 21st century surgeon.

John Bozinovski was educated at Queen's University, Kingston, Ontario. He earned a BSc (Honours) in 1992, MSc (Pharmacology) in 1995 and MD in 1998. The University of Alberta (Edmonton) provided CVT Residency with FRCS(C) in 2004. A Fellowship year Baylor University was split between St. Luke's Episcopal and Methodist Hospitals, under the preceptorship of Joseph Coselli. In July 2005 he became Attending Surgeon and Assistant Professor of Surgery at Baylor, based at St. Luke's (Texas Heart Institute). His scientifc papers and multiple book chapters have centred around aortic surgery techniques, the biochemistry of preservation, and complications of aortic surgery. In January 2007 Bozinovski joined Royal Jubilee Hospital as Attending Surgeon; he chairs the Quality Assurance Committee and continues to make international presentations.

Lynn Fedoruk obtained BSc in Medical Sciences from the University of Alberta, Edmonton in 1984, and MD in 1988. After internship at Royal Columbian Hospital, she did ER and General Practice, then dedicated herself to surgical assisting, initially at Children's Hospital and later at VGH and Royal Columbian. In July 1999 she finally entered the UBC CVT programme and was granted FRCS(C) in Cardiac Surgery in 2005. One year as a Fellow at the University of Virginia, specializing in non-transplant CHF Surgery, led to an appointment there as Attending Surgeon and Clincal Instructor with responsibilities for resident education and clinical research. Fedoruk was lured back to BC and joined Royal Jubilee Hospital in Victoria as Attending Surgeon in February 2007. She continues to work towards a Master's Degree in Public Health/Clinical Investigation and has qualified in aortic endovascular device deployment.

Supporting the Surgeons—the Unsung Heroes

Research Funding

The early development of cardiac surgery in British Columbia would not have been possible without financial support. The BC Heart Foundation (established prior to the Canadian Heart Foundation) was seminal; the grants through BCMRI and St. Paul's allowed early,focussed research to proceed. The P.A. Woodward Foundation and other granting agencies were generous with their funds. In return, the cardiac surgeons would volunteer for public relation events to aid these groups in their fundraising. Fortunately, support from Heart and Stroke is still generous, as are research funds from CIHR, NRC, The Michael Smith Foundation, BC Health Care Research Foundation, Vancouver Coastal Health Authority, BC Children's Hospital Foundation, VGH/UBC Foundation, BC Lung and Cystic Fibrosis, BC Transplant Society, pharmaceutical and medical device companies, and many generous private foundations.

Pacemaker Clinic

The earliest open procedures were corrections of congential anomalies, and a common, serious post-operative problem was complete heart block. On January 30th,1957, Lillehei used myocardial wires and an electrical system developed by William Weirich in a VSD case with heart block (see Chapter 1); this temporary use was rapidly widely adopted. Permanent cardiac pacing was first instituted at VGH in early 1960 with epicardial wires placed by minithoracotomy and abdominal implant of the large pulse generator. With advances in lead technology and generator refinements, the first transvenous infraclavicular subcutaneous implant was done by early 1962.

Cardiac pacing became the purview of the surgeons, who gradually assumed long-term follow-up of the patients in addition to managing complications after implantations. The often rapid failure of the early "hearing aid type" battery-powered generators, with its dire consequences, led to the development of long life batteries such as the lithium iodide cells. An interesting and novel battery was the plutonium-238 power source in the Medtronic Model 9000 pulse generator. The first "nuclear powered" pacer in Canada was implanted at VGH in 1972 by Trapp and Burr.

The St. Paul's Pacemaker Clinic was started by Kavanagh Gray and Peretz in 1966, and in 1971 Clinic Director John Boone pioneered the use of trans-telephone screening and pacer follow-up, enabling better care of the patients from the far reaches of rural BC. With the careful follow-up of their patients, the St. Paul's Clinic has continued to expand with the advent of the Electrophysiology Program, including ablations, ICD implants and the transfer from VGH of the lead extraction program.

As management of follow-up in each surgeon's office required multiple programmers and other equipment, the VGH Pacer Clinic was founded in 1978 by Frank Tyers. Here we could consolidate documentation of implants, centralize pacer programmers, store information regarding old leads and generators, and above all, offer regular documented post-implant analysis of pacer functioning and longevity. All the surgeons participated in the Clinic, with medical records freely shared. Most importantly, the clinic created dedicated positions for nurses (led by Pauline Mills) and technicians (led by Jacquie Clark), encouraging the development of their specialized skills, membership in NASPE, and certification of electrophysiological achievements.

Hyperbaric Oxygenation

In 1960, Bill Trapp read an article by Ite Boerema regarding the potential uses of a hyperbaric environment for surgery. Investigations revealed that some cardiac procedures might be performed at reduced risk in an oxygen-rich environment. Hyperbaric oxygenation (HBO) had already been used for decompression illness in divers and caisson workers. By 1965, a functioning 8 foot diameter chamber, 24 feet in length, was installed at VGH and in use, masterminded by Trapp and Commander Thompson, an ex-Navy perfectionist. Over time, a variety of uses has developed for the chamber: treatment of carbon monoxide posioning, gas gangrene, air embolism, transient neurological disorders and wound healing (both peripheral from arterial insufficiency and central, such as mediastinitis and radiation tissue injuries), and the bends. In the late 1960s and early 1970s, a number of cases of cyanotic congenital heart disease were corrected or palliated in the "tank", all as non-pump cases. The Hyperbaric Unit could be set up to become a sterile field, with facilities for invasive and surface monitoring. It was fascinating to see a "blue" child turn pink as it was introduced to higher concentrations of oxygen and the blood became saturated with oxygen as we "dove" in the tank. Two or three children per month were operated upon over a time span of 4-5 years by Ashmore and Fraser, with anaesthesia provided by Bill Dodds, with excellent results. Some adult cases were performed in the tank, mostly massive pulmonary embolism with shock.

There were many interesting anecdotes in the tank. As the treaments took several hours, mostly to slowly decompress, people would talk, read or play chess. One elderly gentlemen being treated for a non-healing arterial leg ulcer was also suffering from mild cerebral atheroma. On the "bottom" (at prescribed depth and pressure) he played excellent chess; as he "surfaced", and his oxygen saturations returned to normal, his playing became spotty, and then quite poor. Nothing like oxygen to the brain cells to ensure functioning!

The Professional Assistants

Cardiac surgery requires skilled operators, both as primary and assistant surgeons. The dedication of the professional first or second assistants has been crucial to the smooth conduct of surgery in British Columbia.

At VGH is the "Dean" of Assistant Surgeons, Andrew Thompson MD, FRCS(C). Drew has been a constant influence for many years,and as a qualified surgeon provides a major continuing benefit to the surgery programme. Other assistants over the years include:

Clayton Robinson FRCS(C)	Edward Gentis FRCS(C)
Maged Mikail MD	Marek Karolek MD
Henry Litherland FRCS(C)	Roderick March MD
Morgan Brache MD	Alan Currie MD

The Royal Columbian Hospital has been fortunate to have Karen Fry, MD assisting since the inception of the program. Other assistants at RCH include:

Michael Bendall FRCS(C)	Simon Wong MD
Teresa Hogarth MD	Nima Rabbani MD

St. Paul's Hospital was able to secure the services of Claudio Merler as a valuable assistant on the early cases. Other assistants include:

Alexander Cserpes MD	Mary Lynn Brumwell MD, FRSC(C)
Roy Semlacher MD	Dan Brossuek MD
Ercole Leone MD	Matt Mosher MD
Philip Sinanan MD	Ali Kazami MD
Alex Russell MD	Susan Dawson MD

In Victoria, the "Dean" of Assistant Surgeons at the Royal Jubilee Hospital is Bud Faulkner MD,who assisted on the first Victoria case. Other assistants include:

Dave McNaughton MD   Geoff Homer FRCS(C)
Philip Huggett MD   Don McAdam MD

Into The Future

And where do we go from here? Further progress with less invasive procedures including robotic surgery; better valve repair techniques and materials; improved replacement cardiac valves with fewer adverse reactions; more catheter-based valve procedures; better protection of heart and body during surgery; sophisticated pacer/ICD electronics and multi-lead implants; anti-rejection drug improvement tailored to each person's immune system; peri-operative pharmacological stabilization/optimization of the patient—the wish list is endless. And here in British Columbia? A new Cardiovascular Surgery Unit at the Kelowna General Hospital, projected to open in 2012-2014.

Bibliography

Allen, Peter: *Better Lucky Than Good,* Private Press, 2001.

Ashmore, Philip: "The Early Development of Heart Surgery in British Columbia." In Goldman, Bernard, and Bélanger, Susan: *Heart Surgery in Canada.* 2005, ch. 9.

Gerein, Alfred: *Pioneering of Open Heart Surgery at St.Paul's Hospital,* 1991.

Lemon, Käthe: *Spirit of Discovery,* St. Paul's Hospital, 2001.

CHAPTER 12

SURGICAL OPTIONS FOR END-STAGE HEART DISEASE INCLUDING MECHANICAL CIRCULATORY SUPPORT AND CARDIAC TRANSPLANTATION—A CANADIAN PERSPECTIVE

Harpreet Grover and Vivek Rao

Introduction

Throughout history, the human body has always been a source of fascination and mystery. Driven by this allure, man has been able to investigate and operate on virtually every organ in the human body, including the brain, eye, lungs, bone, and kidney. The heart, however, remained one of the last organs to be successfully repaired by pioneering surgeons. For almost twenty centuries, it was considered to be an impossible undertaking that provided no benefit to patients. Today correcting a cardiac complication is no longer a daunting task and such procedures have greatly improved the lives of thousands of individuals around the world.[1] This surgical triumph has given cardiac patients another chance at life and would not have been possible had it not been for the work of innovative surgeons who had a profound desire to learn, the wish to improve the lives of others, and the courage to explore a vital organ which was not well understood. Many of the early accomplishments in the field of cardiac surgery are credited to Canadian surgeons. This chapter will focus on the surgical treatment of end-stage heart disease, including mechanical circulatory support and cardiac transplantation. The relevant Canadian milestones will be highlighted.

It was once believed that operating upon the heart was beyond the capability of any physician, no matter how qualified or skilled. During the nineteenth century, at a time when the limits of medicine were being tested, many leading surgeons in Europe considered heart wounds inoperable and invariably fatal.[2] In the late nineteenth century, Theodor Billroth, a prominent European surgeon, stated, "The surgeon who attempts to operate on the heart cannot wish to preserve the respect of his colleagues."[3] Fortunately, there were those who did not share this belief and forged ahead, trying to develop new techniques to successfully operate on the heart.

Critical to the success of any modern cardiac operation is the ever evolving field of myocardial protection. Canadian leaders in the field include Dr. Tomas Salerno (St. Michael's Hospital in Toronto), Dr. Richard Weisel (Toronto General Hospital), Dr. Ray Chiu (McGill University) and Dr. G. Frank O. Tyers (Vancouver General Hospital). Several major contributions by these investigators led to substantial reductions in perioperative morbidity and mortality attributed to inadequate myocardial protection. Improving results in "low-risk" individuals encouraged surgeons to perform increasingly complex operations on patients previously thought to be unsuitable for surgical intervention.[4]

Surgical Alternatives To Transplantation

Currently, patients with end-stage heart disease are evaluated for a wide variety of surgical options as an *alternative* to cardiac transplantation. While many of these interventions have yielded only transient improvements in symptomatology, many have obviated the need for subsequent transplant. The use of synchronized biventricular pacing has been pioneered by the efforts of Canadian cardiologists including Dr. Paul Dorian (St. Michael's Hospital in Toronto) and Dr. Anthony Tang (Ottawa Heart Institute). The concept behind this device lies in the resynchronization of co-ordinated contractile activity in patients with intraventricular conduction defects. Surprisingly, the results of the MIRACLE (Multicenter Insync Randomized Clinical Evaluation) study demonstrated that this form of pacing can result in reduced systolic and diastolic volumes, improved left ventricular ejection fraction and attenuation of mitral insufficiency.[5] Many Canadian centers were active participants in the MIRACLE study.

Mitral valve repair for congestive heart failure was popularized by Dr. Steven Bolling from Ann Arbor, Michigan (a Canadian by birth!).[6] Bolling's series defied the conventional teaching that patients with severe systolic dysfunction would not tolerate a surgical intervention on their mitral valve. Unfortunately, the four-year survival following MV repair in this forty-eight-patient cohort was only 50 percent and Dr. Bolling has not yet updated his series with either enhanced follow-up or increased sample size. In our own experience, we agree with Dr. Bolling that these high-risk patients can survive surgical intervention. However, the long-term results are less than satisfactory and we prefer cardiac transplantation in eligible patients.

A similar outcome was observed following the clinical experience with the Batista* procedure.[7] The theory of the Batista procedure, alternatively known as partial left ventriculectomy, is to reduce the diameter of the dilated left ventricle in order to reduce wall stress and hence improve overall systolic function. Again, the concept that patients with severe systolic dysfunction would not tolerate such an intervention was refuted by Batista's clinical results. However, a more rigorous evaluation of the medium term results following this procedure was published by McCarthy et al. from the Cleveland Clinic and documented an unacceptable rate of both early and late failure.[8] The experience at Toronto General Hospital (Dr. R. J. Cusimano, personal communication) was similar to that of McCarthy and most patients redilated within two years, developed recurrent symptoms requiring transplantation or died with progression of their heart failure.

A version of Batista's technique is currently under evaluation by the STICH investigators. The STICH (Surgical Therapy for Ischemic Congestive Heart Failure) trial is evaluating the role of surgical revascularization and/or left ventricular reconstruction in patients with congestive heart failure and left ventricular systolic dysfunction. In contrast to the Batista operation that uniformly resected anterior myocardium, the concept behind surgical ventricular restoration (SAVER) is to modify akinetic or dyskinetic areas of myocardium while concomitantly improving myocardial perfusion by surgical revascularization.[8] The STICH trial is currently in progress and several Canadian centers are active participants (Toronto General Hospital, Laval University,

---

* Dr. Ron Batista trained in part in Toronto. —Ed.

Queen Elizabeth II in Halifax and Montreal General Hospital).

Although the goal of all of the above interventions is to delay or even prevent the need for heart transplant, cardiac transplantation remains the gold standard for the long-term treatment of end-stage heart disease. One of the greatest triumphs of cardiac surgery was realized when the first human-to-human heart transplant was successfully completed. This single event, however, represented the culmination of research spanning over sixty years, conducted by medical scientists from all over the world. Experimental cardiac transplantation began at the turn of the twentieth century. In most of these early experiments, the heart was used as an accessory organ or an auxiliary pump in heterotopic transplantations in canine models. The first of these experiments was conducted in 1905, by Alexis Carrel, a French scientist, and Charles Guthrie, an American physiologist. Carrel later won the Nobel Prize in 1912, for his groundbreaking research in organ transplantation and vascular suturing techniques. It was not until after the Second World War, however, that surgeons and researchers began to consider the idea of orthotopic cardiac transplantation in human patients.

Cardiac Transplantation

In 1955, Vladimir Demikhov, a Russian scientist, performed the first orthotopic heart transplantation in two dogs, without the use of hypothermic conditions or a heart-lung bypass machine. Although the animals died shortly after the procedure, this experiment showed for the first time that it was possible to sustain life using a donated heart.[10] In the years that followed, several similar experiments were carried out, but unlike Demikhov's initial experiment, a circulatory bypass machine and systemic hypothermic conditions supported these operations.

In 1960, Richard Lower and Norman Shumway, two American surgeons, further modified Demikhov's experiments by introducing a localized hypothermic environment for the donor heart. Under these conditions, they were able to significantly prolong the life of their canine subjects, but with the poor immunosuppressive agents available at the time, the animals rejected the graft between six and twenty-one days after the operation.[11] Nonetheless, this technique was a major discovery in transplant research, because, for the first time, a transplanted heart remained functional for more than just a few hours. In January of 1964, Dr. James Hardy performed the first cardiac xenotransplantation on a patient who was grievously ill. Since there was no human donor heart available at the time, Dr. Hardy attempted to save the patient's life by replacing the human heart with one from a chimpanzee. Although the patient died shortly after the operation, his death was not in vain. Rather, this extraordinary event set the stage for the first human heart transplant, which would occur nearly four years later.[12]

On December 3, 1967, Dr. Christiaan Barnard, a surgeon in Cape Town, South Africa who had been a surgical resident with Dr. Shumway, performed the first human heart transplant. He replaced the diseased heart of a fifty-four-year-old man by the name of Louis Washkansky, with a healthy one from a young woman who had passed away earlier in a car accident. Although Washkansky lived for only eighteen days after the operation, his death was not due to cardiac complications; rather, he succumbed to a lung infection. Up until his last moments, the transplanted heart maintained a normal circulation and was functioning remarkably well. A month later, another heart transplant was performed by Dr. Barnard, and this time, the patient survived for more than eighteen months.[13] The dream of one day replacing a diseased heart with one from a healthy donor had at last become a reality.

Six months later, on May 31, 1968, Dr. Pierre Grondin performed Canada's first heart transplant at the Montreal Heart Institute. Later the same year, on November 17, Dr. Clare Baker and Dr. James Yao of St. Michael's Hospital in Toronto, operated on Charles Perrin Johnston, who survived for over nine years, becoming the first long-term heart transplant survivor in Canada and the longest in the world in the pre-cyclosporin era.[14]

During the initial years following this surgical milestone, patient mortality due to acute graft rejection remained unacceptably high. The early excitement of heart transplantation quickly diminished and the number of procedures performed globally decreased dramatically from 102 in 1968, to less than twenty in 1970.[15] Advances made during the 1970s, however, helped overcome several of the barriers to cardiac transplantation, and confidence in this procedure was once again restored. Newer and more effective therapies for suppressing the immune system were developed (particularly the discovery of cyclosporin in the mid-1970s) and more efficient methods for monitoring early posttransplant rejection were established, including ventricular endomyocardial biopsies, immunological monitoring, and electrocardiography.[16] Consequently, the number of heart transplants performed throughout the world soared to 190 in 1982 and to over 3,000 in 1996. In Canada alone, the number of heart transplants performed annually increased from 2 in 1981 to 172 in 2000.[17] There are currently twelve cardiac transplant programs in Canada including three that offer pediatric transplantation (Hospital for Sick Children in Toronto, Ste. Justine in Quebec and University of Alberta Hospital in Edmonton).

The one-year survival of heart transplant recipients has risen significantly from 22 percent in 1968 to over 85 percent in 2002, with a median survival of nearly nine years.[18]

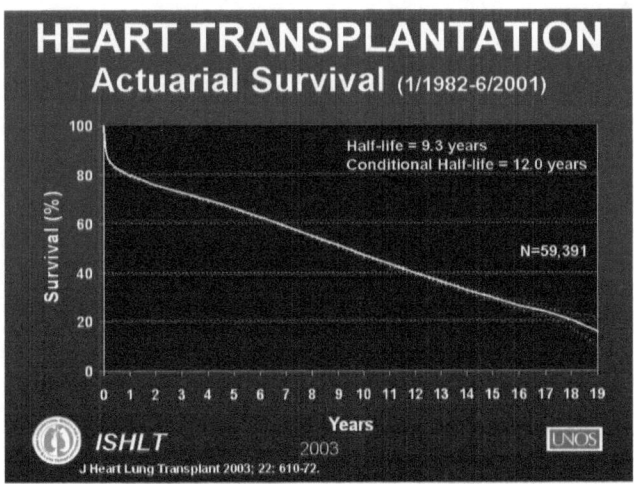

Fig. 12:1 Actuarial survival following heart transplantation.

Thus, orthotopic heart transplantation has become an effective approach for treating patients with end-stage heart failure and remains the gold standard for definitive care.

Unfortunately, most programs in Canada and around the world suffer from an inadequate supply of donor organs to meet the needs of their recipient lists. In 2001, the mortality on the Canadian cardiac transplant waiting list was 19 percent. Thus, almost one in five candidates died before a suitable organ was found. Therefore, most of the larger transplant centers in the country have turned to mechanical circulatory support to bridge their transplant candidates until a donor organ becomes available.

Mechanical Circulatory Support

In the 1960s, there was tremendous excitement about the potential of mechanical devices that would either assist a failing heart in its natural function or replace it entirely. Drs. Willem Kolff, Domingo Liotta and Robert Jarvik led the research in the development of the total artificial heart (TAH).[19] This device was first used as a bridge to cardiac transplantation in 1969. Many patients who received the TAH, however, suffered adverse complications including massive infection, strokes, and multiple organ failure which ultimately resulted in death. A modified version of the original Jarvik TAH is now available as the Cardiowest TAH and has been successfully employed at the Ottawa and Montreal Heart institutes.

In 1962, during the time the TAH was being developed, three American surgeons, Michael DeBakey, Denton Cooley, and Arthur Beall, began developing the left ventricular assist device (LVAD). Four years later, Dr. DeBakey successfully implanted the first LVAD into a patient who was suffering from acute heart failure following a surgical procedure. The LVAD kept the patient alive for ten days and was subsequently explanted once the patient's heart recovered. In 1969, Cooley used a TAH to support a patient until transplantation, but the patient died of acute graft failure. Norman was the first to successfully bridge a patient to transplant with a left ventricular assist device.[20] In the years following these accomplishments, LVAD insertion has become accepted therapy for the treatment of both acute and chronic heart failure.

In Canada, long-term mechanical circulatory support is now offered in six centers with additional centers expected to initiate programs within the year. At present, only existing cardiac transplant centers have expressed an interest in establishing assist device programs. However, the advent of "destination therapy" or the use of LVADs as a permanent therapy for heart failure may result in more cardiac surgical centers offering this highly expensive and resource-intensive service.[21]

There are several commercially available devices currently being employed in Canada for mechanical circulatory support. The paracorporeal devices include the ABIOMED BVS5000 (Abiomed Corp, Danvers, MA) and the Thoratec Assist Device (Thoratec Corp, Pleasanton, CA). The implantable devices include the Cardiowest TAH (formerly Jarvik) and the HeartMate (Thoratec Corp) and Novacor (World Heart Corp, Ottawa, ON) LVADs. Table 1 displays the Canadian VAD centers with the devices currently available at each site.

Table 1: Canadian Centres for Extended Mechanical Circulatory Support

Site	City	ABIOMED	THORATEC	HeartMate	Berlin Heart	Novacor	Cardiowest
Hôpital Laval	Quebec City	+	+			+	
Hospital for Sick Children	Toronto				+*		
Montreal Heart Institute	Montreal		+				+
Ottawa Heart Institute	Ottawa		+			+	+
Queen Elizabeth II	Halifax					+	
Royal Victoria Hospital	Montreal		+	+		+	
St. Paul's Hospital	Vancouver		+	+			
Toronto General Hospital	Toronto	+	+	+		+*	
University of Alberta	Edmonton			+*			

Available devices at each Canadian Institution (asterisk indicates that device is available but not yet implanted at that site)

The Ottawa Heart Institute has the longest and largest Canadian experience with circulatory support devices with over seventy-five implants to date. On May 1, 1986, Dr. Wilbert Keon inserted a Jarvik 7 TAH into a forty-nine-year-old woman with post-MI cardiogenic shock. The woman was successfully supported for several days until she was transplanted and remains alive and well today. Shortly thereafter, Dr. Michel Carrier implanted a Jarvik TAH at the Montreal Heart Institute. The first Thoratec LVAD was implanted by Koshal at the Ottawa Heart Institute on June 5, 1991. The first Thoratec BiVAD was implanted by Hendry on October 31, 1991, again at the Ottawa Heart Institute. In addition, the first Thoratec portable driver in North America (enabling patients to be discharged from hospital) was used by Hendry in 1999. Hendry also performed Canada's first Novacor implant on January 15, 1998, and the patient remains alive and well today after successful transplantation.

We performed Canada's first HeartMate implantation on November 3, 2001, in Toronto. The patient was a forty-seven-year-old man with dilated cardiomyopathy who was in refractory cardiogenic shock despite a sixty-day (!) CCU admission for tailored hemodynamic therapy. At the time of assessment, the patient was unable to speak complete sentences and was bedridden.

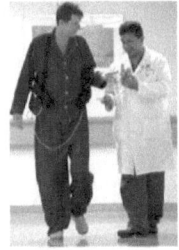

Fig. 12:2 Canada's first HeartMate LVAD recipient four days postimplant with Vivek Rao

He is now ambulatory on the ward. He was transplanted after 166 days of support and remains alive and well today.

Canada's second HeartMate recipient was a twenty-nine-year-old female with a peripartum cardiomyopathy. She underwent LVAD insertion for acute cardiogenic shock on December 1, 2001, in Toronto. She was successfully supported on the device for a hundred days. During her routine follow-up, we noticed substantial recovery of LV function. We elected to explant the device and she remains alive and well over two years from the time of device explantation. She continues to have moderate LV dysfunction, but is well managed on medical therapy and is not currently being considered for heart transplantation.[22]

The Future

The future of cardiac surgery with respect to heart transplantation and mechanical assist devices is extremely promising. Smaller and more lightweight devices that are completely implantable have been developed and several are already being evaluated in clinical trials. These devices also have the potential to be used on a long-term basis as an alternative to transplantation (destination therapy). The ABIOCOR total artificial heart remains under clinical investigation and represents the first generation, totally implantable TAH. To date, no Canadian center had implanted an ABIOCOR device as the initial clinical trial has been carefully limited to a few American sites. Although the preliminary clinical experience was discouraging due to a high incidence of thromboembolic events, the technological advance is a remarkable feat of engineering. Interestingly, it was just over a century ago that many physicians believed that the limits of heart surgery had been reached. In 1896, Stephen Paget, an English surgeon, wrote: "Surgery of the heart has probably reached the limits set by nature to all surgery; no new method nor new discovery can overcome the natural difficulties that attend the wound of a heart."[23] During the twentieth century, however, cardiac surgery evolved to the forefront of medical science and research. What began as a radical medical procedure that no surgeon dared to perform has now been transformed into a well-defined specialty with far-reaching benefits for patients. The development of cardiac surgery was made possible by innovative ideas, skilled researchers, and most importantly, profoundly dedicated individuals who were willing to take calculated risks and tread in unknown waters. Several prominent Canadians have contributed significantly to our field. Advances in technology, which afforded researchers and surgeons the opportunity to put their ideas into action, specifically facilitated progress in heart transplantation and in the development of circulatory support devices. Thus, it would seem that the only obstacle to further advances in transplant surgery and mechanical devices would be man's creativity and ingenuity. Unfortunately, this is not the case. Transplant surgery remains severely limited by the number of available donor organs. As the incidence of heart failure continues to rise, so does the demand for cardiac allografts, which far outnumbers the available supply. In Canada alone, the number of patients awaiting a heart transplant has risen 37 percent since 1991, while the number of heart donors has remained relatively constant. An infinite source of organs, such as mechanical hearts or cardiac xenografts, may someday provide the solution to this problem, but barriers to these therapies, including hyperacute and chronic rejection, have thus far been difficult to overcome. While at present these solutions appear impossible, the same was said about cardiac transplantation only thirty years ago. Heart failure remains the only cardiovascular diagnosis increasing in prevalence in North America, yet the role of surgery has yet to be defined. Canadian surgeons are at the forefront of innovative new technologies and surgical procedures that will likely alter the current management strategies for patients with end-stage heart disease.

Notes:

1   Hugh McLeave, *The Risk Takers* (London: Frederick Muller Limited, 1962), pp. 9-18.

2   Martin Duke, *The Development of Medical Techniques and Treatments: From Leeches to Heart Surgery* (Madison: International Universities Press Incorporated, 1991), pp. 179-86, 201-6.

3   McLeave, Opus cited, Ref. # 1.

4   J. S. Ikonomidis et al., "Myocardial protection for coronary bypass surgery: The Toronto Hospital Perspective," *Ann Thorac Surg* (1995), 60: 824-32.

5   MIRACLE Study Investigators, "Cardiac Resynchronization in chronic heart failure," *NEJM* (2002), 346: 1845-53.

6   S. F. Bolling et al., "Intermediate outcome of mitral reconstruction in cardiomyopathy," *J Thorac Cardiovasc Surg* (1998), 115: 381-88.

7   R. J. V. Batista et al., "Partial left ventriculectomy for end-stage heart disease," *Ann Thorac Surg* (1997), 64: 634-38.

8   A. Franco-Cereceda et al., "Partial left ventriculectomy for dilated cardiomyopathy: Is this an alternative to transplantation?" *J Thorac Cardiovasc Surg* (2001), 121: 879-93.

9   C. L. Athanasuleas et al. for the RESTORE Group, "Surgical anterior ventricular endocardial

restoration (SAVER) for dilated ischemic cardiomyopathy," *Sem Thor Cardiovasc Surg* (2001), 13: 448-58.

10   Duke, Opus cited, Ref. # 2.

11   Ibid.; Robert G. Richardson, *The Surgeon's Heart: A History of Cardiac Surgery* (London: William Heinemann Medical Books Limited, 1969), pp.295-332.; "The Healthy Heart: A Brief History of Heart Transplantation," Columbia University Department of Surgery, *http://www.columbiasurgery.org/programs/ tx_heart/healthy_history.html.*

12   Columbia University Department of Surgery, Opus cited, Ref. # 11.

13   Duke, Opus cited, Ref. # 2.

14   J. E. Wynands, "The contribution of Canadian anaesthetists to the evolution of cardiac surgery," *Can J Anaesth* (May 1996), 43(5, pt.1): 518-34; Toronto *Globe & Mail,* June 1, Nov. 18, 1968.

15   W. J. Keon, "Heart transplantation in perspective," *J Card Surg* (Mar-Apr 1999), 14(2): 147-51.

16   Duke, Opus cited, Ref. # 2.

17   Keon, Opus cited, Ref. # 15.

18   J. D. Hosenpud et al., "The Registry of the International Society for Heart and Lung Transplantation: Eighteenth Official Report— 2001," *J Heart-Lung Transplant* (2001), 20: 805-15.

19   Y. Nose et al., "Development of rotary blood pump technology: past, present, and future," *Artif Organs* (June 2000), 24(6): 412-20.

20   P. Hendry, "Developments in mechanical support as a bridge to cardiac transplant," *Can J Cardiol* (2004), 20: 443-46.

21   E. A. Rose et al., "Long-term use of a left ventricular assist device for end-stage heart failure," *NEJM* (2001), 345: 1435-43.

22   D. H. Delgado et al., "Explantation of a mechanical assist device: assessment of myocardial recovery," *J Card Surg* (2004), 19: 47-50.

23   Raymond Hurt, *The History of Cardiothoracic Surgery: From Early Times* (New York: The Parthenon Publishing Group, 1996), pp. 32-33, 399-408.

CHAPTER 13

CONTEMPORARY STATUS OF HEART SURGERY IN CANADA

Shafie Fazel

The landscape of contemporary cardiac surgery in Canada has changed dramatically over the past two decades. Pediatric centralization, adult surgery quality control issues and the major contributions of Canadian surgeons in the fields of coronary artery disease, valvular surgery and laboratory research will be discussed.

The Bigger the Better: The Pediatric Centralization Story

Within the span of just a few years the number of tertiary pediatric cardiac surgical centres in Canada could have potentially fallen from eleven to six. The Winnipeg pediatric program closed in the mid-1990s, the Saskatoon and London programs ended in the late 1990s, the Halifax program closed temporarily in 2002, and the Ottawa program was scheduled to shut down in April 2003. The current eight programs are located in Halifax, two in Montreal, Quebec City, Ottawa, Toronto, Edmonton and Vancouver. The closures were brought about by events in Canada as well as abroad that highlighted the risk of performing complex congenital corrective operations at centres without adequate experience, support personnel or system infrastructure. Reviewing the events that led to the precipitous closure of several Canadian centres is indeed instructive as we begin to shift the care of adult patients away from the traditional experienced academic centres to smaller community based nonacademic hospitals.

The events that led to the closure of smaller pediatric cardiac surgical programs were triggered by the death of twelve infants in 1993-94 at the Winnipeg Health Sciences Centre; their deaths were thought to be mostly avoidable. The hospital temporarily stopped the delivery of pediatric cardiac surgical services to allow an external review team to examine the circumstances that led to the death of these infants and to identify system deficiencies that required correction. The program was suspended for at least six months. Parents of the children, however, requested that the province conduct a public inquiry and on March 5, 1995, the chief medical examiner for the Province of Manitoba began an inquest into the deaths of these children. In the fall of 1998, the inquest was completed.

Pediatric cardiac surgery epitomizes the problem of the learning curve in connection with complex surgical procedures. The more difficult a procedure the longer the time required to achieve technical proficiency, with a correspondingly greater need to perform such procedures on a regular basis to maintain skills.

The inquest into the death of the twelve children therefore had to determine whether the hospital's relatively high mortality was in keeping with the results of other new programs or whether the death rate was disproportional. The complexity of congenital cardiac defects and their repair, the fragile physiology of infants, especially newborns, and the immense perioperative challenges require not only a skilled surgeon but an entire team of experts to ensure an acceptable outcome. The inquest brought to the fore society's role in dealing with its most vulnerable members, the children. Some argued that society should mandate that children be looked after by an experienced and well established program and that the learning curve should thus be minimized or completely eliminated. In order to achieve this goal the necessary requirements were that every young pediatric heart surgeon be a member of an experienced team that included more senior surgeons. It also required that the case load at any institution should be adequate to maintain the skills of the senior surgeon and to develop the skills of the junior surgeon. The final findings of the inquest were as follows:

> *The available information suggests that the limited number of cases that can be undertaken in a province like Manitoba, with a population of just over one million, represents an increased risk of morbidity and mortality; particularly in the case of high-risk surgery. Even if the catchment area were expanded, the base population would still not be large enough to support a full service program.*

The inquest concluded that the program should remain closed and only be reinitiated in Manitoba as part of a regional program in Western Canada.

Similar developments took place in the United Kingdom in what became well known as the "Bristol Affair." On July 18, 2001, the report of a public inquiry into the deaths of nearly thirty infants at the Bristol Royal Infirmary in the late 1980s and early 1990 was published. The *Canadian Medical Association Journal* (*CMAJ*) ran the headline

"Eerie parallels between British, Canadian inquests into infant deaths." In Britain, television networks showed images of tiny coffins being laid out by aggrieved parents outside the General Medical Council's (GMC) offices in London and of Bristol doctors who were found guilty of professional misconduct. Importantly, the report identified a "club culture" that was pervasive among senior staff in the hospital, and implicitly pointed the finger at the physicians for the delay in recognition of unacceptable outcomes.

In the aftermath of the Bristol inquiry, Dr. Gabriel Scally, the regional director of public health in South West England wrote for the *CMAJ*: "There are undoubtedly parallels between events in Bristol and those in pediatric cardiac surgery in Winnipeg. The combination of the stark nature of the crude outcomes—survival or death, the highly complex nature of the surgery and the patient group involved—all contribute to making this an area of clinical practice that will almost inevitably engender massive public and political feeling."

The Winnipeg and Bristol public inquiries sparked a reexamination of programs across Canada, and the reported morbidity and mortality rates for individual operations, for surgeons, and institutions—all came under heavy scrutiny. In many instances, in spite of acceptable outcomes, provincial governments moved to close the smaller pediatric cardiac surgical centres, possibly to prevent further undermining of society's confidence in the delivery of congenital cardiac surgical services.

One such program was at the London Health Sciences Centres (LHSC). The LHSC had a relatively long history in pediatric cardiac surgery. Drs. Alan Lansing, John Coles

Sr., Martin Goldbach, and Alan Menkis had maintained the program since the 1960s. In the mid-1990s, LHSC recruited Dr. John Lee, who had finished his general surgery and cardiac surgery training in London, prior to a Fellowship at one of the preeminent pediatric centres in the world, the Children's Hospital of Pennsylvania (CHOP). With his recruitment, the institution began expanding its pediatric program and undertook increasingly more complex congenital repairs. Although the catchment area for London was somewhat small at nearly two million people, Dr. Lee led an experienced team that had developed the infrastructure and expertise to conduct complex congenital procedures. In the aftermath of the Manitoba inquest, however, the LHSC decided to close the pediatric program. The number of cases performed by Dr. Lee was deemed insufficient to maintain the skills of the surgeons and the rest of the team in dealing with very sick infants with complex congenital cardiac anomalies.

In May 2002, the report of the Specialized Pediatric Services Review of Ontario was made public. Following the Manitoba inquest, the Bristol inquiry, and the closing of the LHSC tertiary cardiac center, the review recommended that all tertiary pediatric cardiac surgery services be consolidated by April of 2003, at one large, world-renowned facility, the Hospital for Sick Children in Toronto. This decision, naturally, was met with some resistance for fear that centralizing all care at one centre increased the risk for the severely ill infant located a long way from Toronto. It is important to note that the plan to close the Ottawa program has not been, and is not likely to ever be implemented.

The Specialized Pediatric Services Review Committee included representatives from the province's five specialized pediatric centres (Children's Hospital of Eastern Ontario in Ottawa, Children's Hospital of Western Ontario at LHSC, Children's Hospital at Hamilton Health Sciences Centre, Kingston General Hospital, and the Hospital for Sick Children). The purpose of the committee was to review the national and international data available on pediatric cardiac surgical services in the wake of the events in Manitoba and Bristol, to determine the safest and most efficacious manner in which to delivery tertiary pediatric cardiac surgical services in Ontario.

The committee found that in both adult and pediatric surgery there is a strong relationship between low procedure volumes and increased patient risk, echoing the findings of the Manitoba and Bristol inquiries. The Bristol inquiry, in fact, called for the development of "standards that should stipulate the minimum number of procedures which must be performed in a hospital over a given period of time in order to have the best opportunity of achieving good outcomes for children." Toronto's Hospital for Sick Children is the only hospital in Ontario that actually meets the minimum requirements set out by the committee. The Ministry of Health, having agreed to the implementation of all of the committee's recommendations, concluded: "The decision to move children's heart surgery to a single world-class facility is all about doing what's best for children across the province. It's about acting on the recommendations of experts to provide children with the best care and best outcomes possible."

In light of these developments the pediatric cardiac surgery story in Halifax is of interest. Dr. David Murphy, who trained many of the East Coast cardiac surgeons, retired from practice to pursue, in his retirement, a degree in sculptural arts. Dr. David Ross was left at the helm of a one-man pediatric service. Outcomes reported from the Halifax cardiac surgical service remained impeccable—a tribute to Drs. Murphy and Ross. In 2001, Dr. Ross, the residency program director in Halifax at the time, was recruited to join Dr. Ivan Rebeyka in Edmonton. Thus pediatric cardiac services in Halifax were interrupted for a short while until Dr. John Lee from London joined and restarted the program. Halifax has since recruited two new pediatric surgeons—Drs. C. Hancock-Friesen and Stacy O'Blenes. Dr. Hancock-Friesen completed her residency in cardiac surgery in Halifax and then a Fellowship in pediatric surgery at Harvard University. Dr. O'Blenes received both residency and pediatric fellowship training at the University of Toronto. Their performance will obviously be under scrutiny for years to come as junior surgeons working in a well established centre.* Through the process of centralization then, it has become clear that a population of five to ten million people is required to support a successful pediatric heart surgery program, that ideally it should have two or more surgeons and that pediatric cardiac surgery be part of a larger program that includes experienced cardiologists, cardiac anaesthesia, specialized nurses, and allied health professionals. Canada therefore can support six major programs at most. Considering our geography, however, the centralization of pediatric cardiac surgical services is logistically difficult to achieve with only six centres. A final important aspect of pediatric surgery in Canada is that the Congenital Heart Surgeons Society (CHSS) database, established by a group of seventy pediatric heart surgeons across North America, is currently

---

*   To complicate matters, Dr. O'Blenes has since left Halifax.—Ed.

maintained at the Hospital for Sick Children (HSC). The initial data collection began in 1985 under the direction of Drs. John Kirklin and Eugene Blackstone. The data centre at HSC employees 3.5 full-time people and has two physician/surgeon consultants with funding provided by the institutions of the surgeon members with substantial support by HSC. The data accumulation has been significant in determining the success of various procedures over time.

Cardiac Surgery and Quality Control

Ontario's teaching hospitals have had an enviable record of academic leadership in cardiac surgery. By the late 1980s, however, a number of factors conspired to create a crisis in the delivery of cardiac surgical care. The efficacy of coronary bypass surgery in providing both symptomatic relief and prolongation of life was by then scientifically established. Well-trained cardiologists had migrated from the core teaching hospitals to the community with every expectation that their patients would have timely and appropriate access to revascularization surgery. However, resource allocation did not meet need and waiting list pressures mounted. Public and physician criticisms inevitably spilled over into the media, especially after the much publicized death of a patient following coronary bypass surgery at St. Michael's Hospital. His admission had been cancelled numerous times.

It was readily apparent that there was no system for managing waiting lists, triage practices were informal and referring physicians had no access to waiting list information. Wait lists were haphazard, lengthy, nonuniform between institution, and cancellations were frequent. Other deaths of patients on the waiting lists became known and led to increasing pressure on the provincial government. The realization that some Ontario residents were actually funded to have surgery performed in the United States, e.g., those from Windsor, added fuel to the public anger. Ultimately the Ministry of Health responded with a series of initiatives which led to the establishment of the Provincial Adult Cardiac Care Network (later renamed Cardiac Care Network or CCN), a milestone in the development of cardiac care in Ontario.

The St. Michael's Hospital inquiry was initiated in 1988 to identify the hospital, local, regional and provincial factors that drove the long waiting times, cancellations and deaths, with publication of the final report in 1989. The recommendation of the three-person team were: (1) to develop a Metro triage program, and expand it to the provincial level, (2) establish a provincial forum of care providers, (3) gather standardized data on all patients awaiting surgery in the province using an objective ranking system with common terminology, and (4) develop public education programs that establish a hospital-based nurse-practitioner to provide cardiovascular health advice for patients awaiting surgery.

The CCN was created in a step-wise fashion through the collaboration of many agencies and leaders. Its birth can be traced to the Metropolitan Toronto Triage and Registry program, established in 1988 by Drs. Ron Baigrie and Bernard Goldman at the request of the Ministry of Health, the Metropolitan Toronto District Health Council, the CCU Directors' Club, and the University of Toronto. Its initial role was to provide "one number to call" for physicians in the greater Toronto area to access advanced cardiac care resources and to facilitate physician to physician contact. It also established a fledgling database to address, for the first time, the burden of waiting for cardiac surgery.

An urgency rating consensus panel was struck under the auspices of Metro Triage to identify clinical factors that predicted a likely outcome for a given patient. An expert panel, comprised of cardiovascular surgeons, cardiologists, clinical epidemologists, and other academic representatives was formed under the leadership of Dr. David Naylor, then inaugural CEO of the Institute of Clinical Evaluative Sciences (ICES). Through a formal Rand process seven clinical factors were identified, which when combined and weighted, constitute the Urgency Ranking Score (URS). Maximal recommended waiting times for surgery were linked to the URS. The URS was not intended to supplant clinical judgement or the triage practices of an individual cardiac surgical centre, but was provided as a guide to ordering the queue. It represented for the first time the development of a provincial cardiac surgical database which emphasized the problem of waiting and the impact of urgency on outcome.

In response to the recommendations of the St. Michael's Hospital inquiry, the Ministry of Health assigned Dr. Wilbert Keon, head of cardiovascular surgery with the Ottawa Heart Institute, to lead a provincial working group on cardiovascular services. The mission for the Keon Committee was to develop a plan for a comprehensive provincial cardiac program and in July of 1990 the Provincial Adult Cardiac Care Network (PACCN) was established, later to become the CCN in 1995. Key responsibilities of CCN were divided into five broad areas: (1) coordinate the provision of adult cardiovascular services in Ontario, (2) develop strategies to ensure universal access for all patients and physicians in Ontario, (3) develop and maintain a computerized database, the CCN Registry, of patients, urgency score, waiting time, surgical outcome and other important clinical information, (4) create and support the role of regional coordinators in each of the advanced cardiac care facilities to act as the primary patient contact as well as to monitor the wait list and maintain data, and (5) support access to the registry data for research studies with a view toward improving outcomes for Ontario's cardiac surgical patients.

At its inception CCN included the nine existing "full service" cardiac centres and the four hospitals providing "stand-alone" cardiac catheterization facilities. Currently it includes seventeenmember institutions as the cardiac system has expanded. Much of CCN's initial work was concentrated on cardiac surgery but the database now extends to cardiac catheterization and angioplasty as well, with nearly forty thousand patients registered each year. Future plans for CCN include other cardiac-related procedures such as valve surgery, pacemakers, implantable defibrillators and cardiac rehabilitation.

CCN has received national and international recognition as a model for disease specific system management. It provides a forum for dialogue between front-line clinicians, program managers, administrators, scientists and ministry officials. The link with ICES has allowed epidemiologic evaluation with comparisons to other jurisdictions and the setting of population based minimum target rates for catheterization, angioplasty and cardiac surgery. The collection of this data has enabled ICES to objectively and scientifically evaluate cardiac surgical wait times and outcomes, e.g., in its report entitled "Wait and Rates: the 1997 ICES Report on Coronary Surgery Capacity for Ontario, October 1997." Thus, in 1989 it was estimated that there were nearly 1,800 patients per month awaiting cardiac surgery with approximately six hundred cases being performed monthly. Over the subsequent decade, the number of cases being performed rose to nine hundred per month with 1,200 patients awaiting surgery. The careful data tracking clearly demonstrated rising wait times for bypass surgery by 1996-97 to levels deemed unacceptable by the ministry. In response, the opening of new cardiac surgery centres and expansion of others allowed the median wait time for elective patients to decline from a high of nearly eighty days in 1996, to just under forty days in the year 2000. Currently nearly 80 percent of patients undergo coronary bypass within the recommended maximum waiting times based on the urgency score, and deaths on the waiting list thereby declined from 0.6 percent in 1996 to 0.3 percent in 2000.

Through its partnership with ICES scientists, CCN has contributed significantly to a body of knowledge which relates to cardiac services at a system level. Credibility and accountability to both consumers and government has thus been provided. Annual report cards, institution specific, on the outcomes of cardiac surgery, are made public. Surgeon specific outcomes are made available to the individual hospital for quality improvement initiatives. Comprehensive reports on case volumes, wait times, and wait list mortality are produced monthly and distributed to the key stakeholders as well as being posted on the CCN website for public access.

Given the record of success is the CCN model generalizable? The question is posed in the Tommy Douglas Research Institute publication "Revitalizing Medicare: Shared Problems, Public Solutions" (January 2001): "If the Ontario Cardiac Care Network's approach to the management of waiting lists is so admired world-wide, why is it still only the Ontario Network?" In truth, formal waiting list registries are now present in a number of Canadian jurisdictions and CCN has been contracted to provide a support role for a neighbouring province (Quebec). This is consistent with the position of the Canadian Cardiovascular Society Consensus Conference on Indications for and Access to Revascularization, whereby "a national observational database should monitor: patient selection for revascularization; procedural waiting times and determinants of events in queue; clinical and cost outcomes and changing resource needs resulting from population [changes]."

With the political desire to drive waiting times as low as possible, adult cardiac surgery in Ontario is becoming increasingly decentralized. In the recent past, a number of smaller community hospitals have opened full cardiac services including angioplasty and surgery, as well as the opening of new diagnostic centres, even with stand alone interventional therapy. These newer centres have not always been created with CCN input but rather arose as a response to local patient and cardiologic referral pressures as well as political influences and hospital Board aspirations.

Valvular Surgery—A Canadian Paradigm Shift

By the 1970s valve replacement had become a relatively routine operation and was associated with a reasonable morbidity and mortality. The artificial valve industry was undergoing a robust growth, and various companies were producing several types of both prosthetic tissue and mechanical valves. Despite collagen preservation of both pericardial and porcine tissue valves and new anti-thrombotic and fracture resistant materials for mechanical valves, complications continued. Canadian surgeons played a pivotal role in standardizing the reporting of valve-related complications. This was partly because cardiac surgery in Canada was then exclusively performed in major academic institutions with the infrastructure to collect and maintain data on a large series of patients in a standardized manner. Collaboration between cardiologists, echocardiographers, and cardiac surgeons involved with high-volume caseloads as single institutions allowed for the development of local expertise in the analysis and interpretation of valve-related incidents. Canada has been privileged to achieve such excellence at numerous centres, in particular the Quebec and Montreal Heart institutes and the Toronto General and Vancouver General hospitals.

In Toronto the presence of two world renowned cardiac pathologists, Drs. Avrum Gottlieb and Jagdish Butany was instrumental in documenting mechanisms of failure in both tissue and mechanical valves. Their input into the processes of failure influenced both how surgeons implant valves and how manufacturers design the next generation of valves. Some manufacturers continue to send valves with structural failure to Toronto from all over the world for expert evaluation by Dr. Butany.

Dr. Richard D. Weisel from Toronto General Hospital and chairman of the division of cardiac surgery at the University of Toronto, in close collaboration with Dr. Craig Miller of Stanford University, spearheaded a project to develop careful and comprehensive guidelines on reporting valve-related complications and structural failure. The other Canadian intimately involved was Dr. W. Eric Jamieson from Vancouver who had a long interest and involvement in valve surgery outcomes. The proposed guidelines were published simultaneously in all the major thoracic surgical journals, were adopted worldwide, and constitute the gold standard for reports on outcomes of valve replacement. These precise reporting guidelines finally enabled surgeons to compare outcome results from different institutions with different prostheses in a similar manner.

The contributions of Canadian cardiac surgeons have also influenced valvular surgery worldwide—a remarkable achievement for a nation that currently boasts only 130 active cardiac surgeons. Dr. Tirone David of Toronto General was influenced by the seminal work of Alain Carpentier in Paris regarding mitral valve repair. A combination of intuitive understanding of valvular function, an inquisitive mind, and wonderful manual dexterity enabled David to become a world authority in mitral valve repair surgery. His contributions to the field have been significant and have made Toronto General Hospital almost as important as Broussais Hospital in Paris. David evaluated mitral annuloplasty with fixed versus flexible rings, chordal preservation and/or replacement and aortic valve preservation, the David I and David II aortic root sparing reconstructions. Tirone David developed the subcoronary stentless porcine valve as a result of his inquiry into and understanding of aortic root physiology, pathology, and the influence of stented prostheses. Canadian surgeons were extremely supportive of David and were significantly involved in the FDA submission that allowed for release of the Toronto valve to U.S. surgeons (Halifax, Quebec, Toronto General and Sunnybrook hospitals). In addition, considerable inquiry into patient prosthesis mismatch resulted most notably from the Quebec Heart Institute under the direction of Drs. J. Dumesnil and D. Doyle. At Sunnybrook, under the direction of Drs. George Christakis and Bernard Goldman, clinical studies of valve sizing, stented versus stentless aortic valve replacement and patient prosthesis mismatch, as well as long term follow-up of the Toronto valve subsequently evolved. In Vancouver, Dr. Robert Miyagishima pioneered homograft mitral valve replacement, a procedure that had been done many decades earlier by Dr. R. O. Heimbecker at Toronto General Hospital. Thus, Canadian cardiac surgery has been well-identified with valve repair, replacement and its impact on left ventricular dynamics around the world.

Coronary Artery Bypass Grafting and the Story of the Robot

The Canadian Surgical Technologies and Advanced Robotics (CSTAR) unit was recently established at the London Health Sciences Centre (LHSC) in London, Ontario. This is a premier center for advancing robotic and telesurgical technologies in the field of surgery. It is a world-class center that was made possible through a combination of philanthropic contributions and funding from the Canada Foundation for Innovation, Ontario Innovation Trust, and Ontario Research and Development Challenge Fund. The Richard Ivey Foundation played a major role in the development of the robotic story by providing the funds to the LHSC to purchase the Zeus surgical robotic system. This section details the coming into being of CSTAR and the story behind the first closed-chest beating-heart robotic coronary artery bypass surgery performed in the world, here in Canada on September 24, 1999.

Dr. Douglas M. Boyd, who performed this landmark procedure, was born on the Canadian East Coast. He received his medical degree at the University of Ottawa where he went on to finish his residency in general surgery followed by a Fellowship in cardiac surgery. Being at the Ottawa Heart Institute, he was at the Canadian epicenter for advancing artificial heart and ventricular assist devices. He worked closely with Drs. W. J. Keon, T. Mussivand, and P. J. Hendry (covered elsewhere in this book) where the value of technology in advanced cardiac care was emphasized and actively investigated. In 1996, following his fellowship, he met with Drs. F. N. McKenzie, A. H. Menkis and R. J. Novick at the LHSC. London was already established as a leading cardiac surgery center in Canada. It was here that in 1983, Dr. McKenzie and Heimbecker had begun the first Canadian heart transplant program, and where Dr. G. M. Guiraudon had become a world leader in arrhythmia surgery. Dr. Boyd had at that point expressed his wish to advance minimally invasive cardiac surgery.

These advances have focused on two major areas: limiting the incision through which the operation is performed, and avoiding the heart-lung machine. Canadian surgeons have played an important role in the development of these minimally invasive techniques. For instance, off-pump coronary artery bypass grafting was enthusiastically adopted by several Canadian surgeons. Drs. Raymond Cartier at the Montreal Heart Institute, Yves Leclerc at the St. Michael's Hospital in Toronto and Dr. Gopal Bhatnagar in Mississauga have led the off-pump surge. The group from the Hamilton Health Sciences Centre has recently organized the first national multicentre off-pump bypass surgery registry. The results of data on nearly 1,600 patients were recently reported at the Canadian Cardiovascular Congress by Dr. A. Lamy. Dr. Boyd was at the forefront of minimal access coronary artery bypass surgery in Canada. The operation entails reducing the size of the incision during bypass surgery to allow quicker recovery of the patient. It is interesting to note the results of a recent survey performed by Dr.

Nimesh Desai, one of the residents at the University of Toronto, that documented the extent of off-pump bypass surgery in Canada. He found that we perform significantly fewer off-pump bypass procedures than our American counterparts. The reasons for this difference is presently unknown, but likely the lower cost of off-pump surgery and influences of the manufacturers that build off-pump stabilizers and other required equipment, have had a greater impact on the privately operated American health care system.

The enabling technology that permitted the safe application of surgical robots included video cameras introduced through small incisions and robotic consoles that could translate movements at a distance into scaled down movements in the chest via robotic arms. The AESOP camera is introduced through a keyhole incision into the chest cavity where a single lung would be collapsed. Dr. Boyd initially started using this technology to harvest the internal mammary artery (IMA). With the advanced fiberoptics of the AESOP, it was now possible to visualize the IMA in its entire length through a 0.5 cm incision. I remember scrubbing into the operating room to watch AESOP at work. "AESOP, left" and the camera would move leftward inside the chest. "AESOP, in" and the camera would zoom in. No technology is perfect, and the AESOP would frequently not recognize the commands. "AESOP move freakin' left." The Zeus Robotic Surgical System was developed by Computer Motion Inc. The Zeus platform consists of three table-mounted arms that surround the patient intraoperatively. Two arms act as instrument actuators and the third holds a camera scope. Instruments fulcrum at the chest wall and are capable of many degrees of freedom for surgical tasks: in/out, pitch/yaw, roll, and grip.

On the morning of September 24, 1999, Mr. Joseph Penner of Seaforth, Ontario, a dairy farmer, was taken to the operating room at the University Campus of the LHSC. Dr. Boyd's team was successful in constructing a patent LIMA to left anterior descending artery bypass over the course of the day. Months of practice on pig hearts, in the robotic lab on the eighth floor of the University Campus had been invested to allow such an accomplishment. According to Dr. Boyd, the operation had been divided into nearly fifty major steps. Each step had then been categorized according to the perceived level of difficulty, and over the proceeding year, Dr. Boyd and his team, in addition to their usual clinical, academic and administrative responsibilities, had perfected each step. To make the operation feasible, they had to achieve each step in the shortest time possible. The success of their operation is a tribute to their diligence, and methodical approach to a seemingly insurmountable problem. Mr. Penner was discharged from hospital four days after his operation in good health. A predischarge angiogram showed a perfect IMA to coronary artery anastomosis.

Over the ensuing months, many world-renowned surgeons visited LHSC to observe Dr. Boyd at work behind his robot. I had the privilege to attend one of his procedures. Again, it was a single vessel bypass. Dr. Boyd was sitting about five meters away from the patient who was slightly on his right side, asleep under anaesthesia. His left lung was deflated, and the ventilator was only ventilating his right lung. The arms of the robot entered the patient's body. Dr. Boyd had his microphone on his head, sitting in front of the Zeus console. Dr. Reiza Reyman was at the patient's bedside, making constant adjustments to the robotic arms. On the screen, the left anterior descending (LAD) artery could be seen. It had been cut open by Dr. Boyd. A small intravascular shunt was placed to maintain blood flow across the incision into the distal artery. Dr. Boyd was busy manipulating a very small curved needle with sutures attached to it first through the IMA and then through the LAD. At each step he would have to pause and try various needle angles. His hand motions were being translated by ZEUS into motions of the robotic arm. AESOP was controlling the video camera. It would take a minute or two to complete each bite. To me it seemed extremely tedious, but here was a man pushing the boundaries where no one else had.

In a press release on October 19, 1999, Dr. Boyd stated, "We believe this accomplishment has the potential to revolutionize the delivery of cardiac bypass surgery in this country and beyond. It is our hope that it will become the standard of care for our patients at London Health Sciences Centre and others across North America."

For LHSC, this was a tremendous achievement that had been made possible through the coming together of many individuals at the right time, and in the right place. Tony Dagnone, president and CEO of LHSC, stated: "We are tremendously proud of this team of specialists who have devoted themselves to accomplishing this goal. It is a remarkable, and incredibly significant, achievement . . . . The Ivey's have been tremendous supporters of innovative and progressive medical care, and on behalf of the countless patients who will benefit from this technology and this procedure in the years to come, we sincerely thank them for their caring and generosity . . . . Once again, they have demonstrated unprecedented support to advance Ontario's heart care program."

The robotic team, led by Dr. Boyd** and Dr. A. Menkis*** has gone on to add to their tremendous achievement by bringing robotics to valvular surgery. To date, Dr. Menkis has performed thirty robotic mitral valve procedures using the Zeus Robotic Surgical System. In March 2003, LHSC purchased Intuitive Surgical's da Vinci Surgical System, which routinely permits 3D visualization during robotic cardiac procedures. Furthermore, Dr. Rajni Patel (computer engineering) and other investigators within CSTAR are designing new surgical robots that have the capacity to provide haptic (touch sensation) feedback to the surgeon, thus further enhancing the future potential of surgical robots.

Dr. Douglas Boyd has since left Canada for the Cleveland Clinic in Jacksonville Florida, where he is the head of the minimally invasive surgical unit. Dr. Bob Kiaii, his designated replacement, has joined LHSC's cardiac surgery team after a fellowship in cardiac robotics with Dr. Friedrich Mohr in Leipzig, Germany.

Canada at the Cutting Edge

Other centres across Canada have been active in advancing cardiac surgical technology as well. The following is a quick snap shot of surgical activity across Canada.

In Vancouver, under the direction of Dr. S. Lichtenstein, who at one point practiced out of St. Michael's Hospital in

---

** Doug Boyd was recruited in December 2001 to the Cleveland Clinic Hospitals in Fort Lauderdale, Florida.

*** Dr. Alan Menkis is now Medical Director, Cardiac Services Program, University of Manitoba, appointed August 2004.

Toronto, there is an active program trying to perfect the technology to make suture-less anastamoses a possibility. Such devices would be instrumental in cutting down the operating time in robotic cases. The duration of robotic surgeries remain the Achilles heel of the technology, and such devices would go a long way to bring robots to everyday clinical practice. One such device is comprised of two tiny donut magnets. The device is positioned just inside the coronary artery and at the tip of the bypass conduit. When the two magnets are brought close together, the bypass conduit snaps onto the coronary vessel. The hole in the middle of the donuts would allow passage of blood.

The Ottawa Heart Institute team continues to push forward with their artificial heart program. A recent trial, named the REMATCH trial, showed that patients with end-stage heart failure, too sick for heart transplantation, lived longer with the placement of a left ventricular assist device (VAD). Such devices may become the pacemakers of the future. A small implantable VAD or an artificial heart could potentially add years and quality of life to patients who are debilitated by heart disease.

Montreal remains active in both artificial heart and VAD technology as well as in basic science research. Dr. R. J. Chiu at the McGill University has been successful in implementing a very productive laboratory that investigates alternative nonmechanical solutions to the failing heart. Among their significant contributions, along with our centre, is the advancement in the field of cardiac cell transplantation (see below). The Montreal Heart Institute, whose contributions have been summarized by Dr. C. Grondin, has been at the forefront of tremendous advances in cardiac care.

In Halifax, under the direction of Drs. J. Sullivan and G. Hirsch, a very successful training program has been established. They continue to push forward with research into all-arterial coronary bypass construction to prolong graft patency over the traditional saphenous veins.

At our centre in Toronto, Dr. S. Fremes from Sunnybrook, along with cardiology colleagues, has been able to secure a major Canada Foundation for Innovation grant to build a state-of-the-art real time magnetic resonance imaging system that could potentially allow intracardiac surgery without opening the heart. At the Toronto General Hospital, under the direction of Dr. R. D. Weisel, we have become a leading centre for cardiac surgical basic science research including cell transplantation for heart failure, and beating patches for congenital heart surgery.

The Edmonton team led by Dr. Arvind Koshal, who trained at the Ottawa Heart Institute, has moved to the forefront of cardiac transplantation in Canada. On average they perform fifty heart transplants per year, nearly twice the number as the next centre in Toronto. They have likewise developed a well-funded research program to examine the role of the immune system in allograft (human to human) or xenografts (animal to human) transplant rejection.

Contemporary Cardiac Surgical Basic-Science Research in Canada

The Canadian cardiac surgeons continue to be international leaders in the basic science of cardiac surgery. The purpose of this section is to briefly highlight some of the contemporary achievements of Canadian surgeons in the fields of gene and laser mediated angiogenesis, as well as cell-transplantation.

Complete blockage to blood flow resulting from clot deposition in a coronary artery, which supplies blood to the heart muscle, will cause a heart attack or death of the heart muscle. Traditional methods of dealing with heart attack victims have been to reestablish blood flow through the occluded artery. This may be accomplished with a variety of techniques that include administration of "clot-busting" agents, coronary angioplasty and/or stent placement, or coronary bypass surgery. The concept of angiogenesis, the process of growing new blood vessels, is becoming increasingly relevant to coronary surgery. If we can induce angiogenesis at the same time as restarting blood flow to a region of the heart which was previously not receiving enough blood, we may be able to improve the patient's clinical status above and beyond what could be accomplished with bypassing that territory alone. We have known for a very long time that injured tissue is able to repair itself by generation of what we call granulation tissue. Granulation tissue is a highly vascular tissue that enables healing. The new blood vessels that are formed there are an example of angiogenesis. Tumors are able to grow because they can induce angiogenesis. Over the past two decades we have seen an exponential growth in our knowledge of molecular and genetic factors that allow and promote angiogenesis. It became clear that inflammatory cells recruited into damaged tissue express growth factors that initiate angiogenesis. Some of these factors are the Vascular Endothelial Growth Factor (VEGF) and Fibroblast Growth Factor (FGF). The obvious question is then whether clinicians can induce angiogenesis by increasing local tissue levels of some of these growth factors. Certainly as the concept of gene-therapy became better understood, such advances have become clinical reality. It is a burgeoning field that is growing very rapidly.

Canadian scientists, cardiologists, and cardiac surgeons have become active and leading members in the field of therapeutic angiogenesis. Notable among these physicians are the members of the Terrence Donnelly Heart Centre at St. Michael's Hospital in Toronto. Dr. Duncan J. Stewart, a cardiologist, has been the major Canadian figure in this experimental field and his laboratory has made major contributions. In fact, in collaboration with the cardiac surgeons at St. Michael's Hospital, Dr. Stewart has helped organize a clinical trial assessing the effect of EGT therapy at the time of coronary artery bypass surgery. The VEGF gene was directly injected into the portion of the heart muscle in which blood flow was severely restricted and which was not amenable to other revascularization procedures. The initial results suggest that this method of delivery is safe. There were an inadequate number of patients in the trial to allow conclusions to be drawn regarding the clinical efficacy of this procedure. However, this sort of safety trial allows the planning of major trials to test the clinical applicability of gene-induced angiogenesis.

In the mid-1990s, it became apparent to investigators that by inducing minimal and controlled damage to the heart muscle, just as in other injured tissue, a certain degree of angiogenesis could be produced. In particular, the investigators had turned to poking tiny holes in the heart muscle using Laser technology. In fact, the original data remains convincing that a certain amount of angiogenesis occurred. Later clinical trials documented that the patients who had undergone the procedure were more likely to be asymptomatic. Although the benefit of Transmyocardial Laser Revascularization (TMLR) remains unproven, Canadians have played a part in its history. Apart from participating in the clinical trials of TMLR, such as in Halifax's Queen Elizabeth II Hospital,

two young surgical residents have made significant
contributions to the field.

The angina relief offered to coronary artery disease
patients by TMLR is significant. This relief may constitute
a placebo response, a well-known phenomenon in which
an intervention may cause—independent of its clinical
effect—symptomatic relief, perhaps because of the
patient's psychological expectation to feel improvement;
or a true clinical effect. In the latter case, the TMLR
either induces enough angiogenesis and increased
blood-flow to eliminate the stimulus for angina pain, or
causes the cardiac nerves not to feel pain (denervation).
Through a series of detailed experimental work, which
has been subsequently presented at the American Heart
Association meeting and published in the *Journal of
Thoracic and Cardiovascular Surgery,* Dr. Rakesh Arora has
shown that the nervous input to and output from the heart
are intact after TMLR. This work was conducted in the
laboratory of Dr. J. Armour in Halifax, Nova Scotia. The
results from this body of work suggest that TMLR either
induces a placebo response, or that it actually works. Dr.
Marc P. Pelletier, who was a staff cardiovascular surgeon
at Sunnybrook and Women's College Hospital[****], is the
other Canadian who has contributed to this story. While
a surgical resident at the McGill University, he joined the
famous laboratory of Dr. R. Chiu, then chief of cardiac
surgery at McGill. Together they questioned whether a
laser was required to induce the controlled damage or
whether it couldbe replaced. In the work that won him

[****] Pelletier accepted a position at Stanford University and
left Sunnybrook in early 2004. He subsequently returned
to Canada as Head, Cardiac Surgery, New Brunswick Heart
Centre, Saint John, N.B.—Ed.

the American Association of Thoracic Surgeons' Resident Award in 1998, Pelletier showed that making holes using a simple needle can be equally effective. Indeed, three needle holes appeared to induce the same degree of angiogenesis as one laser hole. This observation obviates the need for very expensive laser technology and is an example of how clear thinking can avoid the clutter that can, at times, be created by advanced laboratory science.

Organ transplantation has now become routine. When a heart fails, there is the possibility of transplanting the heart of another human being who has died of other causes into the patient. Transplantation is an old concept, but it did not meet clinical reality until the mid-1960s, and did not gain popular acceptance until the early 1980s with the advent of cyclosporin, a potent immunosuppressant. Cellular transplantation is the new frontier that has resulted in talk of organ regeneration as opposed to organ replacement. This is an exciting field of research. In international meetings such as the Scientific Sessions of the American Heart Institution an increasing number of sessions are dedicated to the field of cell transplantation and cardiac regeneration. Two major academic centres in Canada, namely the University of Toronto and McGill University, have been involved and are true pioneers in this field. The underlying concept for cellular transplantation is that all organs come from one cell, and hence are all different manifestations of the same cellular programming. In a simplified manner, the liver has connective tissue in the same way that the brain or heart or skin does; blood vessels exist in the lungs and the great toe. There exists, therefore, the theoretical possibility of regenerating organs by transplanting cells into dead tissue. Of course, transplanted skin cells will not form heart tissue, but transplanted muscle cells can, theoretically, be programmed to beat in synchrony with cardiac muscle. Indeed, evidence has come from both Toronto and Montreal that cellular transplantation helps to stop the progression of heart failure in a variety of models. The cells that have been shown to work include fetal heart cells, skeletal myoblasts (muscle stem cells), smooth muscle cells, and bone marrow stem or progenitor cells.

It is interesting to note that cell transplantation appears to work even when the procedure does not repopulate the dead heart muscle with a significant number of beating cells. This observation is puzzling and is the source of active research. The transplanted cells also induce a significant amount of angiogenesis and prevent the destruction of the extra cellular scaffolding that holds the heart muscle cells together. The later hypothesis is currently being investigated by Dr. Paul Fedak under the supervision of Drs. R. Weisel and R. K. Li. Another possibility in cell transplantation is to transplant genetically modified super-cells, which can then be guided to perform certain functions. For instance, transplanted cells could express vascular growth factors in order to induce a greater degree of angiogenesis as proven by Dr. Terrence Yau of the University of Toronto.

The last frontier of cell transplantation that is beginning to be studied in the Weisel/Li lab is the possibility that cell transplantation and healthy cell engraftment may potentiate endogenous repair mechanisms that are initially overwhelmed by massive myocyte death. Cardiac stem cells or stem cells from bone marrow may be recruited to the transplanted area and may be responsible for differentiating into new cardiomyocytes. It has previously been held that generation of new heart muscle cells is not possible because mature cardiomyocytes have exited the cell cycle permanently. Increasing evidence, however, is accumulating that suggests a subset of bone marrow stem cells and cardiac-resident stem cells is capable of giving rise to new cardiomyocytes. If such is the case, regeneration of cardiac tissue should be possible.

Conclusion

This chapter has highlighted the clinical, basic science, and administrative accomplishments of the current generation Canadian cardiac surgeons. The magnitude of these accomplishments is particularly impressive when one considers the number of surgeons that actively practice in Canada today as around 130. We have been world leaders in surgical innovation, data analysis and standardized reporting of outcomes, surgical training, and laboratory research. The landscape of cardiac surgery is rapidly evolving as interventional cardiology increasingly assumes the care of routine coronary artery disease patients. The pediatric centralization and adult decentralization developments directly impact on the training of young cardiac surgeons. As the Canadian population ages and the prevalence of heart disease climbs, ensuring access to cardiac surgical expertise may become an important issue in the near future.

CHAPTER 14

TRAINING PROGRAMS IN CARDIAC SURGERY

Gilbert Tang, David Latter, and Richard Weisel

Canadian Surgical Training before 1950

The history of cardiovascular and thoracic surgery training in Canada presents an interesting, albeit complex picture of how cardiac surgical programs evolved into their current state. Traditionally, surgical training is similar to apprenticeship in other skilled professions, where senior surgeons would serve as mentors to junior trainees. Through years of close supervision, the surgical resident would develop the knowledge, technical ability, surgical intuition and clinical experience necessary for independent practice. As early as 1931, Professor William Gallie, chairman of the department of surgery at the University of Toronto from 1929 to 1947, perceived the need and developed a systematic course to train surgical residents in the basic science and surgery necessary for their certification examination. The "Gallie Course" was the first of its kind in Canada and was ahead of those in England and United States. Training was three years in duration, beginning with the initial year in medicine and pathology, followed by a year in general surgery and six months each in two of the three specialties: neurosurgery, urology or pediatric surgery. Residents rotated among the Toronto General Hospital, Toronto Western Hospital and St. Michael's Hospital. During the early part of the twentieth century, cardiovascular surgery was in its infancy. Thoracic surgery emerged as a primary treatment modality for bronchogenic carcinoma and pulmonary tuberculosis. In light of the growing demand for thoracic surgeons, training programs developed in Canada and the specialty of thoracic surgery became certified by the Royal College of Physicians and Surgeons of Canada (RCPSC) in 1946. By the 1940s, surgical training in Canada followed a five-year model, with the first year being a general internship. Afterwards, thoracic surgery, plastic surgery, neurosurgery, general surgery, urology, orthopedics, and obstetrics and gynecology required four additional years of residency training. Residents who completed training in general surgery could spend two to three additional years to obtain certification in thoracic surgery. Cardiovascular procedures were limited in scope at that time and formal cardiac surgery training did not exist.

Birth and Early Development of the Canadian Cardiac Surgery Residency Program

Following development of the heart-lung machine and systemic hypothermia in 1953, cardiac operations became a reality. In 1958, Dr. Bigelow of the University of Toronto created the first university program in Canada to train cardiovascular surgeons. Limited expertise in this specialty meant that cardiovascular operations were performed at selected locations across Canada. Academic hospitals provided the experience necessary for trainees to develop their career as cardiovascular surgeons. Dr. Bigelow's program aimed at providing its residents with a strong foundation in research and clinical training. Subsequent training programs would follow a similar goal of preparing residents for academic practice.

With the increasing volume of cardiovascular operations and need to train cardiovascular surgeons, the Royal College of Physicians and Surgeons implemented a combined fellowship program in cardiovascular and thoracic (CVT) surgery in 1961. Thoracic surgery certification was subsequently discontinued in 1964. The Royal College Committee in Thoracic Surgery initially requested the direct-entry CVT program to be six years in length, including one year of laboratory training to acquire knowledge of cardiovascular hemodynamics and extracorporeal circulation. However, that training model was not approved by the Royal College Credentials Committee and instead a five-year clinical program was implemented. General surgeons who wanted to pursue CVT surgery could also spend two to three additional years to obtain certification. By that time, a number of centres in Canada had an active cardiovascular surgery program: Vancouver, Edmonton, Calgary, Saskatoon, Winnipeg, Sudbury, London, Ottawa, Kingston, Toronto, Montreal (McGill, Laval), Halifax, and St. John's.

Although surgical residents were able to pursue a career in CVT surgery via either pathway, most of them chose to complete general surgery before continuing CVT training. Dr. William G. Williams, recent chief of cardiovascular surgery at the Hospital of Sick Children and past chairman of cardiovascular surgery at the University of Toronto from 1992 to 1997, was one of the few who completed the five-year CVT program during the 1960s and 1970s, as did Dr. Bernard Goldman, previously chief of surgery at the Sunnybrook Hospital and head of its cardiovascular surgery division. According to them, cardiac surgery was still an emerging specialty at the time and most surgical residents wanted the option of being able to practice general surgery if they could not sustain a CVT surgical practice full-time. Having completed general surgery training also offered CVT residents the flexibility of taking the American Board of Thoracic Surgery examination. Residents' preference towards the general-CVT surgery pathway prompted most institutions to have their residents follow the seven to eight-year training model before becoming certified as CVT surgeons. Residents interested in CVT surgery could rotate in those services earlier as junior residents and the duration of CVT training following general surgery depended on the number of prior CVT rotations completed.

Specialization of Cardiac, Vascular and Thoracic Surgery Training: 1966-1992

During the late 1960s, the volume and complexity of cardiac and thoracic surgery procedures exploded and the two specialties became increasingly divergent. It became apparent that a resident would need to subspecialize in cardiovascular or thoracic surgery in order to master either subject. Through the leadership of Dr. F. Griffith Pearson, the thoracic surgery service and its training became separate from cardiovascular surgery at the University of Toronto in 1966. In centres without a dedicated cardiovascular-thoracic surgical unit, a significant number of general surgeons also practice thoracic surgery. However, those general surgeons did not have specialty recognition in thoracic surgery. To provide quality assurance in thoracic surgery training, the Royal College of Physicians and Surgeons in 1976 devised two pathways whereby thoracic surgery could be certified. One was the five-year program in CVT surgery, with at least six months of training in thoracic surgery. The other was based on prior certification in general surgery and two years of further training, of which eighteen months would be in thoracic surgery. A Certificate of Special Competence in Thoracic Surgery could then be issued.

Rapid advances in research and technology in cardiac surgery afforded increasingly complex and specialized procedures. Cardiac surgeons gradually performed fewer vascular operations and residents in CVT programs were thus getting limited operative experience in vascular surgery, not sufficient for independent practice. Vascular surgery in our institution was primarily under the supervision of Drs. Ronald Baird, Donald Wilson, and James Key. In light of further specialization in cardiac surgery, in 1980, vascular surgery became an independent subspecialty for Certification of Special Competence by the Royal College of Physicians and Surgeons. In 1992, the specialty of CVT surgery was renamed cardiothoracic surgery. For residents specializing in thoracic surgery, the two-year Royal College Certification of Special Competence remained.

Emergence of the Current Direct-Entry Six-Year Cardiac Surgery Program: The 1990s

With evolving changes in clinical practice, cardiac, thoracic and vascular surgery gradually became separated and offered individual training programs. Elimination of the one-year general internship and its subsequent licensure for independent practice occurred in the late 1980s. Shortly afterwards, general surgery training was extended to five years. A prerequisite of general surgery training was necessary for entrance into a two-to-three-year cardiothoracic surgery residency program. This requirement meant a minimum of seven years was needed to acquire eligibility for certification in cardiothoracic surgery.

The long time it would take to train a cardiac surgeon inadvertently became a significant deterrent for medical students interested in a career in that specialty. With surgical residency training being long, intense and demanding, the number of applicants to general surgery residency programs also declined. The more lucrative remuneration in the United States attracted a number of general surgery graduates to move south of the border for cardiothoracic training. All of these factors had a direct negative impact on recruiting top-quality cardiac surgery residents in Canada, and drove the idea of streamlining cardiac surgery training in our country.

In 1994, the Royal College of Physicians and Surgeons with the support of the Canadian Society of Cardiovascular and Thoracic Surgeons reviewed the training requirements for cardiac and thoracic surgery across the country. Cardiothoracic surgery was renamed as cardiac surgery and cardiac and thoracic surgery residency training respectively became separate primary specialties with certification. The direct-entry cardiac surgery program began in July 1995, with Edmonton, Winnipeg, Montreal (McGill) and Toronto as the initial four cardiac surgery training centres. For example, at the University of Toronto, the six-year program is currently outlined as follows:

Postgraduate Year (PGY) One

- One month emergency medicine
- One month internal medicine
- One month cardiology consults
- One month pathology
- One month perfusion and percutaneous coronary intervention (PCI)
- Three months general surgery
- Four months cardiac surgery

PGY Two

- Two months medical-surgical intensive care unit (MSICU)
- One month cardiovascular intensive care unit (CVICU)
- Two months cardiology (one month coronary care unit [CCU] and one month heart failure/transplant)
- One month echocardiography
- One month pacemaker/defibrillator/electrophysiology
- Two months vascular surgery
- Three months thoracic surgery
- Optional: One month congenital cardiac surgery (in lieu of one month in thoracic surgery)

PGY Three to Six

- Six months as assistant resident in cardiac surgery
- Twelve months total as senior resident in general surgery, thoracic and/or vascular surgery
- Six months as senior resident in congenital cardiac surgery
- Twelve months as senior resident in adult cardiac surgery

The first two residency years are termed core surgery training by the Royal College of Physicians and Surgeons. The program was introduced in 1992 in an attempt to standardize the first two residency years in all surgical specialties. However, surgeons from different specialties could not agree on a common set of rotations for all residents. In reality, each surgical specialty has its own curriculum in the first two years of residency. To satisfy requirements of the core surgery program, residents in all surgical specialties are required to pass the Principles of Surgery examination, before becoming eligible for the final Royal College of Physicians and Surgeons certification examination.

The PGY Three or Four is generally designated as the academic enrichment year. It allows residents to further scientific knowledge and/or clinical skills necessary to develop an up-to-date clinical practice in the future. Residents may use that year to pursue specific areas of their clinical interest or in research. At the University of Toronto, most residents take additional time to complete a master's or doctoral degree in preparation for a career in academic cardiac surgery.

Canadian Cardiac Surgery Training: The Current State

There are currently three pathways by which cardiac surgery certification can be obtained in Canada

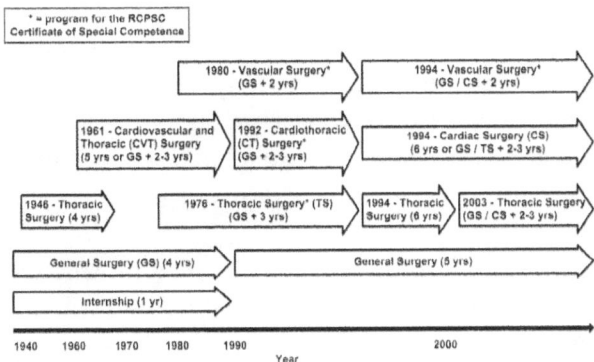

Fig. 14:1 Pathways for certification in cardiac surgery in Canada.

The shortened and more focused direct-entry six-year program allows graduating medical students to complete their cardiac surgery training in a reasonable amount of time. Alternatively, residents having completed general surgery or thoracic surgery training may spend an additional two to three years to pursue cardiac surgery training. Cardiac surgery residents in the six-year program are also eligible for thoracic or vascular surgery certification following an additional eighteen months of training.

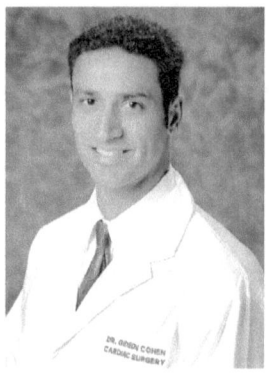

Fig. 14:2 Dr. Gideon Cohen, cardiac surgeon,
Sunnybrook Health Science Centre

Dr. Gideon Cohen, a University of Toronto cardiac surgery program graduate and currently staff surgeon at the Sunnybrook and Women's College Health Science Centre, offered his perspective of the transition from general surgery to the direct-entry cardiac surgery program:

> *My particular experience [in cardiac surgery training] was somewhat unique in that the transition to a direct-entry program occurred during my residency in general surgery, which, at the time, was a prerequisite for cardiac surgical training. Although I was given the option of completing*

general surgery, I chose to forgo such additional training and enter the direct cardiac program at the PGY-5 level. . . . Unfortunately, my training did not allow for other valuable rotations currently available to direct entry candidates, including cardiology, coronary care unit, interventional cardiology, and echocardiography. Having been involved in the teaching of direct-entry residents, I can certainly see the benefits of such comprehensive training. Current residents seem somewhat more mature from a clinical perspective and exhibit an excellent grasp of cardiac physiology, anatomy and pathology, the extent of which seems to exceed that displayed by previous trainees . . . . Having experienced both the old and new training formats, I would certainly recommend the direct-entry program, as I feel that it is extremely advantageous to expose cardiac trainees to cardiac surgical principles as early in their training as possible. Nonetheless, the importance of mandatory general surgical training within the new program cannot be over-emphasized. To develop good cardiac surgeons, we must first ensure that we develop good surgeons.

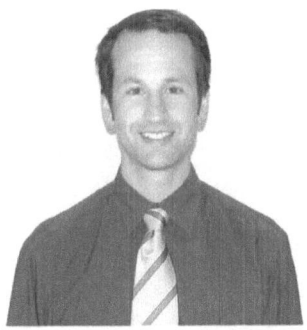

Fig. 14:3 Dr. Michael Borger, cardiac surgeon, Toronto General Hospital

Dr. Michael Borger, another University of Toronto program graduate and now staff surgeon at the Toronto General Hospital, echoed Dr. Cohen's experience:

> *Residents started this new training program in 1995, entering directly from medical school. In addition, several residents transferred from general surgery programs into the new program at a third-year level, in order to facilitate the transition. We were all apprehensive at first, since it was an entirely new program. In addition, the staff cardiac surgeons had to adjust to the nuances of working with residents that are in the very early stages of training. A new set of clear objectives had to be defined, with realistic expectations on the part of both residents and surgeons. Once the initial difficulties were overcome, the program became extremely successful. Residents were happy because they no longer had to spend several years learning general surgery procedures that they would never again perform, and cardiac surgeons were happy because they had a much stronger influence on the early development of their residents. The program has become so successful that there is now significant interest in the United States to adopt a similar curriculum.*

Since 1995, the new direct cardiac surgery training program exists at Dalhousie University, McGill University, McMaster University, University of Alberta, University of British Columbia, University of Manitoba, University of Montreal, University of Ottawa, University of Toronto, and University of Western Ontario.

Table 15A. Summary of cardiovascular and thoracic (CVT), cardiothoracic (CT) and cardiac surgery training programs in Canadian institutions

Institution	History of the Training Program
Dalhousie University	1976 - 1989, 1994 - present
McGill University	1965 - present
McMaster University	1988? - 1992, 1999 - present
Queen's University	Not available
University of Alberta	1960 - present
University of British Columbia	1960s - present
University of Manitoba	1967 - present
University of Montreal	1967 - present
University of Ottawa	1976 - present
University of Saskatchewan	Not available
University of Toronto	1958 - present
University of Western Ontario	1960s - present

Fig. 14:4 Summary of cardiovascular and thoracic (CVT), cardiothoracic (CT) and cardiac surgery training programs in Canadian institutions.

Cardiac surgery residents training in the province of Québec are eligible for both Royal College certification and certification by the Collège des Médecins du Québec. During the 1980s, most Québec trainees took two separate sets of exams to be certified by both colleges, in order to practice anywhere in Canada or in Québec. However, they could still practice in Québec if only certified by the Collège des Médecins du Québec. In 1996, the Collège des Médecins du Québec harmonized the written examination with the Royal College and most recently in 2003 the oral examinations were also harmonized. Québec cardiac surgery residents may now obtain certifications by both colleges with only the Royal College written and oral examinations.

Evolving Changes to Cardiac Surgery Training in Canada

Although the six-year training program in cardiac surgery offers significant advantages, it has limitations. With only a handful of direct-entry residency positions per year, an early interest and commitment to cardiac surgery is often necessary to be competitive in obtaining a training position. Exposure to cardiac surgery is often limited in the first two years of medical school. Only a few students would become interested in the specialty early in their education and fewer would intend to pursue it as a future career. This may have an effect on recruitment of student candidates training to become cardiac surgeons in Canada.

Recent centralization of cardiac surgical services and the evolving clinical practice also pose a challenge to training future cardiac surgeons. Increasing complexity of congenital heart surgery and a limited surgical volume mean only a few institutions in Canada have an active congenital program: University of British Columbia, University of Alberta, University of Toronto, University of Ottawa, McGill University, University of Montreal and Dalhousie University. Several university centres recently formed inter-institutional agreements for residents to obtain their pediatric cardiac surgery training at the selected sites, so as to fulfill the Royal College requirement. This streamlining process means only a limited number of residents may be trained at the above centres at any given time, in order to provide residents with a sufficient clinical experience. The advent of new percutaneous interventional procedures, decline in straightforward operations, centralization of training institutions, decreasing surgical volume at academic centres and increasing volume at suburban nonacademic centres may offer a less ideal training environment for current and future cardiac surgery residents.

Portability of Canadian Cardiac Surgery Training to the United States: problems and lessons learned

For graduating Canadian trainees in cardiac surgery interested in career opportunities in the United States, completing the training requirements of the RCPSC cardiac surgery program does not confer graduate eligibility for certification by the American Board of Thoracic Surgery (ABTS). Until the early 1990s, Canadian residents completing the RCPSC cardiothoracic surgery program were eligible for ABTS certification. During that time, CT surgery residents in Canada were funded from a number of sources, including provincial governments, universities, foreign countries (via governments or academic institutions), and occasionally even by the residents themselves. However, in the United States an accredited CT residency position meant the funding had to come from a hospital or academic institution. This difference in funding requirements might have led to a difference in the range of calibre among CT residents. Institutional evaluation of trainees in Canadian CT surgery programs was not as vigorous as the current standard. A number of borderline candidates who were deemed competent by the training institutions were able to pass both RCPSC and ABTS examinations and obtained certifications. However, after these few surgeons commenced practice in the United States, they led to a multitude of problems that caught the attention of the ABTS and the Accreditation Council for Graduate Medical Education (ACGME) in the United States. This situation prompted a formal review of non-American training programs and their eligibility for ABTS certification. The Residency Review Committee for Thoracic Surgery (RRC-TS), part of the ACGME, was responsible for overseeing and accrediting all cardiothoracic surgery residency programs in the United States. Since the RCPSC cardiothoracic surgery programs had not been accredited by the ACGME, the RRC-TS could not review and recognize Canadian residency training as equivalent to American cardiothoracic surgery training. The disarray of funding sources in Canadian CT surgery programs compounded the difficulty of RRC-TS to properly assess Canadian CT residency programs and their trainees. Because RRC-TS was not able to accredit Canadian programs, the ABTS was no longer able to grant certification to cardiac surgeons having completed the RCPSC training. However, American CT residents remain eligible for RCPSC certification in cardiac and/ or thoracic surgery provided that they have met all the RCPSC training requirements.

The consequence of the decision by the ABTS not to recognize the RCPSC training was significant. According to Dr. Tomas Salerno, chairman of the cardiovascular surgery division at the University of Toronto 1987-1992, prior to early the 1990s, Canadian CT programs had attracted a large number of American trainees. The excellent quality of training, large volume and diversity of clinical material and pleasant living conditions made Canada an attractive alternative to the United States to obtain CT training and subsequent RCPSC and ABTS certifications. Indeed, a number of Canadian-trained American thoracic surgeons have become very successful and currently hold important positions at various American academic institutions and in national and international cardiothoracic societies. The Canadian contribution to training outstanding American cardiac and thoracic surgeons was significant. Furthermore, the American trainees brought to Canada the benefits of their home institutions' philosophy and surgical techniques. Following termination of ABTS certification of RCPSC-trained residents, along with the emergence of direct-entry cardiac and thoracic surgery residency programs in Canada, the attraction for high-quality American candidates to Canadian programs diminished. On the other hand, with limited job opportunities in Canada, Canadian RCPSC graduates who wanted to pursue their career in the United States faced the difficulty of not having ABTS certification. This loss of reciprocity in training recognition made both Canadian and American cardiothoracic residents lose out on getting the best training and career opportunities.

Up until July 2003, only residents in an accredited cardiothoracic surgery program in the United States, with prior American Board of Surgery (ABS) or RCPSC general surgery certification, were eligible for ABTS certification. However, with a steady decline in applications to general surgery and cardiothoracic surgery positions in the United States, American cardiothoracic surgeons are reviewing and considering changing the training requirements to attract better candidates. Beginning in July 2003, ABS certification became optional for ABTS certification, although completion of an approved five-year general surgery residency remained a prerequisite. Alternative training models, such as a six-year direct-entry cardiothoracic surgery program, or a program involving three to four years of general surgery then three years of cardiothoracic surgery, are currently under discussion in the United States. Future policy developments in training programs, accreditation and certification requirements may give Canadian graduates of the RCPSC program eligibility for ABTS certification. Alternatively, the RCPSC certification may in the future be recognized as equivalent to the ABTS certification.

Evolving Cardiac Surgical Practice: Training Nonacademic Cardiac Surgeons

Although coronary artery bypass graft surgery remains the most commonly performed cardiac operation, other cardiac surgical procedures continue to increase in diversity and complexity. Examples include heart failure and transplantation, reoperative surgery, aortic root or complex valvular reconstruction, robotic surgery and congenital heart surgery. Currently, a majority of Canadian cardiac surgeons practice at academic centres. Cardiac surgery graduates intending a career in academia often pursue clinical fellowship training to subspecialize and contribute their expertise to their institution.

Recently, cardiac surgery at the community level has been expanding to match government mandates in raising the volume of cardiac surgical care in various provinces. Cardiac surgery training programs remain at university institutions. Although current residents tend to pursue academic careers, it is conceivable that as the volume of community cardiac surgery increases, residents may want to take up practice at nonacademic hospitals. They may have different training objectives from residents preparing for an academic practice. Efforts will need to be made by training programs to offer the best opportunities for residents planning to become either academic or community cardiac surgeons.

Conclusion

Since the birth of a formal cardiovascular and thoracic surgery residency program in 1961, cardiac surgery has evolved to become a primary specialty with a structured curriculum designed to prepare its residents for a career in academic surgery. The current six-year cardiac surgery program allows residents to explore all aspects of the specialty with the flexibility to pursue in depth areas of clinical and research interests. With changes and advances in the specialty, versatility in cardiac surgery training programs will offer residents a multitude of experiences to conduct different types of surgical practice.

References

Dr. Jaroslaw Barwinsky, personal communication, 2004.

Dr. Irene Cybulsky, personal communication, 2003.

Dr. Anthony Dobell, personal communication, 2003.

Dr. Bernard Goldman, personal communication, 2003.

Dr. Wilbert Keon, personal communication, 2003.

Dr. Neil McKenzie, personal communication, 2003.

Dr. David Murphy, personal communication, 2003.

Dr. Conrad Pelletier, personal communication, 2003.

Dr. Zlatko Pozeg, personal communication, 2003.

Dr. David Ross, personal communication, 2003.

Dr. Tomas Salerno, personal communication, 2003.

Dr. Hugh Scully, personal communication, 2003.

Mr. Michael Thibault, personal communication, 2003.

Dr. William G. Williams, personal communication, 2003.

Royal College of Physicians and Surgeons of Canada. Minutes of Special Committee in Cardiovascular and Thoracic Surgery, 1961, 1976-1978, 1988, 1991, 1994, 1995.

CHAPTER 15

WOMEN IN CARDIAC SURGERY IN CANADA

Terry Kieser

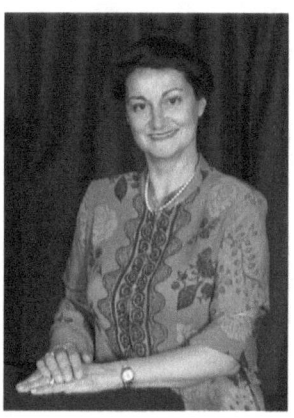

Fig. 15:1 Terry Kieser

I am not sure why there are so few women in heart surgery; it may be the long training required, the difficulty of balancing an intensely responsible profession with the demands of child bearing, or discouragement stemming from societal ideas of careers for women. Whatever the reason, women cardiac surgeons at present number thirteen in Canada out of three hundred men, representing 4.3 percent. What do our male colleagues think of women in their BL (Before Lynda) all-boys club? Times have certainly changed. Nowadays with women reporters interviewing male players in their dressing rooms, and women goalies on NHL teams, women have definitely been branching out. I'm sure that as a group, we can be pretty painful at times—"super women," "male want-to-bes," trying to do it all and never letting any of our male colleagues forget it. In short—men have to tolerate *us*. One sound piece of advice was given by Dr. Lynda Mickleborough, the first woman heart surgeon in Canada: "Don't complain"—nobody likes a whiner. In a world where our male colleagues have grown up being taught that men are the stronger sex and their job is to protect the frail female, it must be quite disconcerting to find out: (1) that they may not need this protection and (2) are interested in same line of work! As difficult as it is for women to climb to the top in this profession, it is just as difficult for men to see us climb. In an ideal world, gender should never be an issue; but we are not in heaven yet, so gender differences and differences in outlook exist. I'd like to think that the perfect human, whether male or female, has just the right amount of assertiveness logic, selflessness and caring.

As any member of a minority group will tell you, whatever one does stand out; that is the very good are very, very good, and the not so good can be thought of as quite bad! Living in a glass house is never easy and carries with it a responsibility for future individuals interested in similar transparent dwellings. This is where Canada has indeed been very fortunate in our first woman heart surgeon, Dr. Lynda Mickleborough.

LYNDA MICKLEBOROUGH

Dr. Mickleborough spent a total of seventeen years after high school, training for her career: four years for a B.Sc. honours in genetics at McGill University, four years in medical school at McGill, one year as a straight surgical intern at the Royal Victoria Hospital in Montreal, and five years in general surgery at McGill, including a research year and two years of cardiovascular and thoracic surgery training at (you guessed it!) McGill under Dr. Tony Dobell (You could say she was definitely a "McGill" girl!). Dr. Mickleborough spent her seventeenth year in training as a cardiac surgical fellow at Toronto General Hospital under Dr. Ronald Baird. So impressive was her surgical meticulousness, dedicated care and feisty "I may be blonde but definitely not dumb" personality, Dr. Mickleborough landed the plum job of staff cardiac surgeon and assistant professor U of T at the Toronto General Hospital in 1981. She is definitely a person that inspires stability of location. After spending sixteen consecutive years training in Montreal, she stayed in Toronto for the next twenty-two years, carving out an illustrious career in cardiac surgery, and leaving a bench mark for all women (and men) interested in this profession.

Always having been interested in research, this bent was recognized very early by her being given the coveted Young Investigators Award of the Cardiovascular Society for "Significance of the Q Wave which Follows the Perfusion of the Ischemic Myocardium" in 1976, only half way through her General Surgical residency. In the next twenty-two years this incredibly productive career would yield fourteen grants totaling $1,566,384 (not including the $16 million grant for the STICH Trial of which Lynda was principle investigator for Canada until her retirement in 2002), eighty-nine peer-reviewed manuscripts, and 115 abstracts/presentations. She has been an invited speaker to fourteen Canadian cities, eighteen centers in the Unites States and multiple times to Italy, Monte Carlo and Japan. She also found time (I don't know where!) to be a member or chair of sixteen local committees in Toronto and arrange cardiovascular teaching for medical and postgraduate students for nine of her twenty-two-year career. In keeping with her international reputation and dedication to the improvement and furtherance of cardiovascular medicine, she has reviewed grants, journals, and abstracts for Canadian, American and European societies, has been a board member of the Heart and Stroke Foundation of Ontario, was on the Editorial Board of the *Journal of Thoracic and CV Surgery* for seven years, and currently holds a position on the editorial board of the *Annals of Thoracic Surgery*. At the top levels of international endeavors, she was on the Council on Cardiovascular Surgery for the American Heart Association, and still is on the editorial board of the *Annals of Thoracic Surgery*, a member of the ethics committee for the American Association of Thoracic Surgery and the NIH study section for surgery and bioengineering, although she retired clinically as of December 2002.

I remember Lynda fondly from my days as a junior resident in general surgery at Toronto General Hospital in 1983. I was always a little intimidated by her—she seemed so confident and not influenced by what other people thought. There was a little envy too—she was where I wanted to be. The thing I most wanted to emulate was her "no nonsense—take no prisoners" attitude. It takes time and courage to develop this attribute but it always serves one well. Lynda, whether she knew it or not, blazed a trail that inspired us all. I don't know if she realized the heavy responsibility she had at the beginning of her career for future women in heart surgery, but ignorance was probably bliss. As is said by Charles Shultz in one of my favorite Peanuts cartoons: (Linus is looking towards the heavens with his blanket in tow) "There is no heavier burden than a great potential!"

How did this wonderful productive career start? How did she pick cardiac surgery for her life's work? Actually it seems to have picked her. Lynda was a new surgical intern, fresh out of medical school, working on a postoperative cardiac surgical ward when she was faced with a tamponading postoperative cardiac surgical patient. Not having had the requisite experience to accurately diagnose the problem, her in-born medical instinct told her something was terribly wrong. Transcending all the usual hierarchy of intern to resident to fellow to senior staff, she knew time was of the essence and went right to the top—Dr. Tony Dobell. Her insistent forthrightness immediately got his attention and the patient was saved. Looking back on this formative experience, the aspect that impressed Lynda most was that Dr. Dobell actually listened to her: "He was a really good guy." Actually, this only attests to Lynda's innate humility: when you're good, honest and caring—you get people's attention. Mentors for Lynda? Dr. Lloyd MacLean, chief of surgery at McGill, Dr. Tony Dobell, who never made her feel any different from her male colleagues and Dr. Ronald Baird, who hired her as the first woman heart surgeon in Canada.

When I asked Lynda what she most wanted to be remembered for as a heart surgeon, again because of her selflessness, she could not answer. Actually her inspiring career is her answer. Only one can be first, after Lynda the rest can only follow. Thank you Lynda, for giving all women who follow, an example that will be forever remarked on as "see it can be done, and done well."

LYNDA MICKLEBOROUGH—A TRIBUTE*

Anthony R. C. Dobell

This is a brief introduction to Lynda Mickleborough who made her reputation through her formidable achievements in twenty-two years at the University of Toronto; but I want to tell you first of her fifteen years in Montreal at McGill.

She came from the Prairies, attending primary school in rural Saskatchewan and high school in Regina, and was accepted into McGill with two prestigious scholarships. She enrolled in the B.Sc. program in 1965 before her eighteenth birthday and graduated with honours in genetics four years later having added two other scholarships along the way.

Thus in 1969 she entered the medical faculty and graduated four years later with the highest academic standing in psychiatry and was voted the graduate with the best qualifications for the practice of medicine.

This self-described farmer was then accepted into the general surgery program at the Royal Victoria Hospital in Montreal. Here I must digress and tell you something of the relationships that then existed in the McGill department of surgery. Cardiovascular and thoracic surgery (CVT) was then a general surgery service at the two adult hospitals, the Royal Victoria and the Montreal General, and this was a happy arrangement due to our close friendship with and support by the two surgeons in chief, Lloyd MacLean and Fraser Gurd.

---

* On the occasion of a Retirement Dinner in Toronto honouring Lynda Mickleborough, May 2003.

Lloyd MacLean had come to McGill from Minnesota as one of Owen Wangensteen's bright, brilliant and confident young men and the McGill department of surgery took off for great heights propelled by him and a bit earlier by Rocke Robertson, followed by Fraser Gurd. Both hospitals began to make most new appointments on a full-time basis and university surgical clinics were established at both sites for experimental surgery.

At the Royal Victoria Hospital where Lynda had her general surgery training, laboratory work flourished in all the specialties under the general surgery umbrella. Hypotheses tested in the lab were brought into the clinical operating rooms. Papers were presented at the surgical forum of the American College and elsewhere. The department flourished. Dr. MacLean rated her "outstanding in all categories."

The CVT service was as I indicated one of the general surgery services. This gave us residents at the junior level who were with us for rotations of three months learning the rudiments of critical care, thoracic and vascular surgery and gave us the opportunity to know and evaluate and encourage the best into our specialty. Lynda of course was one of these. Those headed to our specialty were reassigned to our service for further rotations within the five years of general surgery training before spending two years in the McGill division of CVT surgery as chief resident at each of the four participating hospitals.

One of the general surgery years was spent in research and Lynda studied experimental myocardial infarction, yielding two papers in cardiovascular research and receiving the annual research award of the Canadian Cardiovascular Society for her paper "Significance of the Q wave which follows reperfusion of the ischemic myocardium."

Her four 6-month rotations as chief resident in cardiothoracic surgery, as it then was, were undoubtedly demanding, fatiguing, and probably emotionally draining. I had no complaints from her and she performed as one of our very best. She seemed indefatigable, cheerful, mature, determined and wise. We used to urge residents to always do "the right thing." Lynda always did.

I often assisted our graduates in acquiring an appointment elsewhere. As best I can remember Lynda arranged her appointment in Toronto by herself. She was thirty-three years old, had spent fifteen years at McGill and was ready for the world.

In Toronto, she established her reputation. She did it in part because of elegant, detailed experimental work with a number of co-workers; experimental work that led to clinical innovations that in turn led to superb clinical results in the most challenging cohort of patients: those with heart failure with or without ventricular arrhythmias. This indicates that she worked with individuals in several departments, because the work required expertise in diverse areas and that she impressed with her determination to learn in the laboratory, and to do the experiments with precision. To carry out the complex experiments meant that she was thoughtful and considerate of her associates and impressed on them the vital importance of her work. Finally her written papers were models of precision and conciseness from the abstract to the conclusions, always justified from the observations.

Besides the many outstanding articles published in collaboration with her associates in Toronto she established her unique reputation and expertise starting with the mapping of arrhythmias in 1984 and proceeding to an experimental study of endocardial excision compared to an encircling endocardial ventriculotomy in 1986 that showed that neither had a significant effect on long term structure and function of the left ventricle. This was an extremely complex and elegant study involving as it did cardiopulmonary bypass in an experimental model, studies of left ventricular function and pathologic studies on LV morphology.

She participated as a principal investigator in several papers advancing the technique of intraoperative mapping of ventricular arrhythmias leading to the endoventricular multistudded balloon that she introduced in 1988, showing the superiority of this technique in a series of patients, and in 1990 she mapped thirty-seven consecutive patients successfully with this technique ablating the ventricular tachycardia in 84 percent, an outstanding achievement. Subsequently she showed that the late results were excellent but better in patients with a ventricular aneurysm than in those with an area of dyskinesia.

By 1994, she could report a series of ninety-five excisions of ventricular aneurysms with 86 percent survival at two years and 80 percent five-year survival. In2000 she reported 125 patients with ejection fractions under 20 percent who underwent conventional bypass grafts with a 4 percent mortality when myocardial temperature was mapped after the injection of cold cardioplegia and grafts were first constructed to areas of unsatisfactory cooling even when decent vessels were not seen in these areas n coronary angiography.

These are just some examples of what she has accomplished in Toronto and I have not mentioned her influence on the next generation of surgeons and physicians as a teacher and role model. I congratulate her associates for supporting and encouraging her.

What about the gender thing? She certainly is a remarkable person—a remarkable woman. I think she thinks of herself professionally as a person. True she has considered women's issues, specifically their risk in undergoing coronary surgery, and I'm sure she has been approached for advice by younger women planning a career in medicine or surgery. But she has not made her reputation because she is a woman but simply because she aspired to excellence.

I want to congratulate Lynda directly for her decision to retire. As one now experienced in that state, I can affirm that there is another life out there for this step-grandmother, and I join all her former associates at McGill and Toronto and major cardiac surgical centres everywhere to wish her and Bill well in their new careers, as two former farmers return to the land near Georgian Bay and their island in the Thousand Islands.

Tony Dobell, MD, formerly chief of the division of cardiothoracic surgery at McGill University

STEPHANIE BRISTER

Toronto has indeed been fortunate to have a second woman heart surgeon on staff. In 1998 Dr. Stephanie Brister joined the Toronto hospital team after seventeen years of postsecondary school training and nine years as staff cardiac surgeon at Hamilton General Hospital and associate professor at McMaster University. Another one who had trouble finding the door out. Dr. Brister spent five years obtaining a B.Sc. and master's in genetics from the University of Calgary, three years training in medicine at Calgary, became a general surgeon after five years at McGill, and trained in cardiovascular and thoracic surgery (as was the program at that time) in Kingston, followed by her final year of fellowship training in cardiac surgery at Toronto General Hospital in 1988.

Stephanie wryly points out that she has yet to spend the total number of years in practice as a cardiac surgeon that she spent training for her career. There must be some kind of message here (could it be trial by fire?); however this seems to be the fate of all who choose this specialty, both men and women. When asked if she would do it all over again, whether this career she now upholds is worth it, there was a resounding and definitive yes! I am sure many of us when we stop and think, wonder how we got from point A so long ago to our current position The answer is simply, one step at a time. Remember counting down the number of years on call when we only had three and a half years left? People around us were incredulous as to why the countdown from so long but, having done eight years already of one-in-two to one-in-four call; three and a half years seemed relatively short. When I asked Dr. Brister if she could see herself doing anything else—she replied, "An astronaut." No, not an astronaut doing cardiac surgery, just an astronaut. Dr.

Brister applied for astronaut training the same time as Dr. Roberta Bondar and fortunately for all of us decided on inner space rather than outer.

Mistaken identity is a common occurrence when women choose careers in male dominated fields. Dr. Brister recounted an amusing incident in her first week of practice at Hamilton General Hospital. A senior surgeon Dr. X signed out all of his patients to Dr. Brister's care for his one month of holidays. Dr. Brister was standing on the ward with several of the white coated nurse-practitioners (looking not unlike one herself—who's to know?) when a senior consultant specialist Dr. Y began to give instructions as to the care of Dr. X's patients. When he stated that he was in charge in Dr. X's absence, Dr. Brister had to gently but firmly inform Dr. Y that unfortunately (or fortunately) he was relieved of this duty because she, the new CVT surgeon on staff, had been asked by Dr. X to perform this said care in his absence. Much embarrassment ensued and Dr. Brister tells me that they were fast friends and remain good colleagues many years after!

Role models are necessary for all of us and can be particularly helpful if they are of the same sex. Women wishing to work in male dominated fields may not always be so lucky. However I am not sure that this is necessary. As women in heart surgery, we have all found wonderful mentors who have supported us and nudged us in the right direction in much the same way as our male colleagues have undoubtedly been helped. The key according to Dr. Brister is to find mentors who are self confident and have enough experience to recognize talent and not feel threatened. Dr. Ray Chiu of Montreal was instrumental in steering Dr. Brister toward cardiac surgery and Dr. John Pym eloquently and selflessly instructed her in the art and science of the discipline.

It is indeed fortunate for women to find such mentors who not only recognize talent but are keenly aware of the hard road ahead not least because of gender.

Does gender bias exist in cardiac surgery? Of course it does. It's human nature. I can remember deciding on surgery as a career from the very first operation at which I assisted. As a new third year medical student at the Ottawa General Hospital with Dr. J. B. Ewing, a senior resident was performing a cholecystectomy and Dr. Ewing, getting close to retirement, allowed me to first assist. I was hooked! It honestly felt as if I had done this before (in another life perhaps); however when I announced in my fourth year of medicine, during a surgical rotation, to Dr. Z that I wanted to be a general surgeon, he simply (and I believe quite frankly) asked me, "Who will send you any business?—You are a woman." Being of a more naive and trusting nature then, I thought—okay, I'll do plastic surgery; that's a specialty probably more in line with my gender. Unfortunately, later in my internship year I walked out of the only operation in my life, a nose job. I couldn't stand the blood streaming out of both nostrils, while the surgeon banged away on the conscious patient's nasal bones with hammer and chisel (local freezing only). While I am fully aware today that the specialty of plastic surgery is far more than nose jobs, none the less, one's first impressions can be formative.

Getting back to gender bias, probably one of the few ways to reduce it is to increase the number of women in cardiac surgery. This might actually occur out of necessity. Dr. Fred A. Crawford, president of the Eighty-third Annual Meeting of the American Association for

Thoracic Surgery in Boston, Massachusetts, of May 2003[*] in his presidential address, outlined decreased interest in medicine as a career (medical school applications in the United States were down in 2002 for the seventh year in a row), declining choice of general surgery as a career (12.1 percent in 1981 to 5.1 percent in 2002), and that unless some of the graduating women (now 50 percent of most medical schools in Canada) could be attracted to cardiothoracic surgery, there would be a cardiothoracic surgical *man*power shortage in the near future.

Although the number of women in medical school has increased dramatically, the number of women choosing surgery has remained relatively constant: only about 20 percent of candidates certified by the American Board of Surgery are women. Even more interestingly, since the founding of the American Board of Thoracic Surgery, only 139 of 6748 diplomates (2.1 percent) have been women. Dr. Crawford goes on to comment on the lack of friendliness of the thoracic surgery specialty towards women; i.e., surgical residency programs must be permitted increased flexibility to more easily address medical leave for pregnancy, if the resource of the newly graduating women physicians is to be tapped. Many years ago, it was hard enough for a woman to just get into medical school; now that this barrier has been crossed, it may be easier to go to the next level. One has only to look at recently trained specialists who have been used to female colleagues in their medical school years to see more tolerance of women in the profession. Gender bias may still exist today, but times, they are a-changing; look at Toronto with their second woman heart surgeon—Dr. Stephanie Brister!

---

[*]   F. A. Crawford, "Presidential address: Thoracic surgery education—Responding to a changing environment," *J Thorac Cardiovasc Surg* (2003), 126: 1235-42.

GLORIANNE ROPCHAN

It seems as if there is one woman heart surgeon per centre across the country. I don't think any of us have ever had a female colleague for very long except perhaps during residency. Drs. Brister and Mickleborough were colleagues for a few brief years before Dr. Mickleborough's retirement in 2002. Dr. Glorianne Ropchan has been holding the fort in Kingston now since her graduation from the CVT program in Toronto in 1990. This was after spending seventeen years in university and surgery training programs to become a cardiac surgeon: three years of mathematics, physics and chemistry at the University of Toronto (and one year of French studies in Aix-Marseilles, France), four years of medical school at U of T, a straight surgical internship at Toronto General Hospital (TGH), followed by the requisite (in those days) pond-crossing fellowship in general surgery, a residency in cardiovascular and thoracic surgery and fellowship year all at the University of Toronto. After interviewing many women heart surgeons across the country, the number seventeen arises frequently for the number of years required to train for this specialty. Is this a magic number or does it simply meant that it takes a very long time to prepare for this career?

How did Glorianne become interested in cardiac surgery? In her first year of medical school, her anatomy professor Dr. Brown took his students to watch his classmate Dr. Ronald Baird perform heart surgery at Toronto Western Hospital. The anatomists and surgeons also set up a program for all first year students to spend a day in the OR, so she had the opportunity to see Dr. Clare Baker performing heart surgery at St. Michael's Hospital. At that time, her tutor (assigned to each first year student to provide a connection to clinical/hospital medicine) was Dr. Ernie Michel, a cardiac anaesthetist, who told her that the pharmacology and physiology she was being taught were different from his courses and that what he could do best was to show her the principles in action. She spent numerous hours in and around the cardiac OR at TGH, as Dr. Michel described and explained physiology in "action" during cardio-pulmonary bypass. In second year, she was a lecturer/demonstrator in anatomy for the pharmacy students and she also did an elective in surgery—set up by the department at U of T to expose/interest and attract/entice medical students to consider a career in surgery. It worked! Her first week, she was assigned to spend with Dr. Tirone David. He invited her to come see surgery anytime (as did a number of the surgeons during the elective). Somehow orthopedics, plastics, even neurosurgery (when Dr. Morley had "the girl scrub to help close" and sent the residents off to do "scut") did not have the appeal of the cardiac OR. She missed a few psychiatry lectures (though she dutifully did attend all the clinics) to come and watch and even scrub (!) when Dr. David operated at Toronto Western Hospital (TWH). It was fascinating!—She knew her calling. Then, when as a clinical clerk staying late to watch a left atrial myxoma, Dr. Baird handed her the needle driver to help close the atriotomy, her fate was sealed!

What's bad about being a cardiac surgeon? Basically when you're working, you have no life. Working with two colleagues in Kingston, her days start by seven-thirty and don't finish much before eight or nine at night. Being a woman does make a difference—patients appreciate the feminine touch, although more and more she finds that patients expect that any problem can be fixed. Also the double standard, try as we might to think that we are in the enlightened generation, does still exist. On the humorous side, she has fond memories of working with the calm and professorial Dr. Hugh Scully. As a student, when she saw the resident present a well-harvested, but rather poor relative of the saphenous vein family, he would often say, "We don't make it, we just take it!" The harvested vein used to be attached to a cannula on a glass syringe, made ready for use. One day "vein et al." rolled off a portly patient's abdomen onto the floor, an event announced by the tinkle of the shattering glass syringe. Dr. Scully paused briefly, then calmly asked the circulating nurse, "Would you mind picking that up?" Glorianne and the scrub nurse washed it in antibiotic solutions (just like a valve prosthesis), and the patient did fine! This "sangfroid" was very impressive to an aspiring heart surgeon. Dr. Goldman one day noted her well-worked biceps at the scrub sink—attributable not to any aerobics workout, but to pulling sternums together so there never was any post-op bleeding. Dr. Weisel always had the chest tubes and pacer wires in situ from the left side of the table before the cross-clamp was on. With Dr. Mickleborough, one day the unique event occurred of an OR peopled completely by women except for the patient! Dr. Lipton preferred the classics on "Channel 2" as did Glorianne and had quite a few pointers with pacer leads. Dr. Feindel down in OR Five tried to teach her how to catch flies (in between distal anastomoses).She learned about the intricacies of mitral valve repair and about the "Tirone Factor" from Dr. David. At St. Michael's Hospital where she was assigned for thoracic surgery (!), she was able to see the expertise and experience of Drs. Baker, Hart and Yao and the excitement and enthusiasm of Drs. Salerno and Lichtenstein. Drs. Trusler and Williams were gentlemen pediatric heart surgeons and although the world at Hospital for Sick Children was totally different and enticing, Glorianne eventually decided to remain in adult cardiac surgery. She has memories of the anaesthetists, fellows, residents, nurses, perfusionists and other hospital personnel who made cardiac surgery such a rewarding residency and career. Now she enjoys passing on what she has learned to residents and students, taking them on a tour of the heart, its anatomy and pathology, having them palpate coronary artery disease and pick up the finer points of handling tissues, instruments and patients. She always advises them on their first visit into the cardiac OR, to let their folks know they've seen (and touched) a beating human heart. It's immensely rewarding to be part of the continuum of medical knowledge, to have been a student and now a teacher as well.

When I asked Glorianne would she do it all again? "Probably yes"; when the politics and fatigue get her down, one just needs an elegant case and a grateful patient to remind them of the reason for all the hard struggles. One of her worries for future heart surgeons is the rude awakening many will have when they become staff. Because of their protected lifestyle as a resident, the real world of "staff" may be a brutal contrast. On the other hand, maybe we need to take a leaf out of their book and modify our lifestyle as surgeons—to have a life!

PATRICIA ANN PENKOSKE

Dr. Patricia Penkoske is one of our few imports. Her four years of undergraduate education was spent obtaining a BA in art, history, biology and chemistry at Lindenwood, an American all women's college. Dr. Penkoske broke new ground when she became the first-ever graduate from this college to go to medical school. A summer medical research job at Washington University had enthralled her with medicine. After completing one year of molecular biology graduate school at the University of Wisconsin, she started medical school at Washington University in St. Louis, Missouri from 1970 to 1974. Then followed a general surgery residency at Barnes Hospital, Washington University: four years clinical and two research years on the mechanism of ventricular fibrillation. Her cardiothoracic residency was spent in Boston, Massachusetts, at New England Deaconess Hospital (NED). One and one half years were spent in adult cardiac surgery at NED, but it was her exposure to pediatric cardiac surgery with Dr. Aldo Castaneda at Boston Children's Hospital that shaped her future. From here she did a further year of pediatric cardiac surgery training at the Hospital for Sick Children in Toronto under Drs. George Trusler and Bill Williams, and one year at Barnes Hospital again in clinical and basic research with Dr. James Cox (1983-84). Her clinical and academic career started in Edmonton in 1984, and notwithstanding this busy life, she and her husband Frank had three beautiful daughters.

The call back to home lured our Dr. Penkoske to St. Louis University in 2000 for two years until she went into private practice for the first time in her career in December 2002, in Springfield, Illinois. Patty had some insightful comments on private practice in the

United States; whereas you couldn't beat it for efficiency (patients at a moment's notice are able to have a carotid stent placed the morning of heart surgery), she missed having residents to teach. Having your brain prodded daily by inquiring minds keeps you focused and up to date. In this private practice she performed vascular and thoracic surgery as well as cardiac surgery; she found that the carotid endarterectomy is a very precise and gratifying operation. In Springfield there was a very well developed complementary alternative medicine department at St. John's Hospital. A healing garden welcomed patients and their relatives to relax, heal and be treated amidst waterfalls, tranquility and caring personnel devoted to healing the psyche. Where is Dr. Penkoske now? Back in her beloved St. Louis, training again! She says she is the world's oldest "fellow," in a Critical Care Fellowship Program; she is working toward a life style that will allow some precious time to devote to her three still young daughters, Chloe, seventeen, Elizabeth, fifteen, and Olivia, fourteen years. I asked her if she missed operating—not really, she was replacing it with a life more devoted to her family. Very impressed with the healing effects of the Complementary Medicine Program in Springfield and the fact that this type of medicine predates our "medicine" by millennia, Patty is developing a similar program for the state of Missouri.

When I asked Dr. Penkoske what she wanted to do in life before she knew it was cardiac surgery, she replied "an airline stewardess." However parental persuasion prevailed ("my father forced me to go to college") and hence the path toward medicine and cardiac surgery was set. Very early in her third year of medical school, she knew surgery was to be her career but decided on cardiac surgery after working with Dr. Thomas Ferguson during her general surgical residency at Barnes Hospital. Dr.

Ferguson became a wonderful mentor for Dr. Penkoske encouraging her to go into cardiothoracic surgery. During her residency in thoracic surgery there were some chauvinistic moments: a particular attending physician (better left unnamed!) would tell Patty to scrub out and order some lasagna for the boys, and then laugh. (NTFL).* What was attractive about cardiac surgery for her?—the relative purity of the diagnostic process for most cardiac illness and the technical challenges. Dr. Penkoske finds that the toughest times in the profession are not the hard work or physical demands, but patient deaths which may occur quickly and unexpectedly despite all efforts to the contrary. We think we have failed if we lose a patient, but our role is just different. At these times of loss, family members look to us for help as one wonderful mentor of the writer said "when a patient of yours dies, to the family you represent the last link between this world and the next. You owe them some special time" (author Dr. Gerald M. Fitzgibbon). Fortunately these tough times are few and one has the satisfaction and most gratifying moments in a career when challenging cases such as the many pediatric cases Dr. Penkoske has done over the years, go well. What would she like to see improved upon in heart surgery? Increased compassion in dealing with families. When asked what she would like to be remembered for—treating patients as people, not cases. Therein lies the "art" of medicine.

---

*   NTFL: Not Too F—Likely

IRENE CYBULSKY

Dr. Irene Cybulsky trained in all three specialties, cardiac, vascular and thoracic surgery and has been working as a cardiac surgeon in Hamilton since 1996. She spent a total of eighteen years training and studying after high school to be where she is today: two years in general arts and science at the University of Toronto, four years medical school at U of T, and a surgical internship at Toronto Western Hospital. Then, although Dr. Cybulsky originally intended a career in thoracic surgery, the gods must have deemed otherwise. She spent a year in research at St. Michael's Hospital under Dr. Samuel Lichtenstein, with Dr. Tom Salerno as a supervisor. Then came the requisite four years of general surgery at McMaster University in Hamilton followed by two years training in cardiovascular and thoracic surgery. As part of her CVT training she spent six months at MD Anderson still intending to do thoracic surgery. After this followed four years of refining her surgical skills in Hamilton, interspersed by a one year temporary staff position in cardiac surgery at St. Michael's Hospital in Toronto. Finally, in 1996, a position became available in Hamilton as a staff cardiac surgeon and assistant professor at McMaster. Having trained for so many years, it was good to be able to answer all those well-meaning people (mostly our parents) who said, "High time you got a job!" Newly on staff, Dr. Cybulsky started immediately working on a residency training program for Hamilton—a daunting enterprise for a "long-in-the-tooth" cardiac surgeon, never mind one beginning her practice. She was dogged in her efforts and successfully started the first residency training program in cardiac surgery in Hamilton in 1999. Currently there are five training cardiac surgeons in this program.

When asked what is the toughest thing about being a heart surgeon she answered "not operating"—a true cutter! Possibly all heart surgeons are introverted, narrowly focused individuals liking nothing better than to be in the OR where *nobody* has the right to interfere, where we can devote our entire attention using our hands and brains (contrary to internists' beliefs!) to better one individual's life. It's not that we don't like talking to people but personally I find it more draining to do an 8-11 out-patient clinic for three hours than to operate for eight!

When asked what she didn't like or what aspect she would like to change re: heart surgery, Irene commented on the ridiculous lifestyle. In the olden days, it used to be said that being on call one in two days meant you missed half of the cases. I can remember when I first started operating "for real," how much easier it was than as a resident—my hands were steadier, more precise, my energy much greater and I realized it was due to relative lack of fatigue. I don't know where this martyr-like life originated but it is insane. Once having completed eight heart surgeries, one re-op for bleeding with little or no sleep in four days, my dear husband marched out to my car on my return at 5 a.m., pulled out all the spark plug wires and announced, "You are not going anywhere; you're not competent to drive a car, let alone operate on someone." Is it fatigue that makes us blind to our own humanity, is it a genetic lack of insight, or is it a silly snowball of "I can do this, I am a surgeon, I am weak if I give into fatigue"? All men and women surgeons are guilty of this at one time or another. Realizing that part-time cardiac surgery is not a possibility, there must be a middle road.

Shortly after starting her job Dr. Cybulsky recalls her father calling one day at the office and commenting,

"Well, you're not working today." "Little Irene" had to point out to "Father" that there is a lot more to the work of a cardiac surgeon than operating. There are patients—to be seen before and after surgery or whenever a problem arises. There are blood tests, X-rays and angiograms as well as echoes to review. There are administrative tasks and correspondence to deal with, along with meetings to attend. There are medical students and residents whose education needs to be facilitated. There is research to be done, continuing self-education not to be neglected and of course evaluation and review of one's own work. No wonder the OR is such a haven. She feels one of the biggest challenges is the management of this ever increasing work load. For Dr. Cybulsky the equivalent of two "full" days in the OR per week is a comfortable volume, more than this erodes a "reasonable" life. Hamilton, in order to maximize OR time and accommodate the cardiac surgery wait list, has gone to rotating three case-days. Ideally a surgeon books three relatively short cases in order to finish hopefully within twelve hours—by 8:00 p.m. These can be brutal days. Of course, that leaves the not-so-short cases for the two case day, which also ends up running to 8:00 p.m. (If all goes well . . .) And then—"By the way, are you the surgeon on call today?" comes a-calling the cheery cardiologist. Even her five-year-old son knows about this system and will ask, "Mom, how many cases are you doing today?" Or if she doesn't make it home as forecast he knows, "Mom's having problems at work." He loves the days she doesn't operate because he knows he might actually have his mother's undivided attention while he's still awake. On arrival home, her husband welcomes the late Dr. Cybulsky. Once when Irene came home with a running nose, coughing, and croaking with a hoarse voice, her young son at that time age four-and-a-half years impishly said, "Mom, maybe you need a doctor!"

Our kids keep us humble. A while ago when my daughter Alexandra, aged three, was bemoaning the fact that I was leaving for work; I tried to tell her that I had to go and look after some sick people. She indignantly asked, "Are they sick *again?*" (Why can't you get this right, Mom?)

When asked if she would do it all again, Dr. Cybulsky wasn't too sure, the computer world holds great attraction for her. Perhaps it looks a little more peaceful than her life today. Women definitely face more hurdles and the middle road seems hard to achieve.

Not that we are surgeons interested in "life style," we are simply interested in having "a life."

TERESA M. KIESER

Now about the writer: Like all of my colleagues it took a considerable number of years to finally get to a job: two years Honours biology at the University of Western Ontario, four years medical school, University of Ottawa, three years military service—first two as a cardiopulmonary internal medicine resident and third year as general surgical resident at the Ottawa Military Hospital, National Defense Medical Centre (NDMC). Three more years were spent as a general surgery resident in Toronto with a fourth, the final year, at Ottawa, two years training in cardiovascular and thoracic surgery and one fellowship year in adult cardiac surgery at the Ottawa Heart Institute, followed by a final six month arrhythmia surgery fellowship at Barnes Hospital, Washington University in St. Louis, Missouri. Seventeen and a half years later I finally gained employment with the opening of Foothills Cardiac Surgery Unit September 1988, followed by Royal College examiner 1995-2000 (first woman examiner) and am currently in practice at Foothills Medical Centre (sixteen years) and associate professor at the University of Calgary. This career was contrary to anyone's expectation; my parents actually hoped that I would become a nun and enter a convent for safe-keeping. My only goal in those days was to be a ballerina. However being turned down by the National Ballet School in Toronto, I joined the cardiac circus instead.

Why cardiac surgery? One man: Dr. Wilbert J. Keon. Having trained under Dr. Keon was the greatest single benefit in my formative medical years. Somewhere in my first three months of a cardiac surgery rotation in 1980, I became a convert and disciple. Willy had the gift of bringing calmness to every case no matter how complex.

Along with many of my colleagues, a common thread emerges when asked what is the best and the worst of our profession. It is the saving of lives at the significant cost of our own personal lives, come what may. Wisdom holds that if we saved all of our patients, we wouldn't be doctors (God would be mightily ticked). Imagine if everybody survived? Ever time we operate, the potential for death exists. This aspect of cardiac surgery sets us apart from other surgical specialties and demands a special type of courage and self confidence in all who are called.

What can we as women hope to contribute to this very specialized walk of life? On a basic level maybe there is less "cursing." ("Can't use that word—there are ladies present!") Maybe we can bring understanding and comfort to the women patients and maybe we can encourage other women to enter this most worthy specialty. Most importantly, maybe because our gender is blessed (or taxed) with the bearing of future generations, we can bring more of a nurture nature to cardiac surgery and more humanity amongst our colleagues perhaps?

ADDENDUM

Time, unfortunately, did not permit the following to respond:

Virginia M. Gudas MD FRCSC   Vancouver, British Columbia
Memorial University—1978
FRCSC—Gen Surg, Cardiovasc and Thorac Surg
Cardiothoracic Transplant
Active Staff, Vancouver Hospital and Health Sciences Centre

Camille L. Hancock-Friesen MD MSc FRCSC Halifax, Nova Scotia
Halifax, Nova Scotia
University of Alberta—1992
MSc Science University of Alberta 1995
RCPSC Gen Surg U of Alberta
RCPSC Cardiac Surg Dalhousie University 2000
Fellowship in Pediatric Cardiac Surg: Harvard University
Boston Children's Hospital 18 months
Attending in Adult and Pediatric Cardiac Surgery
Dalhousie University since Oct 2002

Roxane McKay MB MRCS FRCSC   Saskatoon, Saskatchewan
University of Chicago—1970
MRCS (Eng) LRP (Lond) FRCS (Eng)
FRCSC—Cardiothor Surg (Congenital Heart Disease)
Staff Royal University Hospital
Prof, Surg and Peds, University of Saskatchewan
Now at Mayo Clinic

Mary Lee Myers MD FRCSC   London, Ontario
University of Western Ontario—1977
FRCSC—Gen Surg, Cardiovasc Surg
Chief, Cardiovascular surgery
London Health Sciences Centre
Victoria Campus Site
Associate Professor—University of Western Ontario

Denyse Normandin MD FRCSC   Montreal, Quebec
University of Montreal—1974
FRCSC Gen Surg, Cardiovascular and Thoracic Surg
Staff Sir Mortimer B. Davis Jewish General Hospital
Currently in Sabbatical Year

Nancy Poirier MD CVT PQ   Montreal, Quebec
University of Montreal—1992
Cardiovasc and Thoracic Surgery (PQ)
Staff Cardiac Surgery Hôpital Ste. Justine

Nathalie Roy MD FRCSC   Montreal, Quebec
Laval University—1993
FRCSC Gen Surg (Cardiac Surg)
TSFRE Fellowship—2004
(Thoracic Surgery Foundation for Research and Education)
Children's Hospital, Boston, Massachusetts
"Engineering of Conduction Tissue for Cardiac Implantation"

Dorothy Thomson MD FRCSC   Saskatoon, Saskatchewan
Queens University—1979
FRCSC Cardiovascular and Thoracic Surgery
Active Staff, Royal University Hospital, Saskatoon

J. Suzanne Vobecky MD FRCSCC   Montreal, Quebec
University of Sherbrooke—1980
FRCSC Gen Surg, Cardiovasc and Thorac Surg
Active Staff, Hôpital Ste. Justine

Clinical Ass't Surgeon University of Montreal

Acknowledgements:

1. To the women in this chapter, who opened their hearts and provided insight into their intense yet gratifying career: Thank you!

2. To all women heart surgeons for steadfastly maintaining ground in a male domain: Thank you!

3. To Bernie Goldman, who innately uses the right combination of prodding and patience to make writers produce: Many thanks!

4. To my dear husband, for his many hours of review, who knows my mind so well as to be able to express the intent in one succinct word or phrase: A thousand thanks!

5. And finally to those male colleagues who intuitively supported the career paths of their female counterparts described herein: Untold thanks!

CHAPTER 16

PERFUSION IN CANADA

James MacDonald

Cardiopulmonary bypass has been described as "an art trying to become a science" and as such, has continued to evolve to the present-day period of dependability, safety and convenience of use. Over the span of the last thirty-five years, I have witnessed the continued evolution, modification and refinement of this extracorporeal technology called cardiopulmonary bypass (CPB) into what is presently considered to be the "state-of-the-art technology." Presently, surgical efforts have been directed toward a reduction in surgical dependency (OPCAB) so as to eliminate the associated pathophysiology of conventional CPB. Terminology such as "pump standby and off pump" has resurfaced once again. In the late 1960s, as a student heart-lung technician, I had previously performed pump standbys for closed mitral commissurotomies. Sometimes what was old is now new. In that era of mechanical complexity, the thoracic surgeon and pump technician shared a unique and evolving relationship that would foster respect and future professional growth. The learning curve was steep and malfunctions of the heart-lung machine mirrored the surgical challenges of the day. In those early days, the pump oxygenator was without the "bells and whistles" of today and the animal lab was the common testing ground where research was initiated and surgical techniques perfected before being introduced into the operating room.

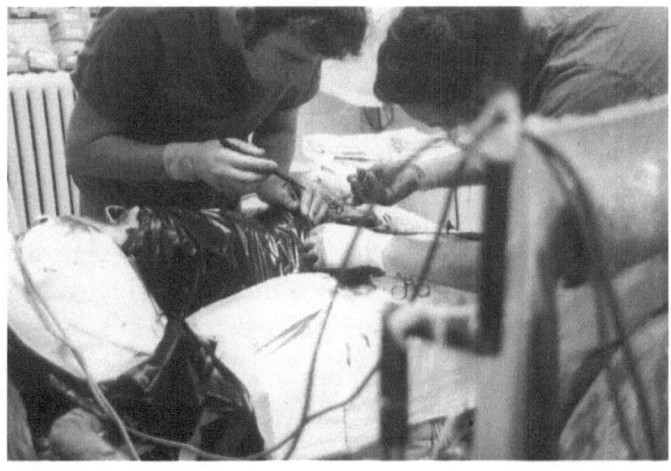

Fig. 16:1 Research Laboratory at Dalhousie University, Halifax, Nova Scotia in late 1960s.

Excessive foam production within the pump oxygenator, caused by excessive cardiotomy suction return, was treated with generous spraying of antifoam-A directly into the open cardiotomy reservoir. Arterial line filtration was in its infancy and frank cerebral injury was an anticipated concern.

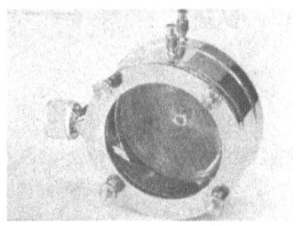

Fig. 16:2 The early Gross arterial line filter used with the Kay-Cross rotating disk oxygenator.

Venting of the open heart was not yet an established protocol and the resulting pulmonary edema was a problem for all concerned. Myocardial protection was in its infancy and "stone heart" was too often a clinical reality.

Across Canada in the early 1960s, open-heart surgery with pump oxygenator support was being performed in a small number of hospitals for the surgical correction of congenital heart defects and acquired valvular disease. The evolution of open-heart technology throughout Canada in the late 1960s and early 1970s mirrored developments throughout the western world. It had become apparent that a more reliable means of supporting the circulation and providing gas exchange would be required for the repair of more complex pathologies. This was the era when the Kay-Cross disk oxygenator and the Mayo-Gibbon heart-lung machine were the tools of the day and their associated mechanical complexities were being realized clinically.

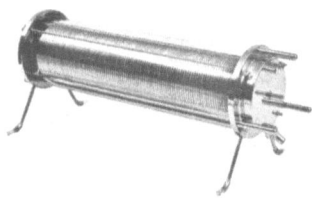

Fig. 16:3 The adult Kay-Cross rotating disk oxygenator

Their inherent complexity required several hours of dedicated preparation and would form a lasting impression on the heart-lung technologist. Early prototypes of bubble oxygenators and membrane technology were then in their infancy and would not be introduced throughout North America for several years to come. I had begun my perfusion career in Halifax in 1968 and began my initial perfusion training on the Kay-Cross disk oxygenator prior to the clinical use of disposable bubble oxygenators in the early 1970s. In 1974, we had began our first clinical use of the Lande-Edwards membrane oxygenator at the

Halifax Children's Hospital under the supervision of Dr. David Alton Murphy and Richard B. Leadon.

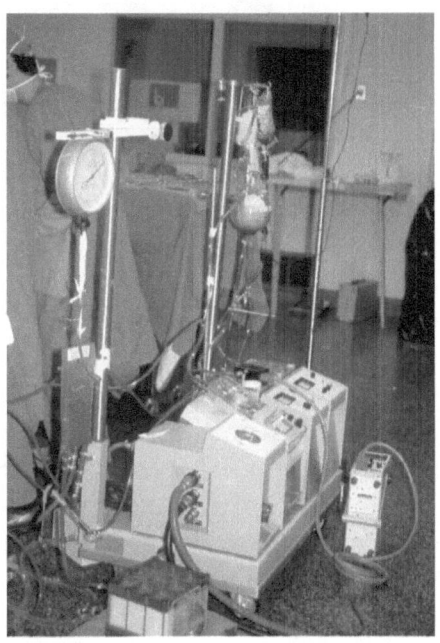

Fig. 16:4 The Lande-Edward silicone membrane oxygenator used at the Halifax Children's Hospital during the mid-1970s for the surgical correction of complex congenital heart defects.

My personal clinical experiences and professional interaction with my perfusion colleagues over these many years, hopefully, would be of assistance to me in attempting to review this initial era of our Canadian perfusion history.

From a historical point of view, one cannot revisit the past without the recognition of several historical milestones. Heparin and its associated anticoagulant effect had been discovered in 1915 by Jay McLean. In 1927, Dr. Charles Best of Toronto proceeded with the further purification

of heparin and reported on his initial research. It would
not be until the 1970s that the maintenance and loading
dose of heparin would be investigated to monitor
activated clotting times. As far back as 1937, John Gibbon
had envisioned the coupling of extracorporeal blood
pumping and artificial oxygenation which, hopefully,
would allow unhurried surgical intervention in the
adult patient. During that same year, Michael DeBakey
had recognized the dependability of the roller pump
as a reliable mechanism for milking large volumes of
calibrated blood along flexible tubing. This positive
displacement pump has remained to the present day as
an integral part of the extracorporeal circuits worldwide.
Polyvinyl chloride tubing had yet to be discovered and
latex rubber tubing was initially used in many of the
pump oxygenator circuits. The exchange of individual
concepts and theories on extracorporeal circulation
had begun to be discussed at surgical meetings in the
mid-1950s. This would provide the fertile soil where
independent theory and isolated research involving
hypothermia, oxygenation and blood pumps were finally
being shared and the vision of cardiopulmonary bypass as
a "tool" for cardiac surgery was about to become a reality.
The dependency of open-heart surgery on this evolving
extracorporeal technology had finally arrived.

History recorded a surgical milestone on May 6, 1953,
when Dr. John Gibbon Jr. of Philadelphia performed the
world's first successful closure of an ASD on an eighteen-
year-old female totally supported by his Mayo-Gibbon
heart-lung machine. His initial research on a heart-lung
machine had begun much earlier in 1937 and his life's
work was chronicled in Ada Romaine-Davis, *John Gibbon
and His Heart-Lung Machine* (Philadelphia: University of
Pittsburgh Press, 1991). Although Dr. F. John Lewis, of
Minneapolis, had closed an ASD one year later without
the use of a heart-lung machine, the trend across North

America to close congenital heart defects under direct vision with mechanical pump oxygenator support, was to continue worldwide.

The Canadian experience in cardiac surgery had its beginnings in Toronto with the pioneering work of Dr. William Mustard and Dr. Wilfred Bigelow. In 1951, Dr. Mustard was performing his monkey-lung experiments by suspending the monkey lung (biological oxygenator) inside bell jars that contained pure oxygen.

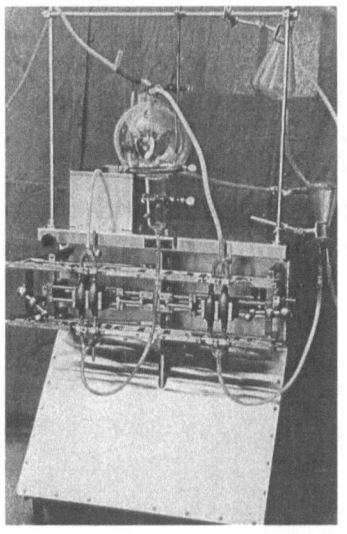

Fig. 16:5 The Mustard Biological Monkey Lung used at the Toronto Sick Children's Hospital in the early 1950s for the correction of simple congenital heart defects.

He next connected the individual monkey lungs in series and attached them to a pumping mechanism. This pump, built at the Banting Institute by Dr. Campbell Cowan, consisted of pressure bulbs and a sphygmomanometer squeezed rhythmically by metal plates. Dr. Mustard would use his biological oxygenator technique between the years 1952 and 1954 on a dozen infants at the Toronto

Hospital for Sick Children. During that time period, Dr. Wilfred Bigelow had spent several years at the Banting Institute working on his surface hypothermia protocol in the dog model. Surface hypothermia served as a link between the period of closed heart operations and the ultimate use of systemic core hypothermia used during pump oxygenator support. The widespread use of systemic hypothermia evolved from Bigelow's discovery that as metabolism slowed in the animal model, the demand for oxygen decreased and, while freezing could kill tissue, chilling the animal would prevent death.

In the early 1950s in Toronto, young surgical residents such as Dr. Ray Heimbecker, Dr. James Key, and Dr. Don Wilson trained under Dr. Bigelow's supervision and were instrumental in the development of an early prototype Toronto heart-lung machine and pump oxygenator. In 1955, Dr. Lillehei of Minnesota and his young physician colleague, Dr. Richard DeWall, began work on the prototype of a simplified disposable bubble oxygenator which was both inexpensive and easy to assemble.

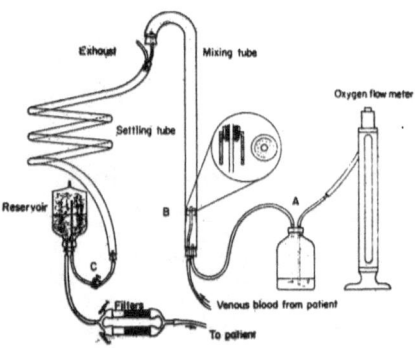

Fig. 16:6 The Original Lillehei/DeWall Helix bubble oxygenator—the first disposable bubble oxygenator used to correct congenital heart defects in Minnesota in the early 1950s.

It consisted of a couple of metal stands, some large diameter beer hose, an oxygen diffuser cork, a reservoir and two gross filters. This Lillehei/DeWall Helix bubble oxygenator had an explosive effect on the worldwide growth of open-heart surgery and opened the door for the commercial introduction and further refinement of a new generation of disposable bubble oxygenators. One year later, in September 1956, Canadian cardiac history would be made when Dr. John Callaghan, of Edmonton, Alberta, performed the first successful open-heart surgery using the Lillehei/DeWall Helix bubble oxygenator to surgically relieve a pulmonary artery stenosis. In 1957 at the Toronto General Hospital (TGH), Dr. Bigelow, Dr. Key and Dr. Heimbecker performed the first successful open-heart surgery in Toronto when they closed an ASD on a twenty-five-year-old female utilizing the commercially available Travenol bubble oxygenator, the offspring of the DeWall Helix oxygenator. Daniel Stanford, a young technologist-engineer, had assisted in the development of the prototype heart-lung machine and may be considered the first perfusionist at the TGH. Stanford and Bigelow did not see eye to eye and, as a result, Stanford was dismissed. Although Heimbecker et al., had developed their prototype heart-lung machine in Toronto, with the assistance of the Canadian Pipe and Steel Fabricators, Bigelow had little faith in this invention and insisted, according to Dr. Heimbecker, that the Travenol bubble oxygenator be used on their first case instead. In 1970, I had made my first visit to the University Wing operating room at the Toronto General Hospital. The invitation was extended to me by the chief perfusionist, Georgina Elliott and her assistant, Gerald Mullis.

Remembering a Typical Day

The year 2003 marked the fiftieth anniversary of the first successful use of the heart-lung machine by Dr. John Gibbon on May 3, 1953. As noted above, only three years later, in 1956, Dr. John Callaghan, of Edmonton performed the first open-heart surgery in Canada utilizing the Lillehei/DeWall Helix bubble oxygenator. In celebration of these anniversaries, the Canadian Society of Clinical Perfusion (CSCP) held a special symposium in Toronto at the CSCP annual perfusion meeting to celebrate the fiftieth anniversary of this event. Several perfusion pioneers came back from retirement to recall and reflect on their initial clinical experiences in several of the original Canadian cardiac centers.

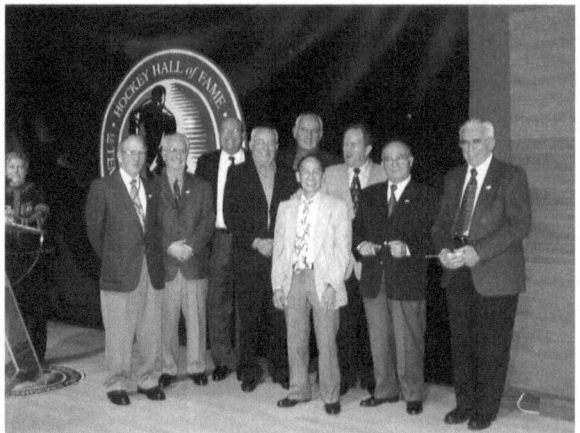

Fig. 16:7 Canadian perfusion pioneers who presented at the CSCP Annual Meeting, Toronto, October 2003. From the left: Roger Sampson, The Montreal General Hospital; Marcel Roy, St. Boniface General Hospital, Winnipeg; Ian Ross, St. John's Regional Hospital, Newfoundland; Richard Leadon, The Victoria General Hospital, Halifax, Nova Scotia; Jim MacDonald, The

London Health Sciences Centre, London, Ontario; Jamie Villameter, The Hospital for Sick Children, Toronto; Dietrich Kemna, The Royal Jubilee Hospital, Victoria; Constantine Fabrikis, Victoria Hospital, London; John Basaraba, Vancouver General Hospital, Vancouver.

Throughout their historical review of the late 1950s and the 1960s, there was a common thread of similarity in their memory recall as they described a typical operative day. The days were long, often times beginning at 0530 in the morning, and were full of anxiety due to the anticipated problems that had occurred in previous cases. Like many of the original heart-lung technicians of that era, I also had trained "on the job," specifically in the use of the American Optical stainless steel heart-lung machine and the Kay-Cross rotating disks oxygenator. The American Optical heart-lung machine consisted of three independent DeBakey type roller pumps. These U-shaped roller pumps were encased in a solid mahogany wood frame, which gave it durability of use and ease of cleaning. Each roller pump had a specific purpose and consisted of the main arterial pump head, a cardiotomy suction pump head and a vent pump head. The entire heart-lung circuit was preassembled, wrapped in muslin wrappers and sterilized by steam autoclaving. One pump technician would scrub gown and glove to assemble each pump component, then pass it off to another technician for instillation. Soft latex plastic tubing, which had been precut and sterilized, was then attached to stainless steel connectors and secured using copper wire tightened with pliers. The adult twenty-five-inch Kay-Cross rotating disk oxygenator had several associated components which consisted of the Gross arterial line filter, venous collection chamber, venous settling chamber and the Brown Harrison heat exchanger. Prior to steam sterilization, the 110 rotating discs would be washed, and preassembled on a horizontal shaft with washer-like spacers separating each disc.

The disc would be placed within a glass Pyrex cylinder with supporting metal end plates on each end to support the shaft. The blood banks of the day had the burden of providing enormous amounts of blood for priming. Up to four liters of whole blood was used to prime the disc

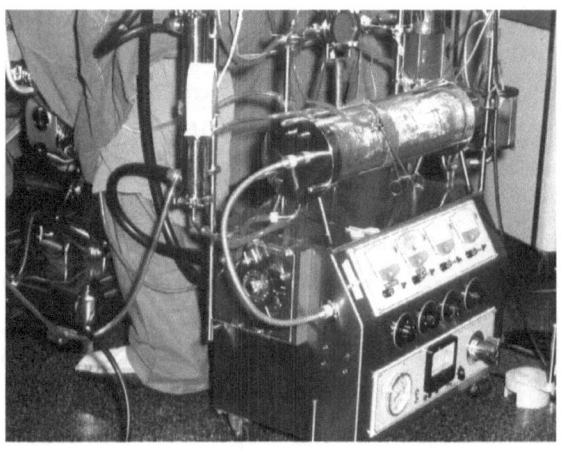

Fig. 16:8 The Kay-Cross rotating disk oxygenator with venous reservoir, venous settling chamber, Brown Harrison Heat exchanger and Gross arterial filter. The American Optical Rotary pump is shown with the main arterial pump.

oxygenator to a level of about one-half inch below the shaft. A film of blood was deposited on both sides of the disc as it rotated up out of the blood prime. The upper portion of the glass cylinder had a mixture of 100 percent oxygen, and 95 percent oxygen and 5 percent carbon dioxide, continuously passing over the rotating discs. The film of blood on the disc was exposed to the oxygen rich atmosphere and the red blood cells would exchange carbon dioxide for oxygen.

As the discs continued their independent rotation, the oxygenated blood films were returned to the stream in the lower portion of the cylinder. This was a continuous process of each disc filming venous blood out of the stream, exposing it to oxygen rich atmosphere and returning the oxygenated blood to the flowing stream. Total oxygenation would then depend on the total number of rotating disc as well as the RPM of each disc rotation. The greater the number of discs, the greater the filming surface, thus the greater the quantity of blood that could be oxygenated in a given period of time. The adult disc oxygenator with all its associated components required a whole blood prime of up to four liters of blood. The pump technician would also prepare the femoral artery cannula prior to the surgeons' arrival and select the appropriate sized venous cannula.

At the end of the surgical day, each pump component and the numerous stainless steel connectors were disassembled, thoroughly washed by hand and then soaked for thirty minutes in a Haemo-Sol solution. Next, they were placed in clean water and washed a second time to ensure that all surfaces were thoroughly cleaned. Each of the 120 discs was independently washed, dried and siliconized. Great care was taken to ensure that each disc was not over siliconized. Excess silicone could be washed off when in contact with blood during surgery with the potential for embolization into the patients' bloodstream. After all the various pump components were dried and preassembled, they were placed in double muslin wrappers, steam autoclaved and placed in a drying cabinet for at least twelve hours. During this same preparation period, each segment of the pump tubing, including the A-V loop, was precut and carefully rolled out and wrapped in muslin wrappers, sterilized and also placed in a drying cabinet to prevent "milking." Milking would render the tubing more opaque after sterilization, which caused the tubing to become cloudy in appearance and, therefore, any air bubbles that might be present would be difficult to see during cardiopulmonary bypass. The thorough washing and preassembly of the various pump components, prior to steam autoclaving, would tale up to three hours after the patient had left the operating room. If any component of this complex extracorporeal circuit was found to be inadvertently left over, this discovery would further extend a long day.

Routine systemic hypothermia was in common use during this initial time period in open-heart surgery and was used as a protective device to allow for extended periods of surgical repair. Monitoring of the patient's body temperature during both cooling and rewarming was essential in the control of a desired temperature, especially during the rewarming phase. The Brown Harrison stainless steel heat exchanger was an integral component of the heart-lung machine and, similar to other nondisposable heat exchange devices of that era, also required a large priming volume in order to afford enough surface area for adequate heat exchange to occur. Any subsequent drop in body temperature, in the immediate postoperative period, could cause myocardial irritability with potential serious cardiac effects. The rectal temperature was initially monitored and was thought to be reflective of core temperature while the esophageal temperature was reflective of the brain temperature, the organ most sensitive to neurological insult. During this initial era, systemic pressure monitoring consisted of measuring arterial pressures with nondisposable transducers that could take considerable time to properly calibrate. The arterial transducer would be attached to pressurized glass bottles and great care was taken to monitor appropriate fluid levels in the bottle so as to prevent inadvertent air embolism. Central venous pressure was monitored by a simplified CVP manometer placed at the patient's heart level. The routine use of Swan Ganz catheters would not be realized until several years later. The monitoring of blood gases was performed by remote machines as were readily available tools to monitor acid base balance. As mentioned earlier, ACT was not available during this era and full systemic heparinization was followed on an hourly basis by repeated heparin doses. The arterial/venous oxygen difference was determined by visual observation only and the arterial line PO2 was often compared to the color of a pack of Matinee cigarettes (Canadian) or Marlboros (U.S.). The heart-lung technician would initiate CPB with their finger on the arterial line in order to monitor the arterial line pressure in the attempt to prevent a retrograde aortic dissection via the femoral artery. Routine inline monitoring of arterial PO2 was not to be realized until the early 1970s.

The Disposable Era

The early 1970s had arrived and, throughout Canada, the complexity and associated concerns of the mechanical pump oxygenators would soon be resolved with the introduction of commercially available disposable bubble oxygenators. As mentioned, the pioneering work and initial clinical success experienced by Lillehei in using the Lillehei/DeWall Helix disposable oxygenator design paved the way for the commercial introduction and further refinement of a new generation of disposable bubble oxygenators that incorporated an oxygenation column, a defoaming chamber and an arterial reservoir. In Halifax, we had begun using our first disposable oxygenator in the early 1970s when we began to clinically use the Travenol disposable soft shell plastic oxygenator produced commercially by Baxter Corporation. It was available in three sizes, the 2LF for infants, the 3LF for pediatric use and the 6LF for the adult patient.

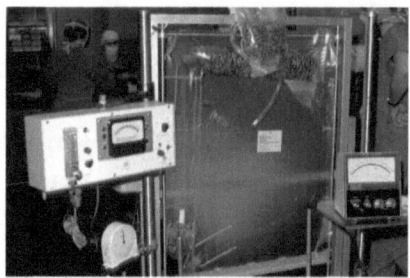

Fig. 16:9 The Travenol Baxter 6LF Soft Shell disposable bubble oxygenator.

It incorporated a simple soft bag design consisting of two sheets of polyvinyl chloride fused together forming segmental channels that resembled the design of the DeWall Helix oxygenator. Although oxygenation was considered to be satisfactory, the Travenol oxygenator did not incorporate an integral heat exchanger. During that time period, the Bentley Temptrol disposable oxygenator, a three-dimensional hard shell oxygenator with incorporating heat exchanger, was being introduced clinically.

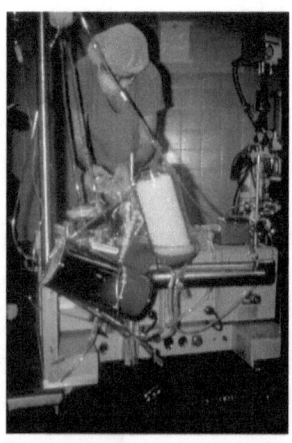

Fig. 16:10 The Bentley Temptrol Hard Shell disposable bubble oxygenator

It too was available in three sizes in order to meet the full spectrum of clinical needs. The heat exchange capacity of the Temptrol oxygenator heat exchanger proved to be less than adequate, so the the Sarns stainless steel heat exchanger was used with the Temptrol oxygenator to facilitate adequate heat transfer. The William Harvey hard shell disposable oxygenator was the first concentric design oxygenator to be manufactured; it incorporated an internal designed heat exchanger that would prove to be very efficient in both oxygenation and heat transfer capability.

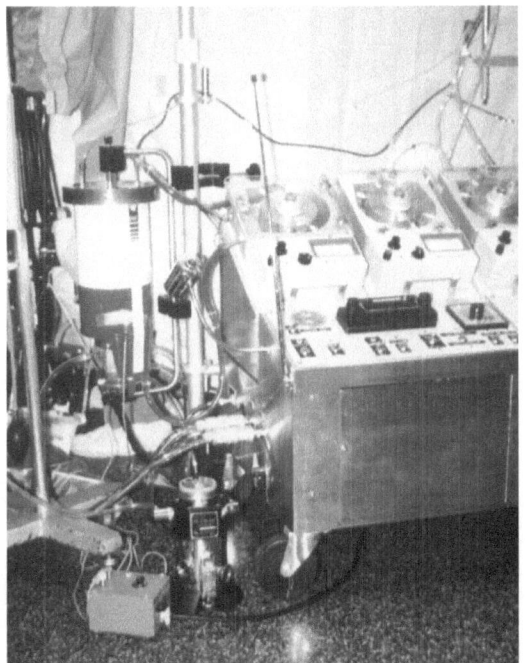

Fig. 16:11 The William Harvey Hard Shell Concentric disposable bubble oxygenator.

During this time period, Shiley Laboratories had also produced two models of their disposable oxygenator for clinical use, the S-100 and the S-100-A. The S-100-A had the same general configuration as the previous S-100 model. The main difference was that S-100 had a heat exchanger coated with polyureathane and the S-100-A used an anodized aluminium coating. This was the era of dependable low prime commercially affordable disposable bubble oxygenators that would witness the growth in open-heart surgery in Canada and elsewhere in the world. In Europe, the soft shell disposable Rygg Kyvsgaard plastic bag oxygenator, initially introduced in 1956, would go through several design modifications and would enjoy limited but successful use within Canada.

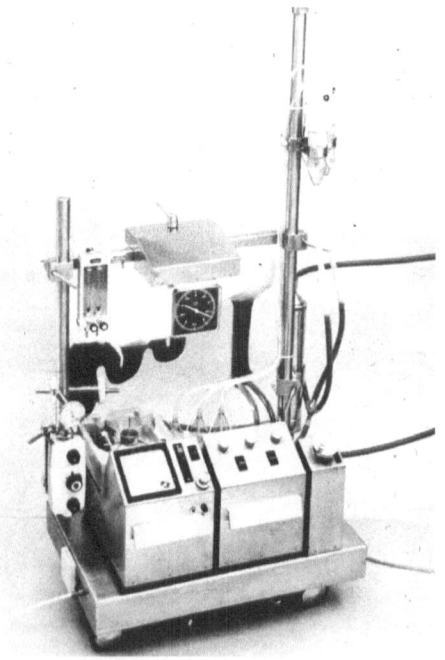

Fig. 16:12 The Rygg Kyvsgaard Polystan soft shell disposable bubble oxygenator with incorporated heat exchanger seen with the Polystan heart-lung machine module.

Summary

In the 1970s, disposable oxygenators and the manufacture of reliable heart-lung machines such as the Sarns heart-lung pump console became the essential adjunct to routinely successful open-heart surgery. The era of dependability in these modern extracorporeal devices had arrived and pump oxygenators would be used without much fanfare within Canada and elsewhere. The subsequent growth of the perfusion profession within Canada will be highlighted elsewhere in this chapter. Of interest, the pump technician of the 1960/1970 era was initially trained "on the job" and often came from various professional backgrounds. Many of these original pioneers were associated with cardiac surgery in such professional roles as physician, operating room nurse, operating room technician, biomedical engineer or lab assistant, etc., and were recruited by individual cardiac surgeons who were familiar with their individual professional backgrounds. During this era, the animal research lab became the training ground where the thoracic surgeon and the pump technician would test the extracorporeal equipment and further refine various surgical techniques. Educational resource material was limited to a few publications. In 1972, Pierre M. Galletti and G. A. Brecher published their cornerstone review of extracorporeal circulation, *Heart-Lung Bypass*, which was considered to be the "bible" for perfusion. One year later, Yukihiko Nose published his *Manual of Artificial Organs, Volume 11: The Oxygenator*, which provided an excellent historical review of various oxygenator configurations and function. Raymond Stofer published *A Technique for Extracorporeal Circulation* which chronicled his initial clinical experience with the Kay-Cross disks oxygenator. Throughout Canada, the thoracic surgeon of the day and the pump technician continued to develop a professional respect that grew out of the need for mutual cooperation within their shared clinical responsibilities. This era of cooperation and dependence on each other would form the foundation of a new specialty called clinical perfusion. One is reminded of the words of Dr. W. G. Bigelow in chapter 5 of his book *Cold Hearts: The Story of Hypothermia and Pacemakers in Heart Surgery.*

> *A new specialty evolved with the advent of the heart-lung pump, that of perfusionist. The responsibility of running the pump was indeed an extremely important one, shared by the anaesthetist. There was the careful cleaning and assembly, adjustments of blood flow, pressure, temperature, balancing blood volumes between the patient and the pump, debubbling, blood analysis and additives. There were hair raising experiences in the early days that taxed their stability, courage and judgement. Modern oxygenators are disposable, with pump and blood cooling devices that are more efficient, but the responsibility is still there.*

HEART SURGERY IN CANADA— A PERFUSION PERSPECTIVE

Kathy Deemar

The addition of cardiopulmunary bypass (CPB) in 1953 greatly increased the scope of cardiac surgery.

The necessity of having perfusionists as part of the surgical team has evolved due to the increased sophistication of technical intervention developed for patients requiring assisted circulation.

The people who operated this new equipment were from different backgrounds, OR nurses, OR technicians, biomedical technicians and others. Formal Perfusion training programs did not start until the early 1970s in the United States, and in Canada the first training program was started in 1979. The program was built on the Respiratory Technology program that was offered at the Toronto Institute of Medical Technology (TIMT). It is a postgraduate program with the requirements being a Registered Nurse, a Registered Respiratory Therapist, or equivalent.

Prior to the training programs, people were trained on the job and the standards varied across the country. The number of people involved was small, making it hard to develop standards. With the rapid increase of cases during the 1970s the profession grew. In the United States, the number of perfusionists was ten times the number in Canada, which helped them to organize and form the American Society of Extracorporeal Technology in the early 1970s, developing national standards and a certification process. At this time, Canadian perfusionists recognized the need to organize as well; although their numbers made this difficult the need was there, leading to the formation of the Canadian Society of Extracorporeal Technology and the development of a Canadian exam. There were only about seventy members, most of whom wrote the exam, but the standards still varied because none of these members had gone through a formal training program. In the end this society fell apart and an association with the American Society was sought. In 1976, the American Society grandfathered all practicing Canadian perfusionists into the American Society, with the only requirement being that the American exam be written within three years. Getting more people to write the new American exam worked well: in addition to increasing the exam's validity, it allowed the Canadians to set a standard for their profession. By 1979, the year the TIMT program started, any Canadians who had not taken the American exam were now obliged to pass it. That year two on-the-job trained Canadians challenged the exam and passed; I was one of those individuals. By 1984 the requirement that perfusionists trained on-the-job write the American exam was dropped and graduation from a recognized training program, which included TIMT, was required. (There are now two Canadian training programs, which are the only programs recognized outside of the United States). The Canadians who have written the American exam have done well and the two Canadian training programs have always scored well.

With the continued growth of cardiac surgery the numbers of perfusionists in Canada grew. By 1989, there were about 150 perfusionists in the country and the Canadian government was talking about professional accountability. At a Canadian meeting that year a group of perfusionists, realizing that if we didn't organize the government could group us with another professional organization, started to work on what would become the Canadian Society of Clinical Perfusion (CSCP). This was accomplished, with a great deal of effort, and in 1990 the first Canadian certifying exam took place.

The society has maintained high standards and today there are about two hundred practicing perfusionists in the country. There are now two training programs, one in BC at the University College of the Cariboo and the original in Ontario, which is now called the Michener Institute of Applied Health Sciences. The CSCP offers the certification exam at its annual general meeting in October every year. The person who hired me was Talara "Tally" Hill who had been an OR nurse trained on-the-job in the late 1960s. She was the head of the perfusion department and ran the animal lab so we worked in the OR and with researchers in the lab. Having developed close ties with her colleagues in the States she was very aware of the need to have professional standards and a training program.

At the time Tally hired me she had been talking to TIMT about training in perfusion. She had looked at the Respiratory Technology program as a base and built on it to develop the perfusion program. I was a Respiratory Technologist before starting my on-the-job training so she found me to be a good test person for the additional skills and knowledge needed for perfusion. The animal lab provided a great part of my training; not only did I learn how to perform the surgery, but also how to build a circuit from scratch and operate the pump.

The technology has evolved as quickly as the profession. In the fifties and sixties reusable disc oxygenators (a screen oxygenator) were used. These devices had metal discs that rotated through a bath of the patient's blood, picking up a thin layer of blood and exposing it to an oxygen rich environment. The number of discs varied depending on the size of the patient. These devices were cumbersome, often leaked, and took a lot of time to be cleaned for reuse. They also required a lot of volume to prime, often using blood as volume to reduce the effects of hemodilution. By the late sixties a disposable plastic "bag" was being used. These oxygenators were large flexible bubble oxygenators that needed to be mounted and wired to a frame. These also required large volumes to prime but had the advantage of being disposable.

In the mid-1970s the first hard-shell plastic disposable bubble oxygenator was introduced. It was much easier to set up; however the heat exchange compartment was on the arterial side of the device, which made de-airing it very difficult. With the introduction of plastic injection moulds to the production line, these devices became easier to make and cheaper. The designs improved, shifting the heat exchanger to the venous side. These devices were easy to use and were very reliable.

Membrane oxygenators have been around since cellophane was first used for an artificial kidney but they were not as effective and inexpensive as the bubble oxygenators. Their main drawback was that the material used was limited by its ability to remove CO_2. The original membrane oxygenators used silicon as the membrane material. These devices were difficult to set up and de-air and were much more expensive then the bubble oxygenators. They were used for long term support or long, difficult cases. Silicon is permeable to both O_2 and CO_2 but is limited by how thin it can be made. By using hollow fibers or sheets made from polypropylene that had micropores of 0.1 microns in size, the new generation of oxygenators were now efficient gas exchange devices. These oxygenators could be made at a cost competitive with the bubble oxygenators, were less harmful to the blood formed elements, and more importantly, were as easy to set up as a bubble oxygenator. With the addition of an arterial line filter and a cardiotomy filter the postoperative ventilation time decreased significantly and ICU stay was shortened.

Myocardial protection is the other area that has changed greatly over the years. Dr. Bigelow is well known for his work with hypothermia, a technique widely used. When I first started, electrically fibrillating the heart or hypothermic anoxic arrest was practiced. The patient was systemically cooled the patient to the range of 28 to 25 degrees Celsius and a cold topical solution was poured over the myocardium. The heart would fibrillate spontaneously. In the seventies we started using cold crystalloid cardioplegia solution (CPS). The next improvement was the introduction in the early eighties of blood cardioplegia. We first used a 2:1 mix, two parts blood to one part crystalloid solution. Then we moved on to 4:1 and now it's 8:1 or greater. These techniques were all used in combination with hypothermia. Then in the late eighties, we started to introduce a terminal warm shot of blood cardioplegia or "hot shot" just before the cross clamp came off. From there started the study of warm versus cold heart surgery. Many centres no longer actively cool patients or use cold CPS. The chemical mix of the cardioplegia varies greatly from centre to centre with various drugs added to the mix to improve myocardial function and to reduce the effects of cross-clamping.

There is constant work being done to decrease the deleterious effects of cardiopulmonary bypass (CPB). The circuits have been made smaller, requiring less volume for priming. Most of the components are now designed on a computer, where flow simulations can be done prior to manufacturing; this has helped reduce the cost of making the components, and has decreased the time between design concept and the product being released to the market. There has been a lot of work on biological coating of the total CPB circuit to make it less reactive to the blood formed elements. The assist devices and artificial hearts have evolved as well. This area will allow us to offer patients alternatives to transplants or give them time to receive a donor heart. In Canada it has always been a challenge to provide the best patient care in a fiscally responsible manner. Some of the evolving technologies are expensive and enough research is needed to prove that patient outcomes improve sufficiently to justify the increased cost. This can be difficult because what we think we can do to benefit the patient may not fit the budget. An example would be biological coating for the CPB circuit: this has shown in some studies to decrease the effects of CPB, but is considerably more expensive then the conventional circuit currently in use.

Perfusionists have become involved in many other areas such as cell saving, plasma sequestration, IABP (intraaortic balloon pump), pacemakers, assisting in OPCAB (off pump coronary artery bypass) surgery, veno-venous support for liver surgery and thoraco-abdominal surgery, hyperthermic perfusion for cancer, and other areas. By broadening our scope of practice the profession will continue to grow.

CPB has changed considerably in fifty years and continues to evolve to better meet our patients' needs. The perfusionist has been very active in that process and will continue to be so in the years to come. The equipment we use today is more sophisticated, better made and safer than fifty years ago. When I started my career in perfusion we were using a plastic bag bubble oxygenator that needed to be wired to a metal frame. This device was large and required a considerable volume to prime it, resulting in patients that were excessively volume overloaded. The patients were induced with morphine and often arrested or became very hypotensive during induction. We used only vein for conduits. The perfusion circuit did not have any filters in it so the patients' lungs were the filters. We did not understand the importance of myocardial protection and we were not able to fine tune variables such as heparin levels, glucose control or even venous saturation. It was not unusual for patients to be ventilated for two days post-op because their lungs were so wet.

Currently the perfusionists are better trained and more knowledgeable then ever before. The equipment we use has improved greatly, as has our understanding of how CPB affects the body. The drugs we use are much safer and we have a better understanding of their use. Our patient outcomes have greatly improved over the years and will continue to do so.

Will the perfusionist still be needed in ten or twenty years? I think the job will change but we will continue to be highly skilled professionals that are an integral part of the cardiac team.

CHAPTER 17

VIEW FROM THE UNITED STATES:
IS THE GRASS GREENER?

Tomas Antonio Salerno

This chapter deals with the health care system and the systems of education and research in Canada and the United States. These are my personal views, based solely on my own experience in Canada and the United States, and do not reflect any political or other interests.

I. Brief Review of the Canadian System of Health Care

Since the nineteenth century, the organization of health and social services in Canada has undergone dramatic changes. What follows is a synopsis of major historical events leading to the current system of health care and the role of the contemporary physician.

Until the end of the Second World War, hospitals and other health care organizations were run by charitable community organizations and churches. Federal and provincial government involvement was limited to the realms of public health and welfare. In 1947, Saskatchewan became the first province to enact universal government financed hospital insurance with the passage of the Saskatchewan Hospitalization Plan.

In 1957, the federal government passed the Hospital Insurance and Diagnostic Services Act, giving it authority to negotiate cost-sharing hospital insurance plans with the provinces. By 1961, all of the provinces had signed agreements providing for free universal diagnostic services and hospital accommodation. Funding was derived from tax revenues, with the federal and provincial governments contributing roughly 50 percent apiece. Physicians' fees were still not covered.

Following the report of the federal Royal Commission on Health Services (1964-65) which recommended a national system of Medicare, the government introduced the Medical Care Act in 1966. Under this legislation it agreed to negotiate a cost-sharing agreement for free access to physician services with each province, subject to five criteria:

1. Universality: public health insurance coverage for the entire population;
2. Comprehensive coverage of hospital and all physician fees wherever incurred;
3. Public management of the system;
4. Portability of coverage from province to province; and
5. Accessibility of all to hospital and physician services without financial or other barriers.

The act came into effect in 1968, and by 1972 all provinces had instituted Medicare coverage agreements.

By the mid-1970s, health care costs were rising and the federal government was no longer able to match the demands of the provinces. In 1977, the original 50-50 cost-sharing arrangement was replaced by Established Programs Financing, a block funding system that provided tax and cash transfers to the provincial governments to finance health care and postsecondary education. Since 1977, the federal government's contribution in these areas has been steadily declining.

Under these new strains, some provinces, in particular Alberta and Ontario, allowed extra billing and user fees for services rendered. In response to concerns that these extra charges were limiting accessibility of health care by creating a two-tier system, the federal government passed the Canada Health Act in 1984. A revised version of the Medical Care Act, this legislation imposed financial penalties for provinces allowing extra billing.

In 2001, 9.7 percent of Canada's gross domestic product was spent on health care—significantly more than the OECD average of 8.4 percent, though considerably lower than the United States., which at 13.9 percent devoted the largest share of its GDP to health expenditures. Canada likewise ranked above the OECD average in health spending per capita, at $2,792 compared with $2,117 (in U.S. dollars), but fell far short of the U.S. figure of $4,887. The per capita GDP for Canada in 2001 was $28,923, compared with $35,179 in the United States.[1]

In an effort to cut costs and streamline services, the Canadian health care system has undergone structural changes. Responsibility for health care planning and management has traditionally rested with the ministry of health in each province. Yet within the last decade, most provinces have downloaded (or "devolved") much of the decision-making power in health care to regional health boards or councils.[2]

Within the province of Quebec, for example, there are currently eighteen Regional Health and Social Service

Boards, which plan and implement services, allocate budgets to health care establishments, and provide feedback to the Ministry of Health and Social Services (*Ministère de la Santé et des Services sociaux*). The regional boards are comprised of an executive director and various community and medical representatives, including a Regional Medical Commission. The membership of the Regional Medical Commission for Montreal-Centre includes three general practitioners, three specialists, the director of public health, the executive director of the regional board, and two members appointed by the deans of the region's faculties of medicine. The role of this commission is to advise the board on the organization of medical services, distribution of manpower, and payment methods for the region.

Cost-cutting efforts have resulted in the decentralization of medical services, hospital closures, mergers of institutions, and the shifting of resources to ambulatory care and day-surgery centers. The increased focus on ambulatory care has allowed more and more health care to be provided outside of the institutional setting.

Physicians have likewise moved increasingly toward private practice where they enjoy easier access to patients and greater professional freedom. Remuneration in private practice is governed in each province by its own health insurance legislation, which details which services are insured, and varies to some extent from province to province. For health-care services that are not covered under a given provincial plan, recommended fee schedules are provided.

Personal Experiences with the Health Care System

I graduated from medical school in 1971 at McGill University in Montreal, and undertook my training in general surgery and cardiothoracic surgery at the Royal Victoria Hospital there. During my undergraduate years at McGill, I experienced health problems that required hospitalization at the Royal Victoria. At discharge, although there was no charge for hospital care, I was faced with a large bill for the medical services provided. This was an intolerable situation since I lived on an annual US$700 scholarship from the Leopold Schepp Foundation of New York, which covered all my school and housing expenses. This was my first experience with the system of health care that existed in Canada before the implementation of the Medical Care Act. I was rescued by the Dean of my school, who was eventually able to persuade the physicians and surgeons involved to waive the medical bills—but not before I had received threats from collection agencies.

Only those who have experienced such a crisis in their lives can appreciate the meaning of universal care as it now exists in Canada. The system is not perfect, and I will attempt to describe some of the problems that I perceive may exist. However, the population of Canada is assured of access to health care without incurring serious financial burden when an illness occurs in the family.

I have had the opportunity to hold positions of leadership in both Canada and the United States. In Canada, I rose to the rank of associate professor of surgery at Queen's University, then undertook a similar position at McGill. In 1983 I was recruited as chief of cardiovascular and thoracic surgery at St. Michael's Hospital in Toronto, and served as chair of the cardiovascular surgery division in the University of Toronto's department of surgery between 1987 and 1992. I then served as chief of the cardiothoracic surgery division at the State University of New York at Buffalo until 1999, when I took up my present position at the University of Miami as Professor and chief of cardiothoracic surgery and chief of the CT Surgery Program at Jackson Memorial Hospital, one of the largest health facilities in the United States. These have all been academic positions. While in Buffalo, I had the opportunity to work with a large number of private cardiac surgeons and was also Chief of the major hospital in the city. My opinions are, therefore, somewhat biased towards the academic life, although I have also had some experience with the private sector in the United States.

During my undergraduate medical training, the Medical Care Act was passed and medical insurance plans were implemented in the various provinces. As I recall, by the mid-1970s the federal government was already experiencing difficulties with rising health care costs; and by the time I finished training in cardiothoracic surgery in 1977, the original federal-provincial cost-sharing agreement had been changed and federal contributions to heath care had begun to decline.

Universal health care is appealing to the general public. Although funds are collected through taxes, care is provided "free of charge" to all Canadians when illness occurs. Physicians initially complained about the control exerted by the government, but this was soon followed by the comfort that, unlike previously, payment for all services provided was guaranteed. Furthermore, a single bill was submitted for each service to one agency (the provincial government) and a cheque was forthcoming at the end of the month.

Yet as I recall, government intervention in health care increased as time went by, including income capping and limits on the resources allocated to the various hospitals. Following the passage of the Canada Health

Act in 1984, extra billing was not allowed and physicians could only charge for services according to the fee schedule negotiated with the provincial government. In the field of cardiac surgery, it became apparent that there were insufficient resources in the Ontario health care system to meet patient demand, resulting in long waiting lists and deaths occurring among patients waiting for surgery. Growing public concern and adverse newspaper and television publicity eventually led to a formal investigation of cardiac surgery at St. Michael's Hospital by a three-member team appointed by the Ontario Ministry of Health.

In their 1989 report, the investigators concluded that there was a province-wide shortage of cardiac-care resources, as well as inefficiencies in triage and allocation of patients. Several recommendations were made which led to increased capacity for heart surgery in the various Toronto hospitals, the creation of an additional cardiac unit at Sunnybrook Health Science Centre, and a triage system that allowed patients to be moved from one hospital to another and, at times, to another city or province. This solution caused inconvenience for patients who had to be transferred from their familiar environment, but dealt with the acute crisis.

Due to long waiting lists, patients with the means to do so frequently opted to have their cardiac procedures performed south of the border in the USA. American hospitals were prepared to accommodate them within a moment's notice. How ironic that the Canadian health care system, in severe need of funds, was losing patients who could afford to pay for services. However, businessmen and others alike, facing serious financial consequences from extended sick leave on rather long waiting lists, found it to their advantage to spend valuable dollars outside the country. It is my impression that, to some degree, this situation still exists today.

The Attitude of Physicians in Canada

Complacency sets in over time in the Canadian health care system. Patient demand is so great that physicians usually do not have to worry about competition for patients. The only limitation for the cardiac surgeon is the availability of operating rooms and ICU beds, always in short supply. With their incomes capped, it seemed to me that physicians lost the incentive to take on additional cases upon reaching the maximum. Hospitals were likewise discouraged from performing more than a fixed number of procedures—at least during my years in Canada—since they were not reimbursed for cases exceeding the quota. I am not sure whether this situation still exists today. Patients with serious coronary artery disease were sent home and, by the time they came back for surgery, one questioned whether the angiogram was still applicable, since so much time had elapsed between the angiogram and the surgical treatment. Surgeons found themselves trying to decide who they should operate upon, taking into consideration the patients' age, work habits and other socioeconomic factors.

In Quebec, physicians initiating their practice received reduced payments unless they agreed with the Regional Medical Commission to practice in institutions designated by the Commission in accordance with distribution of manpower in the province. That usually meant going to work in underprivileged areas for several years. Restrictions were placed in certain areas, especially in the major cities, and physicians entering practice would receive approximately 70 percent of the standard fee in an urban area and approximately 130 percent of the fee if they went into an underserved rural area.

Changes in Medical Education

There have in addition been major changes in medical education within the past decade, which pose challenges to medical students who have to decide very early in medical school what specialty they would like to pursue. Furthermore, unless they complete their specialty training, they no longer automatically qualify for licensing as general practitioners. A physician who abandons specialty training midstream now has to find a position in a two-year family medicine program—all of which are usually taken—in order to qualify for certification by the College of Family Physicians of Canada. All physicians must also pass the two-part qualifying examination of the Medical Council of Canada (MCCQE parts 1 and 2) and become a Licentiate of the Council (LMCC) before obtaining certification in family practice or a specialty, and a license to practice medicine within a given province.

The American Board of Thoracic Surgery (ABTS) no longer recognizes Canadian training in cardiac or cardiothoracic surgery, despite the fact that the Canadian programs are excellent. Requirements for the Canadian Boards are for only three years of general surgery training, whereas their counterpart in the United States requires five years of general surgery in a program approved by the Educational Commission for Foreign Medical Graduates (ECFMG). Since Canadian programs in cardiac and cardiothoracic surgery are not ECFMG approved, residents trained in these specialties in Canada do not qualify to take the ABTS examinations. This severely limits opportunities for trainees completing their postgraduate training in Canada.

Furthermore, a physician who wants to practice in Quebec must undertake at least one year of medical training in the province and pass a French exam. The candidate must also pass the certification exams of the Collège des médecins du Québec and ALDO-Québec, an examination on the "legislative, ethical and organizational aspects of medical practice" in the province. Recruitment to key positions of leadership at universities in Quebec is severely restricted, since most physicians outside the province do not speak French. This limits the recruitment of world leaders to head the universities and their programs. Candidates to an English-language university must attempt the French exam each year but are given a good many years to pass it.

Academic Education

Medical education in Canada traditionally followed the didactic, classroom-based model. However, in recent years, Canadian medical faculties have adopted the contemporary problem-based learning approach. Problem-based learning, essentially a case-based curriculum carried out in small group seminars, was more or less invented during the late 1960s at McMaster University in Hamilton, Ontario, and has been widely copied in Canada and in many American universities, including Harvard. In the United States, the medical student spends a considerable amount of time in hospitals, receiving a clinically based education.

I personally feel that the standard of education is higher in Canada than in the United States. In the area of collegiate sports, for example, American students involved in sports have a lower GPA than their counterparts in Canada. There is tremendous pressure on American college athletes to perform on the field, with lucrative contracts that can undermine the players' education. Class sizes tend to be smaller in Canada, allowing for more personal contact between teacher and student. Universities in the United

States are also on average larger than in Canada, and they are far more numerous: there are currently medical programs in 130 American universities, 17 in Canada.[3]

II. The American Health Care System

The American health care system is considered to be among the best in the world. Although it offers much in the area of advanced technology, innovative treatment and care, it has limitations. The present system of managed care has been evolving for over a decade, a system of cost-containment health insurance plans including health maintenance organizations (HMOs) and preferred provider organizations (PPOs). The system garners many complaints from physicians regarding restrictions on the care that they can provide to their patients, authorization processes, and rates and delays in reimbursement.

In contrast to the Canadian system of socialized medicine, the American health care industry is largely funded by private insurance companies, and includes HMOs, PPOs, fee-for-service plans, and the government Medicare and Medicaid plans. There are also various other government-funded programs providing health insurance for the indigent population. The following is a brief description of the most common types of third party payers and their impact on private and academic medical practice.

Health Maintenance Organizations (HMOs)

HMOs are prepaid health plans in which the health care providers within an HMO group agree to provide specific benefits as needed for a fixed fee per client. Clients are asked to choose a primary care physician or other specialists from a list provided by the HMO. The primary care physician coordinates all of the client's medical care, and has to authorize referrals, where necessary, to a specialist and/or health care facility.

HMOs have various types of contractual agreements with physicians: Group HMO physicians, are either employed by the HMO or receive the bulk of their patients from the plan. "Staff-model HMO physicians" are employed solely by the HMO, limit their practice accordingly, and are paid a set salary. Doctors who enter into an independent practice arrangement with an HMO are paid a fixed fee and reimbursement for services. These physicians usually also have a separate fee-for-service practice. An HMO network model is formed when two or more independent physician groups enter into a contract with an HMO for medical services to its clients. Doctors in the network receive a set monthly fee per client from the HMO.

HMOs have achieved high marks for bringing affordable health coverage to a wide range of consumers, but at what cost? Obviously, patients want the best choices of physicians and health care facilities, and with the wide accessibility of the Internet, many individuals are now researching these options for their care. However, HMOs are prepaid health plans which provide health care from within their own group practices and/or through doctors and other health care professionals under contract. Coverage for most services is usually 100 percent. If a client wishes to be treated by a physician or in a facility outside the HMO's network without prior authorization (which is rarely granted), no coverage is provided. Recently however, a unanimous ruling was made by the United States Supreme Court that the state of Kentucky could "force HMOs to accept any qualified doctors who wants to join."[4] This decision is a significant step in allowing patients greater autonomy and flexibility in choosing their health care provider.

Patient care is traditionally determined mainly by the physician directly involved in the case. With the advent of managed care plans, however, physicians often find themselves hampered by insurance company restrictions as to the types of diagnostic tests, procedures, and even medications that can be prescribed for their patients. "Many doctors across the country say dealing with HMOs has begun to change the way medicine is practiced . . . [and] more than half said HMOs have stopped them from providing treatments and services they considered 'medically necessary.'"[5] Many of my colleagues complain that they have spent inordinate amounts of time arguing with an HMO to obtain approval to prescribe medication and treatment needed by a patient. "'Doctors are working longer for less pay and feeling more frustrated, more fed up with the system and having to qualify additional treatment through representatives of managed care companies who are not physicians,' said Dr. John Grohol, a Texas-based psychologist who oversees mental health content for DrKoop.com."[5] The average monthly payment to physicians in an HMO network is US$10 per patient. In an effort to make their practices financially sound, these doctors are apt to reduce the time spent with each patient, thereby potentially affecting quality of care.

In order to be reimbursed for treating a patient insured by an HMO, an independent physician and/or health care facility must obtain prior authorization. This time-consuming exercise usually requires additional staffing, thereby increasing the cost of doing business. Such requests are usually made to the HMO's utilization department, headed by a licensed physician who has the final say in whether authorization will be granted. HMO subscribers must also obtain a "referral" from their primary care physician for consultation with a specialist, who must also be under contract with the HMO.

Preferred Provider Organizations (PPOs)

The Preferred Provider Organization combines some traditional fee-for-service features with those of an HMO, with providers agreeing to discounted fees for providing care to PPO members. Like an HMO, however, there are a limited number of doctors and hospitals to choose from. When the insured selects a provider within the network, the insurance company pays most of the medical bills. Members can choose to receive care from a provider outside the PPO network, but must then pay a higher deductible and/or co-payment.

Fee-for-Service

This is the traditional kind of health care policy, offering the most choice of doctors and health care facilities to the consumer. Patients are free to choose any provider they wish, and can change provider at any time. In this type of plan, the insurance company pays for part of the care provided, minus a preset yearly deductible, which becomes the responsibility of the insured. Typically this cost sharing is 20 percent payable by the insured with 80 percent paid by the insurance company.

Medicare

Medicare is the federal health insurance program for Americans age sixty-five and older, the disabled, and people with end-stage renal disease. Medicare has two parts: hospital insurance (known as part A), and supplementary medical insurance (part B), which covers physicians' fees and related services and supplies. Medicare does not cover most nursing home care; long-term care services in the home or prescription drugs.

Medicaid

Medicaid provides health care coverage for some low-income people who cannot afford other forms of health insurance. People eligible to receive Medicaid include seniors and the disabled who do not meet the criteria for Medicare eligibility, as well as certain families with dependent children. Medicaid is a federal program operated by the individual states, which decide the criteria for eligibility and the scope of health services offered.

Uninsured/Underinsured

According to the National Center for Health Statistics, approximately 17 percent of Americans under sixty-five, or a little over forty-two million individuals, were uninsured as of the year 2000.[6] Equal access to care is considered extremely important in this country, so in an effort to ensure the availability of equal health care access to the poor, uninsured and underinsured, the government has instituted programs to finance health care for the indigent who do not qualify for Medicaid assistance. Yet since these programs frequently require a co-payment and/or deductible, which the participants often cannot afford to pay, they fail to fulfill the purpose for which they were created. Preventive care is usually not practiced. Health care is sought only when absolutely urgent, usually through a hospital emergency room. These individuals then present sicker than they would have been had they sought care in a more timely manner, thereby increasing mortality, morbidity, and cost.

Many teaching hospitals are county based and are often perceived by the public as offering free medical care. In fact, at Jackson Memorial Hospital in Miami we often experience patients from other countries coming directly from the airport to our emergency room, with their medical records in hand, seeking care. Many private, for-profit hospitals have also being guilty of practicing "patient dumping," a term used to describe hospitals denying treatment to indigent, uninsured or underinsured patients, either by refusing care outright or by transferring them to other facilities. In 1986 the government passed the Emergency Medical and Active Labor Act (EMTALA), to curtail this practice. With the passing of this law, every hospital that receives Medicare dollars is required to provide medical screening and stabilizing treatment to any patient who seeks care in their facility.

Teaching Hospitals

Teaching hospitals in America are the classrooms for the clinical education of physicians and other health care professionals. Statistics show that the cost of care is usually higher at teaching hospitals—approximately 5 percent higher for Medicare patients alone—and insurance companies, citing cost concerns, are reluctant to have contractual agreements with these facilities. In defense of this disparity, teaching hospitals feel that cutting costs too much would damage their mission of training good doctors. At Jackson Memorial Hospital, the teaching hospital where I practice, we have an active Managed Care Department that aggressively pursues contracting with managed care networks and HMOs to help to ensure a good volume of patient referrals to the facility, and therefore to physicians and residents.

III. Comparison of the Canadian and American Health Care Systems

In the previous sections I have given some background on the two systems of health care, along with some views and personal experiences with both systems. This final section provides a summary and comparison of the two health care systems.

Health care in Canada is socialized, providing "free" care for all Canadians regardless of their socioeconomic status. Canadians feel secure that they will receive treatment when in need, and accept long waiting times for services. In each province there is a single fee schedule and a single payer (the government), and with the exception of uninsured services, additional fees are not allowed. Physicians have an abundance of patients to care for, their income is usually subject to some form of capping, and they work in either private clinics or government-funded hospitals.

Medical care in the United States, in contrast, follows more of a free-market model. Most working people and those over sixty-five are assured of some form of insurance, while the underprivileged are looked after by county hospitals under Medicaid. Services are paid for from a variety of sources, with individually negotiated contracts for services. Insurers generally decide how much they will pay for the services rendered. Authorization usually has to be obtained from the insurer prior to giving treatment, and insurers may decline to cover services provided by surgeons or institutions outside their network. They may also disallow claims, such as excess time recovering from surgery that they consider unreasonable. Americans do not accept waiting lists, either short or long. An abundance of hospitals competing in a free market makes access to care readily available for all patients with insurance coverage. It would be inconceivable for an American physician, such as a heart surgeon, to accept income capping. For-profit hospitals seem to do well in the market, although recently some have succumbed to competition.

Data collection and monitoring have been strictly adhered to by some U.S. states, including New York, and by such institutions as the Veteran Administration Medical Centers. As a result, information on say, mortality for cardiac surgery, by center or by a given surgeon, is readily available via the Internet, and is sometimes published in newspapers. Hospitals and surgeons with favorable scores use this data as a marketing tool to attract patients.

Most Canadian physicians have malpractice insurance through one agency, the Canadian Medical Protective Association (CMPA). There is tremendous benefit from this in terms of protection and security. The malpractice climate in Canada, although changing, is much different than its counterpart in the United States. In the United States, there is no equivalent system, and since lawyers have discovered this important source of revenue, the physician is easily sued on a regular basis. Malpractice litigation has reached such proportions that physicians in some states have decided not to carry malpractice insurance. Such is the case in Florida, where annual premiums have reached levels of over US$100,000 for some specialties. Physicians simply advise patients prior to providing services that they do not have malpractice insurance in case of an adverse outcome. This matter has posed a tremendous burden on the health care system, and is one of the issues that will have to be resolved in the near future by means of legislation. Americans are more litigious in all aspects of life, including medicine. The biggest difference, in my view, is that most Canadian medical malpractice disputes are decided in front of a judge, compared to the United States where they are brought before a jury.

The paradigm for the United States in health care is business, with competition and marketing of services provided by the various institutions. In Canada, medical care is government controlled. This is possible due to the small population base in Canada compared to the United States, and different sociopolitical philosophies in the two countries.

The educational system is likewise very different in the two countries. American universities tend to be very large and their number far exceeds those in Canada.

Because of recent changes in Canadian medical education, students completing medical school and internship are no longer eligible for licensing without additional training in family medicine or a specialty. The current Royal College requirements in cardiac and thoracic surgery, and the fact that most Canadian medical schools are not ECFGM approved, mean that the physician will be unable to take the American examinations, thereby limiting their options as to where to find work. Medical education in the United States has also undergone changes, but after internship, physicians can obtain a licence and are free to practice wherever they want, with no government restrictions or penalties as exist in Canada.

What would a heart surgeon moving from Canada to the United States, and vice versa, experience upon arrival at the workplace? Both would have good clinical training, but both would experience psychological and cultural challenges.

The American surgeon would find it difficult to be told where to work, as in Quebec; the penalties for not working in a designated area and for failing to learn French, and to find out that there is an income cap for services provided, with financial penalties once the maximum is reached. The physician would have plenty of patients willing to wait for treatment, with less pressure from malpractice lawyers.

A Canadian heart surgeon moving to the United States would also be well trained and would experience similar problems. He would be free to work wherever he wanted without penalties or second-language requirements. As in Canada, it would be necessary to obtain a licence to practice in each state or province where he wanted to work. Although his Canadian qualifications in cardiac or thoracic surgery are not recognized in the United States, he would likely be sponsored by a university or institution and be able to practice. (Recently, however, this is becoming more difficult due to medico-legal problems.) The surgeon would be free to generate income without quotas or maximums, benefitting from a tax system that allows deductions for a large portion of his expenses. Competition for patients would be fierce, and there would be no delay in providing treatment as patients are unwilling to wait for services. The physician would become more cautious and sometimes wasteful, in treatment practices, since lawyers are always in the lookout for those with malpractice insurance.

In the end, however, as I review my contacts with physicians who have moved south of the border, very few returned to Canada once they adjusted to the life in the

United States. There are a few that decided to return early in their careers, as the system in the United States was not suited to them. And they seem to have done very well in Canada. The majority of physicians who have moved to the United States from Canada, when asked, would not return to Canada. I do not know if there is any message in that last statement. Once one experiences the American system of health care, and adapts to it, one realizes that it has many advantages compared to any other health care system in the world.

Acknowledgements

Ms. Sharon Campbell, nurse-practitioner at Jackson Memorial Hospital, and Dr. Fuad Moussa, my resident in cardiothoracic surgery, have contributed greatly to the preparation of this manuscript.

Notes:

1.   Organisation for Economic Development, *Health at a Glance—OECD Indicators 2003, briefing notes for Canada and the United States of America; Major Economic Indicators* (September 2003), 236: Basic structural statistics, and 243, Gross Domestic Product, all accessed on the OECD website, *http://www.oecd.org*, December 9, 2003.

2.   J. Lomas, J. Woods, and G. Veenstra, "Devolving authority for health care in Canada's provinces: 1. An introduction to the issues," *Can Med Assoc J* (1997), 156 (3): 371-377. By the mid-1990s, 123 regional boards had been established in nine provinces, with only Ontario rejecting decentralized decision-making in health care.

3.   Figure from the Association of American Medical Colleges website, *http://www.aamc.org/medicalschools.htm*, accessed Feburary 2, 2009.

4.   B. Mears, "Justice: States can force HMOs to open networks: unanimous ruling is a blow to managed care," Newsitem on CNN.com, April 2, 2003, *http://edition.cnn.com/2003/LAW/04/02/scotus.court.healthcare/index.html*

5.   T. Porpora, "HMOs: Are they killing us?" Article in *Elan*, an e-zine on African-American women's issues, Sept/Oct 1999, *http://www.geocities.com/~cullars/hmos.htm*

6.   National Center for Health Statistics, *Health, United States, 2002* (Hyattsville, MD, 2002), tables 129, 130, 131.

Addendum: View from the United States; "Is the Grass Greener?"

As I read my chapter in the last edition of this book, and pondered about whether there have been any major changes worth reporting, I came to the conclusion that little has changed regarding the residency training program in CT Surgery. There continues to be a lack of interest by trainees in going into Cardiothoracic Surgery training. As a matter of fact, a large number of programs in the U.S. go unmatched, with positions open each year. The reasons for this are multi-factorial, including the long training period, decreased remuneration, medico-legal issues, and individual preferences.

Regarding patient care, the waiting period for cardiac surgery (or indeed for any type of surgery) in the United States is very short, particularly for funded (insured) patients: We are talking about a delay of hours for cardiac surgery. Special consideration is given to those with insurance, although in the end funded and non-funded patients receive similar treatment once they get into the hospital. All it takes is one phone call to admit a funded patient. Those without insurance coverage usually go to the nearest emergency room and are admitted via that route. An important policy is that all patients must be seen and treated in an emergency situation regardless of their insurance status.

The current financial crisis has had a major impact, mostly on hospitals. While the economy is a matter of concern, the majority of physicians have not yet been directly affected by the recession, apart from those providing elective services which are usually paid for by the patient. Such is the case in cosmetic surgery, performed in clinics or modified hotel rooms as operating rooms. However, with the new Administration in Washington and the promises of changes in health care, the prospect of serious cutbacks in reimbursement will affect physicians in general.

University hospitals, which rely on philantrophy, private donations and other sources of income, have seen their income decline significantly. Many institutions have dismissed employes, while others have frozen their expenditures, including salaries, so that there are no new replacements or new recruits to the University. The near collapse of the stock market has had a negative impact on philanthropy and donations. Plans for construction of new buildings, the development of new programs, recruitment of new leadership and many other activities are on hold at this time. Private universities are concerned about tuition, as students' families may be severely affected by the financial crisis, or may be unemployed.

Hospitals, in general, are desperately trying to curb expenses. Some have delayed payments to suppliers. There is no new recruitment of faculty, nurses, or support staff. Some hospitals have dismissed nurses and non-essential personnel, and are basically trying to survive during this period of transition. The government is threatening to decrease the budget for public hospitals, which are already working under financial stress. The prospects are that this financial situation will worsen. Hopes for end of the recession and for these matters to resolve themselves.

BEEN THERE, DONE THAT

David Latter

The contributions that American cardiac surgeons have made to the profession are undeniable. Canadian heart surgeons can be equally proud of their history. It is true that many Canadian-trained cardiac surgeons have emigrated to the United States to practice and live. Yet, despite all the hype about the advantages of practicing cardiac surgery in the United States and the angst we hear so much of from heart surgeons on the northern side of the Forty-ninth Parallel, I chose to practice in Canada. Not all that you hear on either side of the border is true.

I have trained in and practiced cardiac surgery in both countries. My most recent foray to the United States was intended to be a permanent move, but ended up being only a stage in my career. The reasons why I returned to Canada are myriad, and many of them were personal and family-related. However, some of my reasons were based on the fact that I felt practicing cardiac surgery in Canada was simply better.

There is no doubt that the United States offers more financial remuneration. But this discrepancy is diminishing, and I believe the financial rewards will eventually be similar in both countries. The unrelenting discounting of cardiac surgical services by Medicare and third-party insurers in the United States is well-documented. It has proceeded to the point that when American medical students choose their specialties they see the future of cardiac surgery as one of long training, intense and difficult working conditions, and decreasing financial reward for their trouble. The possibility of such key procedures as coronary artery bypass surgery disappearing in favour of cardiological percutaneous interventions and prevention strategies may also be having an effect on recruitment into the specialty. The result is that approximately 20 per cent of American positions in cardiac surgery went unfilled in a recent residency matching program. This is perhaps the most telling symptom that all is not well in cardiac surgery in the United States. Here in Canada, we are not seeing a similar lack of interest among medical students regarding careers in heart surgery.

It is apparent that in the past ten to twenty years too many cardiac surgeons were produced in the United States. Now, however, it is conceivable that in future not enough will be produced to meet that country's needs.

When I practiced heart surgery in the United States, I was surprised by the number of restrictions on freedom of practice. Every patient's care must be vetted by their insurance company. If a complication arises and the patient's hospital stay is extended the insurer begins calling to push for discharge. Most cardiac surgical centres in the United States have an entire office to "deal" with the insurance companies. In the United States, the individual is not free to choose a cardiac surgeon—their insurance company does that for them—but here, the Canada Health Act allows a patient in any province to receive care anywhere in the nation.

Much is made of waiting times for medical services in Canada acting as a rationing system. To a certain extent this is true, but various provinces have formed, or are in the process of creating, agencies that analyze cardiac service data and make recommendations to the provincial governments regarding service level requirements. In most cases, these recommendations are followed. When waiting times have become too long and patients have suffered as a result, a public outcry has ensued. Elected government officials take quick action if they wish to be reelected. The famous patient who finds he or she must be sent to the United States to have cardiac surgery is often talked about, but I have yet to personally meet one. I suspect their numbers are truly limited.

Another of my concerns about medical practice in the United States is the for-profit nature of the hospitals. American hospitals are businesses. Even the not-for-profit facilities must pay strict attention to the bottom line, for if they fail to be economically viable they soon go out of business. The need to cut expenses, increase productivity, and maximize revenues is omnipresent. While these are laudable objectives, if taken to extremes they can be harmful. In health care the most glaring extreme is the prospect of unnecessary surgery. While I never saw this occur where I practiced, a recent media exposé of a hospital in California performing unnecessary procedures on cardiac surgery patients is condemning proof that this sort of abuse can happen. I doubt that this would ever happen in Canada, where heart surgeons and cardiac surgery departments have more patients than operating room slots available.

The interplay among academic and private-practice cardiac surgeons and cardiologists in the United States was confusing for me at first. Early in my brief stay there I was shocked at being called upon to operate on a patient whose private-practice cardiologist was her interventional cardiologist as well. Over the course of six months, the patient had undergone four percutaneous interventions with the same specialist: an angiogram, a repeat angiogram and stent, a third angiogram with rotablation and stenting, and finally a fourth angiogram following a large anterior wall infarct that had left her in cardiogenic shock. At this point, she was seen for the first time by another physician—me. I was asked to take this lady to the OR for a bypass to the now-infarcted anterior wall. When I arrived to assess the patient, she was in the coronary care unit being cared for by a nurse with no physician in sight. The private-practice cardiologist was at another hospital doing an angioplasty! Obviously one bad physician does not represent an entire profession, but the monetary aspect of medicine is definitely more pronounced in the United States than in Canada. I felt that medicine in general was less of a profession and too much of a business than it is here in Canada.

It is said that Canadian hospitals are much slower than their American counterparts at obtaining the newest technology. This may be true. A large incentive for American hospitals in their pursuit of the latest technology has less to do with efficacy than with marketing and market share. Heaven forbid if a competing hospital can say it is the only facility in the area to offer transmyocardial laser revascularization therapy, even if the procedure has not been shown to be effective. Somewhere between Canadian hospital tardiness (due to financial limitations) and the exuberance of American hospitals (due to marketing considerations) lies an appropriate balance.

Medical malpractice is in a crisis in the United States, and cardiac surgeons haven't escaped its menacing grip. It is true that malpractice concerns continue to grow in Canada, but given the fundamental differences in the judicial systems of the two countries I doubt we will ever reach the state the Americans are in now. State-wide resignations in certain specialties such as the trauma surgeons in Pennsylvania, are a most alarming development.

Another major difference between the two countries is the phenomenon of many small cardiac surgery centres in the United States as opposed to the few, but on average much larger facilities in Canada. I believe there is economy of scale in larger centres, and concentrating cardiac surgical experience in fewer surgeons makes for better results.

For me, the choice was obvious. Despite the deficiencies of the Canadian system, practicing cardiac surgery here offered me more professional freedom and collegiality. A little more financial remuneration is fine; but after all is said and done, it is not just money that makes for a rewarding career.

CANADIAN CARDIAC SURGEONS: SHOULD THEY GO SOUTH?

Claude M. Grondin

Why would a Canadian heart surgeon want to go and practice his trade on American soil? There are several reasons why he might and just as many not to. First and foremost, in addition to considering the possibility, he has to be offered a position! And, in order to be considered, he has to make it known that he is available—and for his own sake, provide that information to the right people, not the want ads!

The surgeon may be asked at different stages in his career and / or invited to assume a different role in his new environment.

In the first instance, the surgeon may be approached in midcareer, after establishing a name for himself in the academic world, or he may leave Canada in the early stage, before any such accomplishment. Hence, he may start in the United States at the bottom or at the top of the ladder. He may also move from a comparatively high position in Canada to a less senior one, academically and otherwise. There is a whole range of possible situations, each different from the next. These varying circumstances will affect not only the decision to move but also, and more importantly, his career.

The surgeon may also wish simply a change of scenery, to try something new, or leave a situation he has outgrown or that no longer offers opportunity for advancement or development. He likewise may do all of this for purely financial reasons or to prove to himself that he can play with the big boys: in the NFL, so to speak, rather than in the CFL. In this case, he may discover that, yes, the money is better in the NFL (and taxes *are* lower), but also that the hits from the larger middle linebackers and cornerbacks can be greater too. And these fellows are *faster.*

As a rule, the earlier he relocates, the less likely the surgeon will be disenchanted, for the simple reason that he has not yet learned the true conditions of the profession here and, therefore, cannot compare them to his new ones. He may think there are no differences but in fact there *are* and there may be major ones. Much depends upon the type of practice one joins in the United States and also, surprisingly, on its location. Some states and areas offer conditions and situations quite like those in Canada, in terms for instance of general neighborhood safety or freedom from medical lawsuits and so on. When it comes to the United States, it is difficult and hazardous to generalize. Some places are little paradises, but others quite the opposite. Generally speaking, the competition is more fierce on the other side of the Forty-ninth Parallel and the stress and strain are at a higher level. Like life itself, the tempo is faster south of the border.

Again as a rule, it may be a mistake to opt for a totally different type of practice, to move, say, from a strictly academic environment to a completely private downtown one, or vice versa. One is better off choosing to do in the United States what one excels at here. That way, there will be less opportunity for failure and for the wolf pack (silently opposed to the new kid on the block or to his arrival in town) to begin howling. The expectations placed on the newcomer's abilities—well-advertised either on his own part or on that of the administrators who hired him (there are always such folks!)—may prove too high to be met and lead to his downfall. For instance, a surgeon may have a proven record of research and publication, yet encounter insurmountable obstacles to research in his new setting and thus fail in his colleagues' eyes, and worse, in his own. In general, it is particularly difficult to walk in at the level of department chief as a foreigner, especially in the academic world. The William Oslers of this world are rare indeed. In this instance, it is probably less risky to go from academia to downtown than to do the opposite, especially if downtown is somehow linked to academia or has residency programs, at least in general surgery.

The above caveats notwithstanding, life and the practice of medicine may be pleasurable in the United States although they do differ considerably in most areas from those in Canada. If, like the author, one relocates in his forties to early fifties and has children, the move will probably be a good one. The kids will like it. In cities of significant size—large enough to have a hospital with open-heart surgery—schooling is bound to be excellent. (Or alternatively, one may go to a smaller place, such as Rochester, Minnesota, or even Marshfield, Wisconsin— population eighteen thousand—and find large and very good hospitals with important heart surgery programs. This-in truth is perhaps the ideal scenario. The author was offered a position at Rochester and let it pass. Regrettably? He will not say.)

School tuitions are high but one gets his money's worth. American schools and society in general reward work, talent, and excellence. Especially excellence. It's one of their trademarks. Children will adapt to a higher caliber of competition much more readily than adults. Intellectually, the United States is a stimulating environment, in fact very much so, contrary perhaps to what some Canadians believe. Even American politics and politicians are interesting. Why? Because they come from a much larger base, for one thing. The Americans know their country;

they're very proud of it. They travel a lot from one end of it to the other, more so than Canadians. Americans also know their history, and their history is fascinating. (In Canada, we have two histories, and as a result, at least some of us seem to forever bicker.) Americans come from a very large melting pot, religious as well as societal. They came to America in search of freedom or liberties of all sorts, to escape tyrants and corrupt kingdoms and political systems. Governments do not intervene much in their daily life: this freedom is readily palpable after a while. Truly!

Medical practice is a different matter.

The American health system is not going in the right direction. Ours has its problems but theirs, likewise perhaps though for different reasons, appear insurmountable. The U.S. system may have been better than ours at one time, one or two decades ago, or at least on a better track, but since the advent of managed care, theirs is far worse, and there seems to be no desire or willingness on the part of politicians and pundits to fix it.

The problem is not—as in Canada—a lack of funds or of capacity to afford a better system. Ten to twenty years ago, the American Medicare system (which applies to everyone over sixty-four) was better than our *current* system, which covers all Canadians, as we are reminded, but not all at the same speed, as we know. The U.S. government's decision to let managed care companies compete for Medicare patients delivered a fatal blow to the system, which in addition has never covered the entire population.

Moreover, to say that the private insurance companies are a nuisance is an understatement. As a case in point, any office of three physicians requires five employees or secretaries to handle the work: one per MD for the regular office load, one for such financial chores as billing and accounting, and one simply to deal eight hours a day with the insurance companies whose only concern is to make and save money.

Malpractice suits are another irritant. They do vary from state to state, however, requiring protection that ranges from $30,000 for a heart surgeon in some (rare) states to over $100,000 in others. But lawsuits and especially interrogations or inquiries leading (usually in less than 10 percent of cases) to suits abound. These consume the physician's time and put everyone on the defensive, often leading to wrong decisions and to unnecessary medical tests and even treatments, in order to protect one's interests. This situation does not exist in Canada.

It is also true that medicine is more of a business in the United States than in Canada. Because it pays so much more, it may be difficult to resist the temptation of performing medical procedures that are more rewarding to the physician than to the patient. This is usually not a problem for the heart surgeon, who gets referrals from another physician who has already made the decision to opt for surgery and has convinced the patient who has complete trust in him. But it may influence the referring physician if, as is often the case, the same person does everything: cardiac catheterization, diagnosis and indications for treatment, including the multiple angioplasties which he, may unilaterally judge necessary. Thousands of cardiologists in the United States make incredible amounts of money, far more than their surgical colleagues, who also may overbill. (Yet the discrepancy between American and Canadian cardiologists has become much greater than that for cardiac surgeons.) In some places, there is no watchdog and very little control over practices where the diagnostician, the decision-maker, and the treatment provider are the same individual. This problem does not exist in Canada either. Proper surveillance would eliminate these profiteers.

Nevertheless, physicians are still well thought of and admired by the American public. And, by and large, they deserve it. In the eyes of hospital administrators, physicians are looked upon as gold because they bring in money and therefore reinforce their position, as opposed to Canadian administrators who may look at MDs as contributing to perennial hospital deficits (as in a sense, we do). The absence of a deficit makes the administrators look better in the eyes of the health minister.

In summary, moving to the United States may be a blessing or a mistake for a Canadian heart surgeon, depending on the circumstances. These may vary considerably. Those who have returned after a short stay obviously did not fall into the right set up, often through no fault of their own, for situations sometimes change or are difficult to assess beforehand because some salesmen do such a good con job. There are possibly as many disappointed early returnees—and their number may be growing—as there are successful and enthusiastic U.S. converts and citizens. Most, however, probably fall somewhere between these two extremes. These individuals have learned to live with the drawbacks and irritants of practicing in the United States, or have encountered more favorable situations and been able to compensate better. The success or failure of the venture also depends on the family. A lot depends on the family. The experience for the children proved very rewarding in our case. Following our return to Canada (to retire, in our case; Canada is the best place for retirement if one does not mind the weather and the politicians), our four children all succeeded in entering medical and law schools, two in each field. Three have now completed their educations—but sorry, no heart surgeons.

Did I personally enjoy the experience? Would I recommend it or repeat it today? As concerns the family, I obviously would. Did I find or do I believe that the practice of medicine and heart surgery are superior in the United States? Frankly, no. In fact, absolutely not in my case, for I had left a nearly ideal situation. I had left for personal reasons. They were primarily financial but also, though to a much lesser extent, professional. Perhaps, in retrospect, I was wrong on the second count—I shall never know—but, like the decision regarding the Minnesota opportunity, that's Monday morning quarterbacking. It serves no purpose.

I would nevertheless hesitate recommending relocating to the United States unless it were for somewhat similar reasons. Today, in all likelihood, the financial incentive would no longer hold as the gap between the two countries has diminished considerably. The family opportunities, on the other hand, remain the same if one has the right circumstances, including a bunch of children, a penchant for adventure and, above all, a loving life-companion. And then, after the fact, there is always the unanswerable question: was one right in making such an important decision at that point in one's life? My own answer is that had I not moved to the United States, I might always have wondered whether I had the guts or, at age fifty, the energy to move south and "just do it." The opportunity arose. I seized upon it. *Carpe diem*, simply.

CHAPTER 18

THE FUTURE OF HEART SURGERY: A RESIDENT'S PERSPECTIVE

Paul W. M. Fedak[*]

Prologue

In the late nineteenth century, William Halsted established fundamental operative principles that enabled the progression of surgery. Halsted postulated that adequate exposure and careful hemostasis would provide for orderly conduct and clear thinking in the operative field. Yet the prospect of gaining access to the interior of the human heart and operating under direct vision presented a unique challenge to surgeons. Both the continuous motion and the vital role of the heart in maintaining the systemic circulation appeared to preclude a straightforward, direct approach to intracardiac lesions. The Halsted principles did not seem applicable and progress in the field of cardiac surgery was slow and cumbersome.

Notably, the origins of successful cardiac surgery lay in the rise of twentieth-century technology.[1] Key technological

---

[*] Paul Fedak is currently a cardiac surgeon and clinician/ researcher at Foothills Hospital, University of Calgary

advances and subsequent applications in cardiopulmonary bypass as well as anaesthesia and coagulation allowed for the rise of cardiac surgery. Cardiac surgeons developed and applied technology to triumph over a seemingly insurmountable surgical frontier.

After the long-standing pessimism surrounding cardiac intervention had been largely eliminated by the routine palliation provided by the Blalock-Taussig shunt, bold surgeons explored the possibility of the direct repair of intracardiac lesions. Extracardiac (i.e., Blalock-Taussig shunt) and indirect-vision intracardiac approaches (i.e., closed mitral commissurotomy) only served to support the growing concern that curative heart surgery could only be performed if the heart was opened in a quiet, bloodless field. Artificial cardiopulmonary bypass held the most promise but was fraught with complications and secondary systemic ill-effects. While this technology evolved, Bigelow's applied hypothermia and Lillehei's controlled cross-circulation facilitated the first series of curative intracardiac operations under direct-vision, namely atrial septal defects repair. These "physiologic" methods were developed by brilliant surgical scientists who used their knowledge of biology, physiology, and anatomy to circumvent one of histories' greatest surgical challenges. These early surgical scientists combined clinical observation and experience with extensive laboratory investigation on animal models before undertaking human trials. Notably, Canadian cardiac surgeons played a key role in developing and introducing these advances based on translational laboratory work. Bigelow studied hypothermia in Toronto and developed the technique that allowed the first successful human intracardiac repair. Also in Toronto, Gordon Murray applied heparin to vascular surgery and was able to perform significant achievements such as the first aortic homograft valve replacement in the descending thoracic aorta.

The surprising results obtained with these early techniques encouraged surgeons to approach more complex intracardiac repairs. However, the inherent limitations of these physiological techniques to protect the organs from prolonged ischemia encouraged researchers to intensify efforts to develop a safe and practical artificial cardiopulmonary bypass apparatus. In so doing, a "machine" would ultimately allow surgeons the opportunity to operate on the heart for extended periods with direct-vision in a motionless, bloodless operative field.

Once the technology had matured, artificial cardiopulmonary bypass became the method of choice for the vast majority of open-heart operations and enabled important achievements in the field. This usurpation of physiology by technology is characteristic of the twentieth century, wherein the "machine" has become a vital component of daily life. One of the key developers of the artificial cardiopulmonary bypass circuit, John W. Kirklin, makes reference to this rather peculiar circumstance:

> I have to conclude that controlled cross-circulation was the most physiological technique that has ever been used for cardiac procedures. It is rare in the history of surgery to do what Walt Lillehei did then, that is, abandon a nearly perfect technique physiologically and adopt one that, at least up to now, has been less physiological than was controlled cross-circulation.[2]

On the other hand, the introduction of technology to cardiac surgery was not a solution without risks. At present, despite the extensive experience and evolution of artificial cardiopulmonary bypass, complications such as stroke, neurological dysfunction, trauma to blood elements, and altered inflammatory pathways continue to defy our modifications of the technique. New and unique challenges arise with the use of technological approaches to physiological problems, and while we examine the great possibilities and immense challenges to be faced in the future of cardiac surgery, this theme will be further explored.

Indeed, what is past is prologue. Technology continues to advance at a rapid pace and at the turn of the millennium, cardiac surgery is at a crossroad. Dr. Delos Cosgrove, when giving his presidential address to the American Association for Thoracic Surgery (AATS) in 2000, referred to the current status of cardiac surgery as "the best of times and the worst of times."[3] The twenty-first century offers enormous opportunities and difficult challenges for the future of the profession. In a similar presidential address to the AATS in 2002, Dr. Timothy Gardner offered a measured perspective:

We must focus on our heritage, its lessons, and its inspirations and see what that history teaches us, not just about the here and now but also about our future.[4]

Accordingly, the following chapter will explore the possibilities and challenges facing the future of the profession and practice of cardiac surgery in the context of our rich surgical heritage. The areas of clinical practice, research, and education are examined.

The Future of Heart Surgery: Clinical Practice

1. Coronary Bypass Surgery

Perhaps the most important lesson to be learned from our rich history is that the clinical practice of cardiac surgery will continue to be shaped by the development and introduction of new technologies. When new technology is introduced, it will inevitably change the way we do things. What we do now is not necessarily what we will do in the future. In fact, new technology will not only change what we can do but also who will do it. For example, coronary bypass grafting is one of the most frequently performed and most studied operations in the history of surgery. Coronary bypass grafting has been the mainstay of cardiac surgical practice since its rise in the 1980s and has improved over time with exceptional short and long-term results. Why should it be done differently? Technology has been developed and now applied in many novel ways for revascularization of the heart. The introduction of advanced interventional catheters and coronary stents has eliminated cardiac surgeons from a large subpopulation of patients with coronary artery disease that would otherwise been treated surgically. The rates of coronary bypass surgery are falling. Technology will always beget new technology and cardiac surgery will continually evolve or someone else will find a different way to do it.

Traditional coronary grafting is invasive and the early concerns about artificial cardiopulmonary bypass support to permit cardiac standstill and bloodless operative field creating secondary systemic ill-effects have never been completely resolved, despite half a century of its use. Enabling technology has now been developed to facilitate coronary grafting without the use of cardiopulmonary bypass: "off-pump" surgery with a minimally invasive approach is possible with the use of specially designed platforms. The proposed advantages of an "off-pump" approach include increased operative speed, lower costs, reduced perioperative complications (i.e., cerebral emboli and renal failure) and shorter hospital stays. While the proposed advantages are not entirely validated to date, it is a technically feasible approach that will likely benefit selected individuals.

2. Surgical Robotics

Similarly, surgical robotics has been introduced to further minimize the invasiveness of the approach and allow coronary grafting via port incisions. It is conceivable, although not clear to date, that a robotic-assisted minimally invasive internal thoracic (mammary) graft to the left anterior descending coronary artery will be superior to a coronary stent and equally acceptable to patients.[5] The development of robotics for cardiac surgery is exciting and the technology is highly functional. Computer imaging and modeling can be applied to enhance direct-vision and minimize technical "noise" in microscopic hand movements. Robotic systems have a clear advantage in allowing magnified direct-vision with the ability to simultaneously control and eliminate physiologic tremor and inherent limitations in human hand motions. Halsted would be very impressed. However, the application of this technology has not been as rapid and widespread as one might imagine. Why? Is this the future of clinical practice? Unfortunately, the current technology is being directed to do things the way we always have been doing them, only through smaller incisions and on a beating heart. In my opinion, the future of cardiac surgery for coronary disease will not be sewing bypass grafts in place with a needle and thread, whether by a needle driver in an open chest or a voice-controlled robotic arm through a micro-port incision. The future will be using technology to do things in ways that we have not yet imagined. Innovative methods have been proposed to create a sutureless anastomosis,[6] and when combined with robotics, the future for minimally invasive beating heart coronary grafting is encouraging.

3. Imaging

Perhaps the most important future technological advances are the rapidly developing areas of robotics and noninvasive cardiovascular imaging. For example, real-time MRI allows a detailed examination of the beating heart as well as intracardiac structure and function without opening the chest. Similarly, the recent application of real-time three-dimensional (3-D) echocardiography has provided new insights into valve function that almost immediately resulted in the application of innovative new surgical procedures. [7,8] We are seeing relationships in the heart that we could never appreciate before. Surprisingly, even at the turn of the millennium, the dynamic anatomy and physiology of the cardiac valves and coordinated contractile function of the myocardium are not entirely understood. Our knowledge of cardiac anatomy and its proposed functional effects on cardiovascular physiology is ancient and is largely based on cadaveric dissection and crude animal experiments. As demonstrated by Buckberg and colleagues, cardiac surgeons have not even appreciated and applied all of the concepts established in the past by the early work of anatomists.[9] We have yet to understand the coordinated efforts of the heart. For example, biventricular pacing has been well documented to improve heart function and represents a dynamic relationship that was previously unrecognized.[10] With advances in real-time cardiac imaging we will be afforded a unique opportunity to understand cardiac anatomy in its dynamic form, directly observing its three-dimensional configuration during the cardiac cycle. This information will uncover novel anatomic and physiologic relationships in the beating heart. Using these data, cardiac surgeons will be able to more scientifically remodel and reshape the heart to optimally restore its function. In so doing, reconstructive cardiac surgery will become more of a science and less an art. By establishing new principles, applying novel techniques based on these principles, and subsequently having the ability to accurately measure the outcomes of the procedures, results will drastically improve and their use will become more widespread and more easily implemented in the global cardiac surgery community.

Importantly, the new robotics and enhanced imaging will profoundly shape surgical practice when used in combination. It is conceivable that in the near future, we will have the tools necessary to enter the heart with highly articulate robotic instruments that we can use to operate under direct-vision without stopping the heart and without the use of any cardiopulmonary bypass techniques. We will fulfill the tenets of Halsted without opening the chest, without opening the heart, and without stopping the circulation. When robotic articulating hands are added to the end of a catheter that "glows" in real-time MRI or real-time 3-D echocardiography, the possibilities are then endless for intracardiac repairs of valves, intracardiac shunts, and the implantation and replacement of micro-pacers and defibrillators that require no leads. These technologies will also be available to facilitate the application of catheter-based prosthetic valve implantations.

4. Artificial Intelligence

The practice of cardiac surgery is indeed at an important crossroad. The "man" versus "machine" controversy is popular at the turn of the millennium. In 1997, the world's greatest chess player, Grand Master Garry Kasparov, was defeated by a computer with artificial intelligence engineered by IBM. People were shocked by the ability of a machine's clear superiority over the human intellect in the complex endeavor of chess. We have yet to apply the potential of artificial intelligence to the care of our cardiac surgical patients. However, there is clearly a momentum and desire in contemporary cardiac surgeons who see the need for continued progress. For example, imagine that implantable devices could also send wireless signals that surgeons and cardiologists could monitor, providing constant beat-to-beat data on cardiac dynamics at a molecular and whole organ level. Not only will these devices enable us technically but with added artificial intelligence it may even guide us as to when and how we should intervene in an individual patient. Consider the following thought experiment. Imagine a smart-card implanted into the left ventricle that communicated with the world-wide web and simultaneous monitored the patient's cardiovascular physiology and compared it to ongoing clinical trials and databases enriched with global clinical outcomes. Imagine that your heart was linked to your laptop or handheld computer and with continual real-time analysis, it told you when to take your heart medications and how many to take on a given day. Imagine as a surgeon doing a consult that you had access to this smart-card and it helped guide you to when and how you should operate on that patient. Imagine it again because it may happen in the future.

5. Artificial Heart

Perhaps the most striking contemporary example of the rise of technology in the field of heart surgery is that of the artificial heart. Left ventricular assist devices are used routinely in some clinical centers and totally implantable artificial hearts have been evaluated in series of patients.[11] Efforts to make the devices smaller, more efficient and less thrombogenic are underway. There are significant challenges in this endeavor, particularly in the enormous costs involved. At the other end of the spectrum, the lowly intraaortic balloon pump never made the cover of *Time* magazine but it is a marvel of our ability to employ a keen knowledge of cardiovascular physiology with advanced technology and computer-assisted function to benefit our surgical patients. This is an example of applied technology that is simple, efficient, and highly effective.

> The techniques used in cardiac surgery should be based upon clinical experience with emphasis on simplicity, knowledge of cardiac anatomy, and the desire to accomplish the most good for the patient, with the least risk. New techniques are reported in a steady stream in the surgical literature. Trainees in the specialty of cardiac surgery must learn to judge the potential merit of new methods. Advice to the neophyte cardiac surgeon should be—modify, simplify, then apply. Enthusiasm for a new procedure must always be tempered by cautious and considered judgment. [12]

> —Denton A. Cooley, MD

The use of advanced technology, particularly the artificial heart, is resource intensive and expensive. In a universal heath care system like Canada's, cost effectiveness and widespread applicability are essential. In the twenty-first century, progress in cardiac surgery will no longer be limited by the availability of technology, but by the costs inherent in the evolution and implementation of our great inventions. The future challenge will no longer be how to intervene, but in whom and when.

> With its emphasis on technology, the juggernaut of medical science has often strained and frayed the traditional personal bond between doctor and patient. It has presented medicine with a tangle of ethical dilemmas, bringing moral implications ever closer to daily life— and death. And, if that were not enough, it confronts society and government with the urgent problem of just how to pay for it all.[13]

The Future of Heart Surgery: Research

Historically, progress in the field of open-heart surgery involved an intensive research effort to develop the technology of artificial cardiopulmonary bypass to surpass the physiological limits imposed by the beating heart. However, current research in the field of molecular and cellular biology may offer similar promises as do future advances in technology. These are equally exciting and parallel the advances in the birth of the field of cardiac surgery. Interestingly, the code underlying DNA was uncovered at the same time that artificial cardiopulmonary bypass was introduced. Since that time—also echoing the expansion of the field of cardiac surgery—research in molecular biology has evolved and now allows investigators to manipulate genes, molecules and cells at will. We can manipulate the genome and create new species. In this way, transgenic animals have been developed to answer fundamental questions in biology and physiology. Our ability to modify, simplify, and then apply in molecular biology has enormous potential that offers great promise in the field of cardiovascular medicine and surgery. I propose that the historical dichotomy of technology versus biology in the field of cardiac surgery will merge in the twenty-first century and offer possibilities for surgical reconstruction and repair previously inconceivable to the pioneers of the twentieth century.

Cell Transplantation

Accordingly, the future of cardiac surgery offers the promise of powerful new biological therapies using modified cells and tissues. [14, 15] The concept of "biosurgery" has been proposed and regenerative medicine—although in its early stages—will dominate all aspects of medicine and surgery in the twenty-first century. Emerging cell-based therapies include cell transplantation for myocardial injury and the creation of bioengineered cardiovascular tissues to enhance surgical repairs of myocardial defects. These are novel biologic approaches to restore and regenerate failing myocardium that may enhance the rapidly developing technological interventions for patients with cardiac disease. For example, the ability to successfully isolate, purify, and expand mammalian cells *in vitro* offered the possibility of altering diseased tissues by way of cell transplantation. Cardiomyocytes have been isolated and cultured at various developmental stages from the hearts of many different species including humans. Cell transplantation involves isolating these cells from tissues, expanding them in culture, and subsequently implanting them into injured myocardium. In 1994, cardiomyocytes from transgenic fetal mice were first isolated, expanded in culture, and transplanted into syngenic mouse hearts. The implanted cells survived the procedure and engrafted into the host myocardium. Importantly, cell engraftment did not compromise cardiac function or rhythm and chronic immune rejection was not encountered. Stable engraftment of transplanted cardiomyocytes was also observed in cardiomyopathic canine hearts without adverse effects, establishing the concept of cardiac cell transplantation in diseased hearts. In 1996, a Canadian cardiac surgeon Richard Weisel, and his colleague Ren-Ke Li, provided the proof of concept in animal models that cell transplantation can improve cardiac function after myocardial injury.[16] Transplanted fetal cardiomyocytes formed a cardiac tissue that limited scar expansion and improved the systolic function of cryoinjured rat hearts. The field of cell transplantation for cardiovascular disease was ready for further application in the clinical arena. Not unlike the pioneering work of Bigelow in hypothermia and the clinical application to intracardiac repairs, cell transplantation was soon applied by other pioneering surgeons around the world in patients undergoing coronary artery bypass grafting. Another Canadian cardiac surgeon, Ray Chiu, has also made key contributions to the proof of concept and basic science of cell transplantation as a therapy for ischemic heart disease. [17]

The restoration of cardiac function and regeneration of lost myocardium with cell transplantation and tissue engineering are promising new surgical tools for the growing number of patients with cardiovascular disease. Autologous cell transplantation restores regional and global cardiac function after myocardial infarction or dilated cardiomyopathy by providing myogenesis, stimulating and participating in angiogenesis, and by limiting maladaptive ventricular remodeling. Bioengineered muscle grafting offers the promise of myocardial regeneration by replacing irreversibly damaged myocardium with healthy autologous tissue to facilitate surgical remodeling of the failing heart.

The application of autologous tissue engineering to the repair of congenital cardiac malformations will revolutionize the treatment of these children. Imagine an implantable vascular graft that is dynamic, can grow with the child, and is nonthrombotic and nonimmunogenic. Significant progress has been made already and clinical applications have been attempted.[18] It is only a matter of time before this biological approach to surgical reconstruction is improved and becomes the mainstay of congenital cardiac surgery. Similarly, the ability to create a nonthrombotic and physiological autologous tissue valve will forever change the treatment of valvular heart disease.[19] In addition, even pacemakers may one day be replaced by the targeted regeneration of the cells regulating cardiac conduction.[20]

Gene and cell therapy are rapidly being combined with significant effects of cardiac recovery after injury.[21] The future will likely combine these efforts with tissue engineering to provide a dynamic, autologous, functional tissue that will not only replace diseased tissues after surgical reconstruction but may provide enhanced, or even supernormal function. These efforts will be facilitated by the enhanced imaging and robotic instrumentation. We will likely be capable of performing directed gene-enhanced cell transplantation to diseased myocardium using real-time imaging and appropriate catheters. Efforts in this area are already underway and although in early stages, show significant promise as a proof of concept.

Stem cell research may be the key to this developing field of tissue engineering. If we can understand how an individual cell can differentiate and expand into a mature tissue, such as contractile myocardium, than autologous tissue engineering is conceivable from even a single healthy heart cell or arterial cell. Cardiac surgery and its future development will likely be shaped by developments in stem cells research and its implications on tissue engineering.[22] Cardiac surgeons in the twenty-first century may be uniquely poised to apply the basic sciences discoveries made in this realm of investigation to patients with cardiovascular diseases. If an innate system of cardiovascular tissue regeneration truly exists, as is currently proposed by leaders in the field of stem cell research, than cardiac surgery may one day involve using our surgical skills to reprogram the signaling pathways in the human body rather than opening the chest, stopping the heart, and repairing it with a needle and thread.

The Future of Heart Surgery: Education

With advanced technology comes the inevitability of change and accordingly, the cardiac surgeon must be adaptable and accommodating in clinical practice. The half life of new technology is about three years, shorter than any surgical residency program. In addition, the traditional surgical training dogma of "see one, do one, teach one" where surgical skills have been acquired in the operating room is rapidly becoming obsolete. The complexity of contemporary surgical procedures, the premium placed on surgical time, and the ongoing pressure to minimize error continue to present a challenge to surgical educators. The risk profile of patients presenting for cardiac surgery continues to rise, particularly as technologies allow lesser complex procedures to be performed by percutaneous coronary interventions. We can no longer expect cardiac surgeons to acquire novel skills solely in the operating room. How will surgeons learn to perform these highly technical procedures in the future? Interestingly, the answer is a similar theme that applies to education as it does to clinical practice. Educational technology has been developed that is changing the way surgery is taught to young surgeons. Virtual reality simulators and computerized skills models have been recently introduced at the University of Toronto. For example, the Immersion Endoscopy Simulator is a revolutionary medical simulation platform that delivers realistic, procedure-based content for cognitive and motor skills training. The system consists of a PC, an interface device and software modules. Current modules include colonoscopy and bronchoscopy scenarios. Laerdal's SimMan is a universal patient simulator designed for use as a tool in teaching psychomotor skills as well as cognitive and critical thinking pathways. It is manipulated via a Windows based interactive software package that controls such functions as ECG waveform and rate, NIPB, respiratory rate, temp, vocal sounds and much more. The Hermes voice control interface is a speaker dependent voice recognition system that enables the surgeon to issue spoken commands to the Hermes Control centre. It works in conjunction with the Aesop robotic arm allowing the surgeon endoscopic scope movement via voice control. This is an important adjunct to robotic cardiac surgery. Also, the Stryker telecommunications system is a teleconference system enabling long distance and internal bidirectional audio and video feeds. The system allows for real time video audio interaction for a multitude of educational sessions.

Toronto surgeons have made a commitment to respond to these unique challenges by developing the University of Toronto Surgical Skills Centre at Mount Sinai Hospital. This facility and its team of educators provide a laboratory setting where basic and complex surgical procedures can be learned and practiced. The belief is that surgeons will achieve a higher level of expertise more rapidly in a laboratory setting, where they can employ educational principles of repeated practice with feedback. In addition, educational research is conducted in skills acquisition and evaluation. This research will provide answers to fundamental educational issues and allow testing of innovations in surgery. For example, current efforts will determine if the practice of a vascular anastomosis is feasible with nonliving synthetic models as compared to cadaveric tissues. In this way, optimal models can be developed to assist in the development of exceptional surgical skills before attempts are made in the operating room. Similar models are used for troubleshooting cardiopulmonary bypass problems, without compromising patient care. The University of Toronto Surgical Skills Laboratory is becoming an internationally recognized centre of excellence in surgical education and provides a new training model using advanced technology that has intrigued surgical training programs around the world. This approach will likely become a major component in the future training of highly skilled and technologically adept cardiac surgeons.

Summary: The Cardiac Surgeon of the Future

The cardiac surgeon of the twenty-first century will be a leader of innovation capable of merging and applying available advances in technology and biology to repair and remodel the damaged in heart in ways that were previously inconceivable.

> If we look back at our heroes, those who were instrumental in our decision to become surgeons, what they all had in common was that they were exceptional human beings who inspired respect and either had the charisma of the artist, or the candor and the technical

brilliance of the craftsman. They were true professional leaders.[23]

Perhaps the only predictable event is that the specialty of cardiac surgery will continually be dominated by innovative, progressive, dynamic surgeons who will provide a rich and colorful biography and continue to lead a legacy of achievement.

Notes:

1. P. W. Fedak, "Open hearts: The origins of direct-vision intracardiac surgery," *Tex Heart Inst J* (1998), 25(2): 100-11.
2. J. W. Kirklin, in discussion of C. W. Lillehei et al., "The first open-heart repairs of ventricular septal defect, atrioventricular communis, and tetralogy of Fallot using extracorporeal circulation by cross-circulation: A 30-year follow-up," *Ann Thorac Surg* (1986), 41: 19.
3. D. M. Cosgrove, "Developing new technology," *J Thorac Cardiovasc Surg* (2001), 121(4 Suppl): S29-S31.
4. T. J. Gardner, "Presidential address: Our heritage and our future," *J Thorac Cardiovasc Surg* (2002), 124(4): 649-54.
5. R. K. Wolf, "Where are we going with computer-assisted or robotic cardiac surgery? A piece of the totally endoscopic coronary bypass puzzle," *J Thorac Cardiovasc Surg* (2002), 123(6): 1029-30.
6. P. Tozzi, A. F. Corno, and L. K. von Segesser, "Sutureless coronary anastomoses: revival of old concepts," *Eur J Cardiothorac Surg* (2002), 22(4): 565-70.
7. E. Messas et al., "Chordal cutting: a new therapeutic approach for ischemic mitral regurgitation," *Circulation* (2001), 104(16): 1958-63.

8.   Y. Otsuji et al., "Mechanism of ischemic mitral regurgitation with segmental left ventricular dysfunction: three-dimensional echocardiographic studies in models of acute and chronic progressive regurgitation," *J Am Coll Cardiol* (2001), 37(2): 641-48.

9.   F. Torrent-Guasp et al., "The structure and function of the helical heart and its buttress wrapping. I: The normal macroscopic structure of the heart," *Semin Thorac Cardiovasc Surg* (2001), 13(4): 301-19.

10. C. M. Yu, "New insight into left ventricular reverse remodeling after biventricular pacing therapy for heart failure," *Congest Heart Fail* (2003), 9(5): 279-83.

11. B. Radovancevic, B. Vrtovec, and O. H. Frazier, "Left ventricular assist devices: an alternative to medical therapy for end-stage heart failure," *Curr Opin Cardiol* (2003), 18(3): 210-14.

12. D. A. Cooley, *Reflections and Observations: Essays of Denton A. Cooley*, collected by M. A. Kneipp (Austin, Tex: Eakin Press, 1984), p. 78.

13. S. W. Nuland, *Time* (1996), 148(20): 7.

14. P. W. Fedak et al., "Restoration and regeneration of failing myocardium with cell transplantation and tissue engineering," *Semin Thorac Cardiovasc Surg* (2003), 15(3): 277-86.

15. G. H. Tang et al., "Cell transplantation to improve ventricular function in the failing heart," *Eur J Cardiothorac Surg* (2003), 23(6): 907-16.

16. R. K. Li et al., "Cardiomyocyte transplantation improves heart function," *Ann Thorac Surg* (1996), 62(3): 654-60.

17. R. C. Chiu, "Therapeutic cardiac angiogenesis and myogenesis: The promises and challenges on a new frontier," *J Thorac Cardiovasc Surg* (2001), 122(5): 851-52.

18. T. Shin'oka, Y. Imai, and Y. Ikada, "Transplantation of a tissue-engineered pulmonary artery," *N Engl J Med* (2001), 344(7): 532-33.

19. T. Shinoka, "Tissue engineered heart valves: autologous cell seeding on biodegradable polymer scaffold," *Artif Organs* (2002), 26(5): 402-6.

20. A. Ruhparwar et al., "Transplanted fetal cardiomyocytes as cardiac pacemaker," *Eur J Cardiothorac Surg* (2002), 21(5): 853-57.

21. J. Leor et al., "Gene transfer and cell transplant: an experimental approach to repair a 'broken heart,'" *Cardiovasc Res* (1997), 35(3): 431-41.

22. J. R. Fuchs, B. A. Nasseri, and J. P. Vacanti, "Tissue engineering: a 21st century solution to surgical reconstruction," *Ann Thorac Surg* (2001), 72(2): 577-91.

23. M. R. de Leval, "From art to science: a fairy tale? The future of academic surgery," *Ann Thorac Surg* (2001), 72(1): 9-12.